Ethical Issues in Anesthesiology and Surgery

Barbara G. Jericho
Editor

Ethical Issues in Anesthesiology and Surgery

Springer

Editor
Barbara G. Jericho
Hospital and Health Sciences System
The University of Illinois
Chicago, IL
USA

ISBN 978-3-319-15948-5 ISBN 978-3-319-15949-2 (eBook)
DOI 10.1007/978-3-319-15949-2

Library of Congress Control Number: 2015957686

Springer Cham Heidelberg New York Dordrecht London

Printed on acid-free paper

Springer International Publishing AG Switzerland is part of Springer Science+Business Media (www.springer.com)

This book is dedicated to the memory of my parents,

Norbert and Marsha Jericho

Preface

Ethical Issues in Anesthesiology and Surgery uniquely brings anesthesiologists, surgeons, and clinical ethicists together to address the challenging ethical issues both anesthesiologists and surgeons encounter in their academic and daily clinical practice. Ethical topics arising in pediatrics, research, anesthesiology, and surgery are included in this one book with each topic beginning with a case presentation that readers may relate to real-life ethical situations.

An anesthesiologist and a surgeon, unlike other specialists, are interconnected in the simultaneous care of one patient. The ethical issues that impact one specialty are intertwined with the ethical issues of the other specialty. Whether the ethical issue involves do not resuscitate orders in the perioperative period or the ethical care of children of Jehovah's Witnesses, anesthesiologists and surgeons need to work together and with the healthcare team to address ethical issues of their patients, respecting the wishes and goals of their patients.

The topics covered in *Ethical Issues in Anesthesiology and Surgery* include informed consent issues of pediatric patients, adolescents, and emancipated minors; preoperative testing: ethical challenges, evidence-based medicine, and informed consent; informed consent and the disclosure of surgeon experience; perioperative considerations of do not resuscitate and do not intubate orders in adult patients; do not resuscitate decisions in pediatric patients; ethical care of the children of Jehovah's Witnesses; fatigue and the care of patients; conscientious objection; ethical implications of drug shortages; ethical challenges in high-risk innovative surgery; professionalism in the operating room; honesty in the perioperative setting: error and communication; futility and the care of the perioperative patient; end-of-life issues; ethics in research and publication; and ethics in animal research.

Ethical Issues in Anesthesiology and Surgery is a resource for nursing and medical students, nurses, resident physicians, fellows, attending physicians, educational institutions, and hospital committees for addressing ethical issues in research as well as clinical ethical situations encountered in the care of patients in academic and private practice settings. This book is a valuable tool for ethics education to render clinical ethical principles more understandable and is a resource for those institutions with a scarcity of ethics resources to help address challenging ethical situations critical to the care of patients. By educating practitioners in the practice of bioethics, ethical issues will be more easily identified and resolved for the optimal care of patients.

I would like to acknowledge all of the authors who have generously contributed to this book. I would like to especially acknowledge Gail Van Norman who supported my initial involvement on a committee on ethics that has lead me on a path to where I am today; Stephen Jackson who continues to support my passion for ethics; Jeffrey Jacobs who has been a great supporter of my ethics projects and professional growth; James West for his support and encouragement; Joseph Kras for his contribution to this book and other collaborative projects; Cynthiane Morgenweck for her contribution to this book and our ongoing collaboration on ethics projects since 2009; the surgeons and pediatricians I have become acquainted with during this endeavor and who have graciously contributed to this book; Springer, Julia Megginson and Maria Smilios for their support of this book; and the man who says always reach for the stars.

I hope *Ethical Issues in Anesthesiology and Surgery* brings anesthesiologists and surgeons together to address ethical issues in the care of patients and to support ethical practice in research and publication.

Chicago, IL, USA
Summer 2015

Barbara Gayle Jericho, MD

Contents

Contributors

Kenneth R. Abbey, MD, JD Department of Anesthesiology, Portland Veterans Affairs Medical Center, Portland, OR, USA

Department of Anesthesiology and Perioperative Medicine, Operative Care Division, Oregon Health and Sciences University, Portland, OR, USA

Peter Angelos, MD, PhD, FACS Department of Surgery, MacLean Center for Clinical Medical Ethics, The University of Chicago Medicine, Chicago, IL, USA

Rose J. Campise-Luther, MD, FAAP Department of Anesthesiology, Medical College of Wisconsin-Children's Hospital of Wisconsin, Milwaukee, WI, USA

Logan K. Chastain, MD Department of Radiology, Southern Illinois University School of Medicine, Springfield, IL, USA

Ran Cheng, MD Department of Anesthesiology and Perioperative Medicine, Operative Care Division, Oregon Health and Sciences University, Portland, OR, USA

Christina D. Diaz, MD Department of Anesthesiology, Medical College of Wisconsin-Children's Hospital of Wisconsin, Milwaukee, WI, USA

Alberto R. Ferreres, MD, PhD, JD, MPH, FACS(Hon), ASA(Hon) Department of Surgery, University of Buenos Aires, Buenos Aires, Argentina

Joel E. Frader, MD, MA Department of Pediatrics, Division of Academic General Pediatrics and Primary Care, Medical Humanities and Bioethics, Ann & Robert H. Lurie Children's Hospital of Chicago, Northwestern University Feinberg School of Medicine, Chicago, IL, USA

Sabha Ganai, MD, PhD Department of Surgery, Southern Illinois University School of Medicine, Simmons Cancer Institute at Southern Illinois University, Springfield, IL, USA

Scott B. Grant, MD, MBE Department of Surgery, Rutgers Robert Wood Johnson Medical School, New Brunswick, NJ, USA

Stephen H. Jackson, MD Department of Anesthesiology, Good Samaritan Hospital, San Jose, CA, USA

Jeffrey S. Jacobs, MD Department of Anesthesiology, Cleveland Clinic Florida, Weston, FL, USA

Barbara G. Jericho, MD Department of Anesthesiology, The University of Illinois College of Medicine at Chicago, Chicago, IL, USA

Liza-Marie Johnson, MD, MPH, MSB Department of Pediatric Medicine, St. Jude Children's Research Hospital, Memphis, TN, USA

Richard J. Kelly, MD, JD, MPH, FCLM Department of Anesthesiology and Perioperative Medicine, Health Policy Research Institute, University of California Irvine School of Medicine, Orange, CA, USA

Irini N. Kolaitis, MD FAAP Department of Pediatrics, Division of Hospital Based Medicine, Ann & Robert H. Lurie Children's Hospital of Chicago, Northwestern University Feinberg School of Medicine, Chicago, IL, USA

Joseph F. Kras, MD, DDS, MA Department of Anesthesiology, Washington University School of Medicine, St. Louis, MO, USA

Ross Milner, MD Department of Surgery, MacLean Center for Clinical Medical Ethics, The University of Chicago Medicine, Chicago, IL, USA

Parth K. Modi, MD Department of Surgery, Division of Urology, Rutgers Robert Wood Johnson Medical School, New Brunswick, NJ, USA

Cynthiane J. Morgenweck, MD, MA Center for Bioethics and Medical Humanities, Medical College of Wisconsin, Milwaukee, WI, USA

Chen Nisynboim, LLB, JD University of California Irvine School of Law, Irvine, CA, USA

Michael O'Connor, MD, FCCM Department of Anesthesia and Critical Care, The University of Chicago Medicine, Chicago, IL, USA

Shuddhadeb Ray, MD, MPHS Department of Surgery, Washington University School of Medicine, Saint Louis, MO, USA

Baddr A. Shakhsheer, MD Department of Surgery, The University of Chicago Pritzker School of Medicine, Chicago, IL, USA

Eric A. Singer, MD, MA, FACS Department of Surgery, Section of Urologic Oncology, Rutgers Cancer Institute of New Jersey, Rutgers Robert Wood Johnson Medical School, New Brunswick, NJ, USA

Puneet Singh, MD Department of Surgery, The University of Chicago Pritzker School of Medicine, Chicago, IL, USA

Gail A. Van Norman, MD Department of Anesthesiology and Pain Medicine, Department of Biomedical Ethics, University of Washington, Seattle, WA, USA

James M. West, MD, MA Department of Anesthesiology, Methodist-LeBonheur Healthcare, Memphis, TN, USA

Chapter 1
Informed Consent: Pediatric Patients, Adolescents, and Emancipated Minors

Irini N. Kolaitis and Joel E. Frader

Abstract Permission to perform medical procedures on children poses special ethical and legal considerations. Decision makers must focus on the child's interests and attend to cognitive and emotional factors affecting developing children. As children grow, adults must increasingly include them in decisions about their health care. Decisions made by clinicians with parents or guardians on behalf of children require a higher, more rational basis, than decisions one may make for one's self as an autonomous adult.

Keywords Pediatrics • Informed Consent • Physician-Patient Relationship • Informed Refusal • Assent • Parental Permission • Emancipated Minor • Mature Minor

Case Presentation

A 16-year-old girl has been in the Pediatric Intensive Care Unit (PICU) for 72 hours receiving treatment for presumed sepsis. Four years ago she developed fatigue, fever, rash, and arthritis, eventually leading to a diagnosis of systemic lupus. She has required intermittent treatment with various

I.N. Kolaitis, MD, FAAP (✉)
Department of Pediatrics, Division of Hospital Based Medicine, Ann & Robert H. Lurie Children's Hospital of Chicago, Northwestern University Feinberg School of Medicine, 225 E. Chicago Avenue, Box 152, Chicago, IL 60611, USA
e-mail: ikolaitis@luriechildrens.org

J.E. Frader, MD, MA
Department of Pediatrics, Division of Academic General Pediatrics and Primary Care, Medical Humanities and Bioethics, Ann & Robert H. Lurie Children's Hospital of Chicago, Northwestern University Feinberg School of Medicine,
225 E. Chicago Avenue, Box 16, Chicago, IL 60611, USA
e-mail: jefrader@luriechildrens.org

B.G. Jericho (ed.), *Ethical Issues in Anesthesiology and Surgery*,
DOI 10.1007/978-3-319-15949-2_1

immunosuppressive medications, with a recent flare of symptoms treated with high dose steroids. Just prior to this admission, she developed fever and abdominal pain then had a change in consciousness. She received initial care at a community hospital with subsequent transfer to a tertiary care children's hospital.

In the course of her PICU stay, she developed a tense, tender abdomen. Ultrasound imaging suggested a possible abscess and a large amount of intra-abdominal fluid. Surgical consultants have recommended an exploratory laparotomy and the anesthesiologist has gone to the bedside to speak with the parents. As the conversation evolves, it becomes clear that the parents have a deep fear, based on a previous experience with another relative, of their daughter going to the operating room and believe she will get better with the ongoing medical treatment. The PICU attending, surgeon, and anesthesiologist meet in the hallway to discuss how to handle the parents' lack of adequate understanding of the situation and desire to refuse consent for anesthesia and surgery.

May the parents refuse recommended surgery under these circumstances? What approach should the clinicians take in response to the parents' reluctance to consent? If the parents continue to refuse after additional efforts to persuade them, what steps should the clinicians take?

Introduction

All clinicians need to develop an understanding of the ethical and legal bases for informed consent. While the current doctrine traces its roots in several landmark legal cases, our duty as clinicians engaging in the informed consent process regularly extends beyond the law. Clinicians have a moral obligation to ensure that patients and families make decisions based on their own values, with sufficient information and an understanding of how alternative actions fit those values.

An appreciation of the complexity of the informed consent process develops over the course of a clinician's career. How patients and families arrive at a decision, what information each patient and family need to make a decision, and how religious and cultural beliefs, financial status, and the family dynamic have an impact on decision making will vary from case to case. Working with patients and families to arrive at informed medical decisions builds a trusting and strong patient-family-clinician relationship.

The triadic nature of the patient-parent-clinician relationship changes the process of informed consent for clinicians, especially as the developing child becomes more involved in his or her own decision making. While in most cases decision-making authority rests with the parent or guardian, clinicians must encourage age appropriate involvement of the patient, obtain pediatric assent when necessary, and ensure that decisions made by the parent or guardian represent the best interests of the patient. In this chapter, we discuss the history of informed consent, the current definition of the doctrine of informed consent, and special considerations for the application of the informed consent doctrine in pediatrics.

History of Medical Decision Making

A review of the history of medical decision making reveals a shift in the way patients and clinicians make decisions. In the past, medical decision-making authority generally rested in the hands of clinicians caring for the patient; typically, patients completely accepted the recommendations of their physicians. In the United States, this paternalistic style of medical decision making lost favor in the second half of the twentieth century, propelled by court decisions in malpractice cases and coinciding with the ascendency of civil and individual rights in many aspects of American life (e.g., the release of warehoused mental health patients, the abolition of legal segregation, and the lowering of the voting age). Most patients, clinicians, and society now recognize the importance of patient or surrogate involvement in the medical decision-making process. The idea that patients have a right to be informed about their health information and have a right to accept or reject offered or recommended medical interventions has emerged as the guiding ethical and legal principle in our medical decision making. This shift in the locus of control over decisions respects the autonomy of the patient or the authority of the patient's legally authorized representative. Clinicians must now carefully balance promoting what they believe represents the best interests of the patient with respecting the patient's or surrogate's views about how to proceed. This model of medical decision making has come to be known as shared decision making to distinguish the process from a solely professional or patient-centered process [1, 2].

History of Informed Consent

Our understanding of informed consent evolved as a result of the changes in the medical decision-making process and also in part as a result of several landmark legal cases. One of the earliest cases highlighting the concept of informed consent, *Schloendorff v. The Society NY Hospital,* was decided in 1914. In the case, Ms. Schloendorff presented with abdominal pain and consented to an exam under anesthesia to determine if a diagnosed tumor was malignant. However, she did not agree to surgical removal of the tumor. During the procedure, her surgeons found a large malignant abdominal mass. They proceeded to resect the mass against her wishes rather than put her through another surgery. Ms. Schloendorff sued the hospital and the court ruled in her favor stating that her physicians had committed medical battery in proceeding with a surgery for which they had no consent. The court's opinion included, "every human being of adult years and sound mind had a right to determine what shall be done with his body; and a surgeon who performs an operation without his patient's consent commits an assault, for which he is liable in damages. This is true except in cases of emergency, where the patient is unconscious, and where it is necessary to operate before consent can be obtained" [3]. While the surgeons acted based on what they believed was in the best interests of the patient, the concept of unilateral decision making by physicians was starting to lose favor. Respect for patient autonomy had begun to emerge as an equally important component of medical decision making. Physicians had to promote the best interests of the patient, yet ultimately defer to what the patient believed represented his or her best interests.

This landmark ruling brought the importance of consent to the forefront of medical ethics discussions for years to come. *Schloendorff* gave rise to the notion of simple consent, making the provision of medical treatment contingent on specific consent from the patient or surrogate. However, this 1914 decision did not address the quantity and quality of the information physicians should share with patients. Perhaps clinicians also need to make sure patients understand the indications, risks, benefits, and alternatives to the recommended treatment. In 1957, the case of *Salgo v. Leland Stanford Jr. University Board of Trustees* clarified these matters under the law. Mr. Salgo presented with aortic thrombosis requiring aortography for diagnosis. His post-procedure course was complicated by permanent paralysis. Later investigation found that the intravenous contrast used in the case had not been used often enough to constitute routine practice. Salgo's physicians knew of the risks associated with the procedure, but did not provide that information to their patient. The court ruled that the "physician violates his duty to his patient if he withholds any facts which are necessary to form the basis of an intelligent consent by the patient to the proposed treatment" [4]. Our modern understanding of fully informed consent finds its roots in this case. Simply obtaining voluntary consent from a patient no longer sufficed; physicians had to ensure that patients received the information the patient needed to make a fully informed decision.

The legal discussion turned to how to define adequate disclosure in the informed consent process. Two different types of disclosure emerged in arguments before courts: the professional practice versus the reasonable person standard. The professional practice standard holds that adequate disclosure is determined by the customary physician behavior in a particular professional peer group. From this perspective, the physician should tell the patient what he or she believes another reasonable and experienced physician in the same community would disclose in similar circumstances. A variation on this approach involves disclosure of the amount of information a well-informed physician, current on relevant medical information, judges the patient needs in order to weigh the risks and benefits of the care options. By contrast, the reasonable person standard states that the physician should disclose all information that a reasonable lay person would want to know to make an informed decision. This disclosure standard seeks to shift control from the physician to the patient and family. While courts have largely abandoned the professional practice standard in favor of a patient-centered standard, no universally accepted definition of a reasonable patient exists. Moreover, recent thinking in medical ethics and legal precedent go beyond simple disclosure to an assessment by the clinician of the adequacy of the patient's or surrogate's understanding of the risks, benefits, and alternatives of available interventions (or nonintervention). Discovery of an inadequate or flawed appreciation of the facts should then trigger additional attempts to educate the decision maker or further inquiry into the patient's or surrogate's decisional capacity. In other words, *no valid consent exists if it turns out the decision maker does not have adequate information, does not understand the information, or lacks the ability to make a decision appropriate to the circumstances*. As part of the informed consent process, clinicians best serve patients and protect themselves by determining and meeting the unique informational and decision-making needs and preferences of particular patients and families [5].

Informed Consent: General Concepts in Pediatrics

Goals and Limitations in Pediatrics

The doctrine of informed consent serves the same goals in pediatrics as it does in all other fields of medicine. While the nature of the physician-patient relationship differs in pediatrics, as it includes, in most cases, a parent or guardian, the physician must still ensure that the patient or surrogate develops an adequate understanding of the proposed intervention(s) and makes an informed choice based on the information provided.

Clinicians who care for children face several challenges and limitations in applying the informed consent doctrine in daily practice. The first stems from the complex nature of the triadic patient-parent-clinician relationship. In most cases, clinicians will not obtain consent directly from the patient but seek permission from the child's parent or guardian. As a result, the informed consent process fundamentally differs from adult medicine where a competent adult patient engages directly with his or her clinician. Second, clinicians must take into account the developing autonomy and decision-making capacity of the patient. With adult patients, one can usually assume the patient has adequate decision-making capacity and can act autonomously. In pediatrics, the patient's capacity varies based on his or her age, cognitive ability, maturity, experience, and interest in participating in the medical decision-making process.

Consent by Proxy and Parental Permission

Consent by proxy occurs when a patient lacks decision-making capacity and relies on a surrogate decision maker. In pediatrics, a parent or guardian acts in this role and authorizes diagnostics, treatment, or research participation on behalf of a child. Proxy consent assumes the parent or guardian makes decisions based on "the best interests" of the patient, rather than the expressed or inferred preferences of a patient who previously had adequate decision-making capacity. The American Academy of Pediatrics (AAP) Committee on Bioethics argues that this process involves obtaining informed "permission" rather than proxy consent since the word "consent" implies acting in one's own behalf, based on personal beliefs and values [6]. Clinicians treating children have a duty to protect the best interests of the patient and recognize that some decisions may primarily promote the wishes and desires of the parent or guardian rather than patient's interests. Nevertheless, decisions for children can involve complex matters for patients and families, including such factors as the family's overall financial and emotional-social stability and wellbeing. In other words, a narrow focus on the child's interests may not adequately take into account legitimate competing interests of others.

Assent

When the medical decision-making process involves older children, clinicians should attempt to obtain the assent of the patient in conjunction with the permission of the parent or guardian. In doing so, clinicians respect the child's developing capacities and rights to information about his or her health care, enhance trust in the physician-patient relationship, and empower the patient to begin taking ownership of his or her personal health information and to develop medical decision-making skills [7]. Pediatric assent, like consent, should be voluntary; parents, guardians, and clinicians have to appreciate the potential for coercion or undue influence from family dynamics or financial pressures. Clinicians should engage the patient to the degree that he or she desires to be involved in the decision-making process. Some children may defer all medical decisions to their parents or guardians. In some cases, the parent or guardian may request excluding the child from decisions. Such requests may arise from a genuine desire to protect their child from distressing information or expectations. However, most agree that parents and clinicians routinely underestimate what children already know and understand about their clinical situation, and excluding children risks losing the child's trust in his or her caregivers [7]. Clinicians should generally encourage all patients to participate in conversations about their personal health care, respecting patients' wishes to opt out of receiving information or participating in decisions. Clinicians have an obligation to educate parents and guardians that engaging children in discussions regarding their health care is an important professional responsibility.

The AAP Committee on Bioethics emphasizes that obtaining assent involves an interactive process of sharing information and joint decision-making by all parties. The committee strongly urges against the use of assent forms, which have the potential to make the process feel bureaucratic and impersonal. The AAP notes that the assent process should include:

1. Helping the patient achieve awareness of his or her medical condition.
2. Explaining what the patient should anticipate regarding diagnosis and treatment.

3. Assessing the patient's understanding of the information provided and his or her condition.
4. Obtaining an expression of the patient's willingness to proceed with care.

In some cases, the assent process may elicit conflicts between the child and his or her parent or guardian. Unless the patient is deemed a mature or emancipated minor, the legal responsibility for a child's health care decision making falls on the parent or guardian. When clinicians feel the child's view deserves support and the legal decision maker persists in disagreeing, ethics consultation or appeal to the courts may be appropriate, especially when the clinical stakes are high. This complex and sensitive topic will be discussed in more detail later.

Assessing the Decision-Making Capacity of the Pediatric Patient

Interrogating the adequacy of decision-making capacity poses difficulties in adult medicine and pediatrics, as no universally satisfactory tools accomplish the task. Important considerations when assessing decision-making capacity in a child include: (i) the ability to understand and discuss important medical information, including risks, benefits and alternatives of proposed options; (ii) freedom to choose from the options presented; and (iii) demonstration of consistent beliefs and values [8]. Factors that play a role in a child's understanding of the clinical situation and ability to make informed decisions include the child's age and developmental stage, personal life experiences—including experience in the medical system, religious and cultural background, family dynamics, and experience with decision making [8–13]. While no single age threshold implies decision-making capacity in pediatrics, some research suggests that on average, individuals aged 14 years and older possess rational reasoning capacity indistinguishable from that of young adults with the legal authority to make their own decisions [9]. We do not require adults to make rational and fair medical decisions; a concept that raises considerations and questions about holding out a higher bar for decisions made by minors. That said, our society limits minors access to various privileges (e.g., drinking alcohol or renting a car) based on knowledge that the ability to reason does not fully match the ability to reflect and make mature decisions. Modern neuroscience suggests that teenagers have a relatively high tolerance for risk, focus on short-term consequences of their actions, and tend to make decisions influenced by others, especially peers and family members, rather than make independent decisions.

Components of Informed Consent

Clear guidelines exist to help clinicians engaging in the informed consent process with a patient or surrogate. The guidance emphasizes an interactive process, rather than the act of signing a consent form. The current consensus on informed consent indicates that the following should be included [5]:

1. Providing adequate and clear information in language that both the patient and parent or guardian can understand. This information should include: the nature of the diagnosis, proposed diagnostic and therapeutic options, risks and benefits of reasonable options, and possible alternatives, including that of not pursuing treatment.
2. Assessing the decision maker's understanding of the information provided.
3. Assessing, if only informally, the capacity of the designated decision maker (patient or surrogate).
4. Ensuring that the decision maker articulates a clear and voluntary informed choice from the options presented.

As with all difficult conversations in medicine, the consent process should take place in a quiet place with the clinician having ample time to address all of the patient's and parent's or guardian's questions and with all parties having limited distractions. Unless the patient's condition is emergent, clinicians should initiate the discussion well in advance of the proposed intervention to allow the patient and family sufficient time to digest the information and not feel rushed to a decision. Clinicians should be prepared to engage with the patient and parent or guardian on more than one occasion, since full consent constitutes a process that occurs over time rather than in an isolated event. Time and attention devoted to this process and open and honest communication demonstrate respect for the patient and family, likely enhance trust in the clinician, and improve outcomes and adherence to treatment.

Informed Consent: Age-Based Approach in Pediatrics

The informed consent process and the parties involved will vary based on the age and developmental status of the patient [6–12].

Infants/Toddlers

Very young children lack decision-making capacity and cannot provide assent or consent for themselves. As a result, full decision-making authority rests with the patient's surrogate, usually a parent or guardian. Decisions made by the surrogate to accept or refuse treatment should reflect the best interests of the child.

School-Age Children

School-age children should be empowered by their parents and clinicians to begin taking ownership of their personal health by encouraging them to participate in the consent process. While decision-making authority rests in the hands of the parent or guardian, the clinician should seek and acknowledge the child's views on what has been proposed. Given their lack of fully developed decision-making capacity, these expressions of assent or dissent may not reflect a deep understanding of their medical condition. Requiring formal assent in this clinical setting is problematic. If clinicians and parents are not prepared to accept a child's refusal and would, in any case, override it, soliciting assent runs the risk of incurring anger and resentment. Regardless, children deserve to know age-appropriate information about their clinical situation and have their opinions expressed and appreciated.

Adolescents and the "Mature Minor"

Adolescence constitutes an important time for young patients transitioning from childhood dependence to autonomous adulthood. Clinicians face challenges when caring for adolescents, as noted above: they may possess rational decision-making capacity but lack emotional maturity and legal authority to make good decisions. In most cases, legal decision-making authority for medical decisions involving adolescents rests with parents or guardians. In such cases, adolescents should be offered active involvement in medical decision making, assent should be obtained, and their opinions acknowledged and taken seriously.

Some states grant decision-making authority to minors that do not qualify as emancipated but have adequate capacity to make particular decisions and can thus be deemed "mature minors" [14, 15]. States vary regarding the age at which a child can be considered a mature minor and the process for determining the decision-making capacity of a patient [15]. As with adults, mature minors can accept or reject treatment and diagnostic interventions without the consent or permission of their parents or guardians. However, clinicians should encourage parental awareness of mature minors' decisions and urge patients to involve their parents for appropriate emotional and other support.

Emancipated Minors

In some cases, minors have adult medical decision-making authority given their status as legally emancipated based on: being pregnant or a parent, in the military, self-supporting and/or not living with their parents, marriage, or court determination [16–18]. For these patients, clinicians must obtain informed consent directly from the emancipated minors, who may decline or invite the involvement of adults important in their lives.

Informed Refusal and Dissent

Refusal of consent for recommended medical treatment or diagnostics poses important challenges for clinicians. Adult patients with adequate decision-making capacity can refuse treatment or diagnostic interventions even for idiosyncratic reasons, unless the treatment is legally required (e.g., treatment of tuberculosis or other communicable diseases). Clinicians often find refusals troubling, especially with decisions to refuse life-saving therapies. Nevertheless, allowing capacitated adult patients to refuse diagnostics or treatment shows respect for autonomy, a key tenet of Western medical ethics.

When a patient with capacity refuses to accept medical recommendations, clinicians have an obligation to ensure that the refusal represents a true, voluntary informed decision. The 1980 case of *Truman v. Thomas* highlighted the important concept of informed refusal. In the case, Ms. Truman died of cervical cancer after multiple refusals of a pap smear test offered by her physician, Dr. Thomas. After her death, her family sued Thomas for negligence for failing to perform a pap smear, resulting in her wrongful death. The California Supreme Court ruled that when a patient refuses treatment, the clinician still has a duty to inform that patient of the risks of refusal as rejection of medical recommendations does not mean that patient has the same understanding as the clinician of the risks of refusal [19]. This case raised important questions of what duty a physician has to a patient who refuses testing and what additional information the individual who refuses should receive about the risks of forgoing the recommended intervention.

When encountering refusals of their recommendations, clinicians must attempt to identify the reasons behind the refusal. The process may uncover a failure in communication with the medical team, fear or misunderstanding of the proposed intervention or potential outcomes, or mistrust of the medical system. Addressing these issues may help the patient, family, and clinician come to agreement about what to do. Explaining the risks of deferring treatment or diagnostic interventions is a key element of such discussions.

In pediatrics, refusing recommended care is much more problematic. Parents or guardians must make decisions focused on the best interests of the child and may not decide simply on the basis of personal preference or whim, as they could for themselves. Clinicians have a duty to ensure that decisions made on behalf of an incompetent patient represent the child's best interests. However, determining what constitutes the best interests for an individual child poses substantial challenges and may vary, depending on the personal, religious, or cultural perspectives of the involved parties. In addition, the child's prognosis and likely quality of life post-intervention may have an impact on the family unit, including its finances and other relationships. When presented with a parent or guardian who refuses medical recommendations, the clinician must carefully consider the risks of refusal to the patient and consider how seeking legal intervention will affect the family unit and future interactions with medical providers. Cases of parental refusal do not often end up in court. However, in the majority of such cases the courts have sided with the clinicians, especially for religion-based refusals but less likely for refusals involving life-threatening or potentially disabling medical conditions [20–22].

We conclude this discussion with a reiteration of the issues involved in child dissent. As clinicians encourage the involvement of children in medical decision making, they will encounter cases in which the patient disagrees with the recommendations of the physician or decisions made by his or her parent(s) or guardian. This dissent must be taken seriously, though. Unless the patient qualifies as a mature or emancipated minor, the decision-making authority remains with the parent or guardian. The AAP Committee on Bioethics suggests honoring pediatric dissent when the proposed intervention can be postponed without substantial risk or more time can help the patient reach a better understanding of the clinical situation. In the research setting, especially with studies that will not directly benefit the patient, United States federal regulations require the affirmative agreement of the child to participate [6].

Clinicians and parents must recognize that overriding a child's dissent has implications, principally the undermining of trust, for family dynamics and for the physician-patient relationship. A child's dissent may reflect immaturity or lack of a deep understanding of the clinical circumstances. Courts have recognized that decision-making capacity evolves over years, with most judicial rulings acknowledging the importance of the views of adolescent patients [21]. Even though families and clinicians cannot always honor a patient's choice, her or his views and feelings at all times deserve respect.

Unique Considerations

Jehovah's Witnesses and Blood Consent

Surgeons and anesthesiologists face a special challenge when caring for members of the Jehovah's Witness church. Jehovah's Witnesses possess strong beliefs against accepting blood products. In some cases, individuals or their community will accept non-cellular components of blood, such as albumin, intravenous immunoglobulin, clotting factors, and the use of non-blood primed equipment for extracorporeal circulation or intraoperative scavenging, if the circulation is uninterrupted. Unlike Christian Scientists, Witnesses do not reject most aspects of modern medicine though do request accommodations for their sincerely held religious conviction to abstain from accepting blood products, based upon their interpretation of biblical passages [23, 24]. Of note, clinicians often have misconceptions about Witnesses' beliefs. The church teaches that those who have involuntarily received impermissible blood have been violated in ways that are morally equivalent to rape, and the victims will not suffer religious consequences of the actions of others. Even the deliberate acceptance of blood may be considered a sin, one forgivable by God if the believer properly seeks atonement.

Operating room personnel may struggle with such cases, given inherent surgical risk of blood loss and the potential for lifesaving via transfusions. For many surgical cases, the informed consent process will include consent for intra-operative blood products. Adult Witnesses with adequate decision-making capacity may legally refuse transfusion, even if refusal places them at life-threatening risk. Clinicians must respect the informed refusal of blood by autonomous adults or surrogate's decisions based on a previously competent individual's clearly expressed wishes.

Witness parents generally hold that The Bible calls for refusing blood products for their children, as well as themselves. This conflicts with most clinicians' view that transfusion can serve the best interests of their patient, whose parents should not impose their religious views on a child, as yet unable to consider and endorse the tenets of their parents' faith. In general, United States courts have supported clinicians' petitions to order life-saving transfusions. In dire emergencies, clinicians may take temporary custody of a child in order to provide transfusion, though they must petition the court for review after the fact. In less acute circumstances, clinicians should seek court approval prior to giving blood. The decision to apply to the court requires care, with reflection on the actual need for blood, given possible repercussions for the child's family, religious community, and clinician-family dynamics. If the medical need for blood products is not fully clear and refusal of blood product does not place the patient at imminent, life-threatening risk, clinicians should engage the family, discussing possible alternatives to blood products.

The courts have recognized the evolving decision-making capacity of patients and respected the religious convictions of mature minors. The 1989 court ruling *In Re: EG* provided one example of a decision that favored the religiously-based beliefs of a mature minor. In this case, a 17-year-old Jehovah's Witness diagnosed with acute lymphoblastic leukemia (ALL) agreed to chemotherapy but not blood transfusions, a decision her mother supported. The hospital sought legal custody of the patient, claiming she was a neglected minor and obtained an initial court order to give blood transfusions. The Illinois Supreme Court reversed the decision on the family's appeal. The decision declared the patient a mature minor, with a consistent set of religious beliefs, who possessed a competent adult's right to refuse lifesaving treatment [25]. Such cases highlight the importance of determining if a patient could be considered a mature minor based on a consistent pattern of religious practices and beliefs. See Chap. 6 for a more detailed discussion on this topic.

Trainees

Obtaining informed consent in teaching environments also presents particular challenges, as training programs must balance the obligation to provide expert medical care with the need to educate successive generations of practitioners. Training programs rely heavily on residents and fellows for patient care and administrative responsibilities and, in turn, trainees rely on direct hands-on experience and the guidance of attending physicians and surgeons to develop their clinical skills and medical knowledge. As the competence of trainees grows, they require less oversight and in some circumstances may perform without direct attending supervision. The gradual transition to independent practice has implications for the informed consent process. Most patients and families do not understand the complexity of the medical training system and may believe that a trainee obtaining consent is the attending surgeon or anesthesiologist. The doctrine of informed consent teaches that patients or surrogates have a right to know about all aspects of their health care, including who will perform their procedure and the extent of trainees' involvement. Parents or guardians must provide specific consent if trainees will participate in the care of their child. If parents or guardians refuse trainee involvement, the lead attending should attempt to resolve the issue with the family by explaining the importance of training programs. If no resolution can be reached, the attending needs to explore transfer of the patient to a nonteaching facility or undertake the case without trainees [26, 27].

Emergency Surgery

This discussion of informed consent has presumed that the patient and parent or guardian have ample time to discuss the indications for the proposed intervention, risks, benefits and alternatives, and arrive at an informed decision. In some cases, however, a parent or guardian may be unavailable to provide consent, yet delaying care for a critically ill child solely to obtain consent would place the child at increased risk of harm. In these cases, ethics and law consider consent for medical assessment and treatment presumed, a concept known as the doctrine of implied consent. Clinicians can proceed with necessary, emergent medical care until a parent or guardian can provide consent for ongoing care. This authority to proceed stems from the clinicians' duty to promote the best interests of the patient and the assumption that a reasonable person would consent to emergency care if given the opportunity [28, 29].

An AAP policy statement from 2011, "Consent for Emergency Medical Services for Children and Adolescents" provides guidelines for practitioners facing clinical situations where no parent or guardian is available to provide consent. The statement outlines specific criteria that must be met in order to presume consent and proceed with emergency treatment of the patient [29]:

1. The patient has an emergent condition that places the child at imminent and life-threatening risk.
2. The child's parent or guardian is unable or unavailable to provide informed consent for treatment.
3. Treatment cannot be delayed until consent is obtained.
4. Practitioner will only provide care for emergent conditions.

Informed Consent and Language Barriers

In our multilingual and multicultural society, practitioners must acknowledge the challenges that come with caring for patients and families with limited or no knowledge of English. In such cases, informed consent should be obtained with help of a certified medical interpreter, whether in person or with the use of telephonic or video interpreting. Using a family member as an interpreter raises serious concerns about the accuracy of the interpretation and freedom of the communication from familial or cultural biases. Trained medical interpreters ensure that the patient and family fully understand the nature of the proposed intervention, that the medical team knows about the child's relevant medical history, and appreciates the family's beliefs and values. Ensuring proper communication enhances the physician-patient-family relationship.

Informed Consent When Multiple Physicians Participate in the Case

Many surgical cases require a team of physicians to succeed, including anesthesiologists and occasionally, multiple surgical subspecialists. In such cases, obtaining informed consent involves specifying each physician's role and consideration of overwhelming parents or guardians with multiple similar discussions. The lead surgeon overseeing the case should initiate and control the consent process. This individual should also involve the surgical subspecialists anticipated to play a large role in the case in the informed consent process. The lead surgeon should prepare the patient and family for the possibility of other surgical subspecialists becoming involved if the surgery uncovers a need for additional subspecialty expertise. Openness and honesty about what may transpire in the operating room helps alleviate preoperative anxiety and prepares patients and families for what may occur in the postoperative period. In some cases, the child's critical condition may not allow for intraoperative discussion with new surgeons but team members should attempt to provide frequent and comprehensive updates to the family. Consent for anesthesia should occur separately.

Elective and Cosmetic Surgery

Some types of surgical cases should be deferred until the patient can participate in the decision-making process. Examples include bariatric surgery, gender reassignment, and many cosmetic procedures. These cases rarely involve urgent circumstances and all have potential long-term physical and psychosocial implications for the patient. Their complexity calls for involvement of a multi-disciplinary team, including mental health professionals, social workers, nurses, and physicians, among others, with the likely need for decision making over a prolonged period. For these reasons, efforts should be made to defer such cases until the minor patient can provide assent.

Surgical Innovation and Research

Advancing surgical science and technique, improving surgical outcomes, and increasing efficiency requires innovation and research. In surgery many advancements may be discovered unexpectedly during an operation or new ideas may be tested in the operating room without formal study. Most surgeons feel a continuum exists between surgical innovation and research. Informed consent in such circumstances has considerable complexity and will be discussed in detail in Chap. 10. Here we note that pediatric surgeons should consider how surgical innovation and research might affect the patient. Including children in surgical trials requires parent permission and, when appropriate, pediatric assent. The need for such specific permission does not provide a warrant for conducting uncontrolled surgical innovation outside of formal research protocols. When facing a new and unexpected surgical option in the operating room, surgeons should assess the circumstances of the case, their personal expertise and skill, the expertise and skills of other team members, the potential risks of proceeding with a not yet validated technique, and the potential for conflicts of interest arising from enthusiasm for employing a technique of one's own invention. In most cases, using a new technique should involve speaking with the family and obtaining informed consent. If consent for innovation cannot be obtained from the parent or guardian, the surgeon should proceed with the originally agreed-upon surgery [30, 31].

Conclusions

Learning to obtain adequate informed consent is a fundamental skill all clinicians must develop. Attention to this process denotes a respect for the moral obligation clinicians have to help patients and families arrive at decisions that align with personal values and beliefs. Clinicians caring for children face particular challenges in the application of the informed consent doctrine in daily practice. Instead of directly obtaining informed consent from the patient, clinicians request informed permission from the parent or guardian. In doing so, clinicians have a duty to ensure that decisions made on behalf of an incompetent child serves the child's best interest. However, defining the best interests of a child involves complexities, as parents and patients take many factors into consideration when making decisions for their children. Clinicians must work with the patient and parent or guardian to arrive at a mutually acceptable decision, but cannot accept decisions that place the child at clear, substantial or life-threatening risk. Clinicians caring for children also have a professional responsibility to empower patients to begin to take ownership of their own health care as they grow from dependent, incompetent children into autonomous adults.

References

1. Faden RR, Beauchamp TL, King NM. A history and theory of informed consent. New York: Oxford University Press; 1986.
2. Beauchamp TL, Childress JF. Principles of biomedical ethics. New York: Oxford University Press; 2001.
3. Schloendorff v. Society of New York Hospital. NE1914. p. 92.

4. Salgo v. Leland Stanford etc. Bd. Trustees. P 2d: Cal: Court of Appeal, 1st Appellate Dist., 1st Div.; 1957. p. 170.
5. Berg JW, Appelbaum PS, Lidz CW, Parker LS. Informed consent: legal theory and clinical practice. 2nd ed. New York: Oxford University Press; 2001.
6. Bartholome WG. Informed consent, parental permission, and assent in pediatric practice. Pediatrics. 1995;96(5):981–2.
7. Levetown M. Communicating with children and families: from everyday interactions to skill in conveying distressing information. Pediatrics. 2008;121(5):e1441–60.
8. Brock DW. Children's competence for health care decisionmaking. Children and Health Care: Kluwer Academic Publishers, Dordrecht, The Netherlands and Norwell, MA; 1989. p. 181–212.
9. Weithorn LA, Campbell SB. The competency of children and adolescents to make informed treatment decisions. Child Dev. 1982;53(6):1589–98.
10. King NM, Cross AW. Children as decision makers: guidelines for pediatricians. J Pediatr. 1989;115(1):10–6.
11. Koocher GP, DeMaso DR. Children's competence to consent to medical procedures. Pediatrician. 1990;17(2):68–73.
12. Harrison C, Kenny NP, Sidarous M, Rowell M. Bioethics for clinicians: 9. Involving children in medical decisions. Can Med Assoc J. 1997;156(6):825–8.
13. Alderson P, Sutcliffe K, Curtis K. Children's competence to consent to medical treatment. Hastings Cent Rep. 2006;36(6):25–34.
14. Sigman GS, O'Connor C. Exploration for physicians of the mature minor doctrine. J Pediatr. 1991;119(4):520–5.
15. Coleman DL, Rosoff PM. The legal authority of mature minors to consent to general medical treatment. Pediatrics. 2013;131(4):786–93.
16. Cady FC. Emancipation of minors. Conn L Rev. 1979;12:62.
17. Horowitz RM, Davidson HA. Legal rights of children. Colorado Springs: Shepard's/McGraw-Hill; 1984.
18. Holder AR. Legal issues in pediatrics and adolescent medicine. New Haven: Yale University Press; 1985.
19. Truman v. Thomas. P 2d: Cal: Supreme Court; 1980. p. 902.
20. Saskatchewan (Minister of Social Services) v. P.(F.). DLR (4th)1990. p. 134.
21. Ridgway D. Court-mediated disputes between physicians and families over the medical care of children. Arch Pediatr Adolesc Med. 2004;158(9):891–6.
22. Cronin DC, Squires J, Squires R, Mazariegos G, Lantos JD. Parental refusal of a liver transplant for a child with biliary atresia. Pediatrics. 2013;131(1):141–6.
23. Dixon JL, Smalley MG. Jehovah's Witnesses: the surgical/ethical challenge. JAMA. 1981;246(21):2471–2.
24. Thomas JM. Meeting the surgical and ethical challenge presented by Jehovah's Witnesses. Can Med Assoc J. 1983;128:1153–4.
25. In re EG. NE 2d: Ill: Supreme Court; 1989. p. 322.
26. McCullough LB, Jones JW, Brody BA, editors. Surgical ethics. New York: Oxford University Press; 1998.
27. Jones JW, McCullough LB. Consent for residents to perform surgery. J Vasc Surg. 2002;36(3):655–6.
28. Nwomeh BC, Waller AL, Caniano DA, Kelleher KJ. Informed consent for emergency surgery in infants and children. J Pediatr Surg. 2005;40(8):1320–5.
29. Sirbaugh PE, Diekema DS. Consent for emergency medical services for children and adolescents. Pediatrics. 2011;128(2):427–33.
30. Schwartz JA. Innovation in pediatric surgery: the surgical innovation continuum and the ETHICAL model. J Pediatr Surg. 2014;49(4):639–45.
31. Luks FI, Johnson A, Polzin WJ, NAFT Network. Innovation in maternal–fetal therapy: a position statement from the North American Fetal Therapy Network. Obstet Gynecol. 2015;125(3):649–52.

Chapter 2
Preoperative Testing: Ethical Challenges, Evidence-Based Medicine and Informed Consent

Gail A. Van Norman

Abstract Preoperative medical testing for anesthesia and surgery presents certain ethical challenges. Medical evidence suggests that most preoperative testing is unnecessary and may actually harm patients, violating the ethical principle of non-maleficence. When preoperative testing is done, the anticipated true benefits and possible harms should be disclosed to the patient, as with any medical decision. Certain tests, such as pregnancy and HIV (human immunodeficiency virus) testing require particular care in the informed consent process, because they may be affected by the explicit legal rights of the patient. When patients refuse preoperative testing, the physician should generally respect the patient's decisions unless it would lead to care that is bizarre, futile, or below published professional standards.

Keywords Ethics • Preoperative Testing • Evidence-Based Medicine

Case Presentation

A 71-year-old woman presents to the anesthesia perioperative clinic for a preoperative evaluation for an elective total hip arthroplasty for avascular necrosis of the hip. Her health history is otherwise unremarkable except for a distant history of smoking. The orthopedic surgeon orders her usual battery of preoperative screening tests, including complete blood count, coagulation screen, basic chemistries, and electrocardiogram.

G.A. Van Norman, MD
Department of Anesthesiology and Pain Medicine, Department of Biomedical Ethics, University of Washington, 1959 NE Pacific Street, Seattle, WA 98195, USA
e-mail: gvn@uw.edu

B.G. Jericho (ed.), *Ethical Issues in Anesthesiology and Surgery*,
DOI 10.1007/978-3-319-15949-2_2

Introduction

Ethics of medical testing, such as genetic testing, prenatal screening and paternity testing are widely discussed in the literature. But ethical implications for more "routine" tests, including routine preoperative tests, have been largely overlooked by anesthesiologists and surgeons. This may be due to misconceptions that routine testing is necessary to promote the best medical practices and patient well-being, is not expensive, and has few if any harmful effects. Although there is an abundance of literature and professional guidelines to steer evidence-based preoperative testing, studies show that anesthesiologists and surgeons routinely ignore this information [1]. Not only is this not scientifically and medically sound, it also raises ethical problems.

Physicians generally order preoperative testing intending to benefit the patient through more appropriately directed perioperative care (the principle of beneficence), or to identify and treat correctable problems prior to surgery, and thus avoid unnecessary risks (the principle of nonmaleficence). In some cases, physicians order tests in the false belief that they may be medico-legally protective ("defensive medicine") or to prevent "unnecessary" operating room delays [2]. This strategy is one that pursues self-interest on the part of the physician, and does not have the patient's interests first in mind. In fact, excess costs are passed on to the patient, insurers and society [3]. And such tests generally do not decrease and, if inadequately followed up, often increase the physician's medico-legal risks [4], as well as increasing the patient's medical risks.

Principles of medical ethics include respect for patient autonomy, beneficence (promoting good), and nonmaleficence (avoiding harm). Ethical patient care entails moral obligations to consider whether our actions are compatible with each of these principles.

In this chapter, we will consider general medical and ethical principles of perioperative testing, examine examples of common practices that routinely violate ethical principles, and discuss preoperative tests that have special ethical implications--mandatory preoperative pregnancy testing and HIV and hepatitis testing.

"Screening" Tests Versus "Targeted" Tests

"Routine" or "screening" tests differ from "targeted" tests in the balance of risks and benefits, and therefore they also differ in ethical weight. "Routine" preoperative tests are those that are performed in all or at least most patients and are not directed by individual patient considerations. Until recently, for example, it was common practice to obtain preoperative electrocardiograms (ECGs) in all patients over the age of 50 regardless of the presence or absence of known cardiovascular morbidity. Such ECGs are often justified by anesthesiologists as aiding them in diagnosing perioperative myocardial infarction by providing a baseline comparison before and after a suspicious event. But as we will see, baseline ECGs do not substantially aid perioperative care.

Screening tests do not evaluate a specific complaint of the patient, and are not directed at the individual's particular risk of undetected baseline cardiovascular disease. Such tests are directed at general populations who have a lower prevalence of disease than patients with specific risk factors. The lower the prevalence of a disease in a population, the more likely a test will result in a falsely positive or falsely negative result. Depending on the sensitivity and specificity of the test, a "false positive paradox" can occur in populations with low-prevalence of disease, in which the number of erroneously positive tests exceeds the number of true positive tests (Table 2.1a).

Table 2.1 The False Positive Paradox; testing of a low prevalence population leads to a greater number of false positive than true positive tests

A condition known as "Mysterious Anesthesia Reaction" or MAR is associated with a significant risk of complications upon exposure to an anesthesiologist. The condition affects 0.5% of the population overall. The test has a false positive rate of 5%, and a false negative rate of zero. Your preoperative clinic director decides that all patients must be tested preoperatively for the condition. The test costs $20. You test your first 5000 patients:

(a) Testing in a low-prevalence population

Number of people tested	**Number of people with MAR**	**Number of people without MAR**	**Total**
Positive test result	(True positive) 25	(False positive) 250	**275**
Negative test result	(False negative) 0	(True negative) 4725	**4725**
Total	**25**	**4975**	**5000**

Total cost of testing: $100,000.00

Cost to detect a true positive (true cost of avoiding one complication): $4000.00

Number of people labeled as positive: 275, or 15 × the actual number of people who are positive. 250 of 5000 people will be falsely labeled as having the condition

(b) Testing in a high-prevalence population

It turns out that MAR only occurs in natural redheads, who represent 2% of your clinic population. MAR occurs in 10% of redheads. So you decide to only test redheads. Of the next 5000 preoperative evaluations, the numbers look like this:

Number of people tested	**Number of people with MAR**	**Number of people without MAR**	**Total**
Positive test result	(True positive) 10	(False positive) 5	15
Negative test result	(False negative) 0	(True negative) 85	85
Total	10	90	100 (2% of 5000)

Total cost of testing: $2000.00

Cost to detect a true positive: $200

Number of people labeled as positive: 15, or 1.5 × of the number of people who are actually positive. 5 of 5000 people will be falsely labeled as having the condition

Total savings in testing strategy B: $88,000.00

Total absolute reduction in false positive tests: 345

"Targeted" tests, in contrast, evaluate a specific problem in a particular patient at risk. Myocardial imaging studies may be performed prior to surgery in a patient with a history of chest pain suggestive of angina, for example. Targeted tests have a much higher probability of having true positives and true negative results, since they are directed at patients who have a higher prevalence of disease (Table 2.1b).

All medical tests, whether screening tests or targeted tests, carry significant risks that must be weighed against the probability of the test providing real, relevant, and important information. Furthermore, not all medical tests are ethically equivalent. Some, such as HIV and pregnancy testing, can introduce serious social risks and create specific and avoidable harms that other tests do not.

The Case Presentation, Continued

The anesthesiologist in the perioperative clinic is reviewing charts late one night and discovers that our patient's activated partial thromboplastin time (aPTT) is 56. All other coagulation studies are within normal limits. She finds no evidence of factors that would elevate the patient's risk of bleeding and calls the surgeon to alert her of the results. The surgeon responds that she wants another aPTT drawn in the preoperative holding area in the morning. The next day, the phlebotomist makes 5 attempts before obtaining blood for a repeat aPTT. The blood clots on the way to the lab, and the phlebotomist returns to the patient to make 2 more attempts. The repeat aPTT is 56. The operating room is delayed for 2 h, and the surgeon decides to proceed with surgery despite the second abnormal lab result. With no peripheral veins for access, the anesthesiologist elects to place a central line, causing a large pneumothorax that requires treatment of hypotension and the placement of a chest tube.

False positive and false negative results can label a patient as having a condition they do not have, or falsely reassure that the patient does not have a condition that they in fact do. In the former case, further testing and subsequent interventions may increase expenses and subject the patient to potential complications of the testing, or to unnecessary treatments with more attendant risks. True positive test results may be clinically insignificant but can also lead to unnecessary further testing with its accompanying risks. Further testing always increases cost–through the cost of the test itself and the cost of managing any complications or treatments that may result from it. In our clinical case, further testing had the unintended consequence of exhausting peripheral intravenous access, necessitating a more invasive procedure that was then attended by a potential life-threatening complication.

Systematic over-testing increases the cost of health care to all patients in an already over-burdened health care system. This type of expenditure also diverts funds that might be spent on productive aspects of medical care to enterprises that have little or no hope of being beneficial to this patient or to patients in general.

The Role of Evidence-Based Testing in Ethical Care of Patients: Addressing the Balance of Risks and Benefits

The principles of medical ethics demand that risks of preoperative testing (potential maleficence) be weighed against the importance of the information to be gained (potential beneficence). The modern practice of medicine is firmly rooted in belief in scientific evidence: using scientific data to inform patient care is what distinguished the ancient practice of medicine from that of sorcery. Currently, we speak of practicing "evidence-based medicine" (EBM). In evidence-based practice, clinical experience is inextricably wedded to the conscientious and explicit use of the best available medical evidence when making clinical decisions. Nonsystematic (anecdotal) clinical experience and untested hypotheses are insufficient grounds for determining a physician's actions in all but the rarest of circumstances–and then only when no credible evidence exists. EBM emphasizes respect for patient autonomy, by requiring that the patient be informed about the risks and benefits of proposed tests and therapies. Informed consent and recognition of the patient's values and goals are also emphasized in the practice of EBM [5–7].

Evidence shows that many commonplace medical practices are not only unhelpful, but actually cause serious harm. Examples include administration of albumin for treatment of shock, which has now been shown to increase mortality [8]. Screening mammography prolongs the life of 1 in 2000 women over a 10-year period, but leads to a false diagnosis of cancer and institution of cancer therapy in 10 women during the same period, leading many to question its benefit-risk ratio [9].

Despite strong medical evidence regarding harms, many practitioners are unwilling to relinquish long-standing practices [10]. Patients' expectations of the benefits and harms of screening tests and of treatments are often unrealistic, and may further encourage physicians to be injudicious in ordering them [11]. Reluctance to give up traditional but potentially harmful practices may have deep psychological roots, leading some to propose legislative action to compel doctors to use the evidence presented in such studies [12]. Movements such as the "Choosing Wisely" campaign in the United States (US) are gaining ground, and, "Choosing Wisely" has already identified unnecessary preoperative testing as a target area for practice improvement in anesthesiology and surgery [13].

Once we understand that ethical preoperative testing involves (1) identifying the true benefits to patients and (2) balancing them against evidence of harms, (3) determining which tests actually provide not only accurate, but clinically relevant information (i.e., information that will lead to effective preoperative optimization and perioperative risk-reduction strategies), (4) providing this information to patients in the informed consent process and (5) pursuing in partnership with the patient a clinical strategy designed to maximize potential benefits and minimize potential harms in accordance with their values, we can draw clearer and more cost-effective clinical plans for perioperative care.

What Is the Evidence for Performing Preoperative Screening Tests?

In order to appropriately inform our patients about preoperative tests and rationally determine whether tests should be ordered, all physicians involved in perioperative care are ethically obliged to have at least passing knowledge of the evidence regarding any tests they order, and to use that knowledge in a rational way. Fortunately for anesthesiologists and surgeons, the literature on routine preoperative tests is both abundant, and quite consistent. Sadly, studies show that anesthesiologists and surgeons are commonly ignorant of the evidence regarding the tests usefulness, and/or willfully ignore the evidence at hand. Some studies show that in a significant number of cases, the physician never even examines the results of the tests they order [14].

Electrocardiogram

In 1993, Atkins and Roizen, in an argument prescient to EBM, provided a powerful case for giving up one of our most beloved preoperative screening exams: the ECG [15]. The ECG is an insensitive and nonspecific examination that has little role in preoperative management, and yet is one of the most difficult to convince anesthesiologists and surgeons to relinquish.

Patients with abnormal preoperative ECGs have a greater risk of cardiovascular death than those with normal ECGs (1.8% vs. 0.3%, odds ratio 4.5). Although that may appear to be a meaningful difference, for low-to-intermediate risk surgery, the absolute difference in cardiovascular death is clinically insignificant, and the value of this test as a predictor of negative outcomes is virtually nil [16]. Furthermore, the test does not lead to changes in management that might account for any risk mitigation. In an unselected preoperative population, almost half of all ECGs are abnormal. Coronary revascularization prior to noncardiac surgery is now based on clinical findings and the patient's current medical therapy and not the ECG, and is rarely indicated in the truly asymptomatic patient [17]. A comprehensive literature review found that the predictive power of preoperative ECGs is weak at best and that there is no evidence to support the value of "baseline" ECGs preoperatively [18]. Age over 65 independently predicts the presence of an abnormal ECG, but does not predict a modifiable risk factor for surgical patients. In one study, of 1149 ECGs reviewed, only 0.44% of patients without clinical risk factors had abnormalities on their ECG, irrespective of age [19]. In patients over age 70, up to 75% have abnormalities on a preoperative ECG, but these abnormalities do not independently predict postoperative cardiac complications when other clinical risk stratification is done such as the American Society of Anesthesiologists (ASA) physical status and the American Heart Association (AHA) cardiac risk index [20]. The predictive power of an abnormal ECG for perioperative cardiovascular events is slightly greater for patients with cardiovascular risk factors than those without, but the difference is not statistically significant. In fact, in one study a normal ECG had the same predictive value for such events [21]. According to AHA guidelines, preoperative ECGs are not indicated in asymptomatic persons of any age undergoing low-risk procedures [22]. The ASA Task Force on Preanesthesia Evaluation found no compelling evidence for routine ECG testing for age indications alone, but recommended possible testing for those at risk due to underlying disease, or due to clinical findings at a preoperative visit [23].

The total burden of harm of screening ECGs is not known, but in many patients with either falsely abnormal or clinically insignificant abnormal findings, additional testing is often undertaken with its attendant economic cost and medical risks. How can we argue ethically or medically that ECGs should be routinely ordered in low-to-intermediate risk patients when (1) there is no evidence that the vast majority of patients benefit, (2) there is no evidence that care is changed, and (3) there is evidence at least from an economic standpoint that both individual patients and patients collectively suffer harm?

Electrolytes

Recent literature on routine preoperative screening of serum electrolytes is scant, but results parallel that of ECG testing.

In one study, not only was the incidence of abnormal findings on chemistry tests low, but also in no patient was the anesthesia management modified as a result of the test [24]. In another systematic review, routine preoperative biochemistries discovered unexpected abnormal sodium or potassium levels 1.4% of the time and abnormal creatinine levels in up to 2.5% of patients, but clinical management was rarely modified [18]. A survey of studies from the National Health Service in Britain failed to identify any evidence about the effectiveness of such tests [25]. Furthermore, several studies demonstrated that chronic hypokalemia is not associated with increase risk of perioperative arrhythmias in the noncardiac surgical patient [26, 27]. Fritsch et al. found that abnormal electrolytes occurred in about 1.6% of patients preoperatively, but were not predictors of perioperative complications [28]. Johnson and Mortimer reported that preoperative management was altered in response to only 0.2% of results in 100 patients. No complications arose that were attributable to the test results [29].

Complete Blood Count

In one review of preoperative complete blood count (CBC) testing in otherwise asymptomatic patients, abnormal levels of hematocrit (HCT) or hemoglobin (Hgb) were found in about 5%, but Hgb was rarely below 9 g/dl, well above currently recommended thresholds for transfusion. CBC findings lead to a change of management in 0.1–2% of patients. Unexpected low platelet counts were rare (<1%) and rarely if ever resulted in management changes [18]. Another study of routine preoperative tests found that 60% had no indications and only 0.22% found abnormalities that might have changed perioperative management. However, those abnormalities were never acted on, and no complications resulted [30].

Coagulation Screening

Routine preoperative testing of coagulation parameters in asymptomatic patients in an effort to predict intra- and post-operative bleeding is well studied. For patients undergoing noncardiac surgery who do not have a history or physical findings suggestive of an increased risk of bleeding (Table 2.2), preoperative testing does not identify those at increased risk, is expensive, and exposes patients to the risks of further unnecessary testing.

Multiple studies involving adults and children undergoing low risk ambulatory surgery, major general surgery, major orthopedic surgery, major neurosurgery, spine surgery, endoscopic procedures, and ear, nose, throat (ENT) procedures demonstrate that coagulation screening does not predict bleeding risk and that patient history is at least as effective in predicting perioperative bleeding [31–37]. The ASA Task Force on Preanesthesia Evaluation does not recommend routine coagulation screening [23].

In our case scenario, the most common cause of an isolate elevation in aPTT (after "undetermined") is anti-lupus antibody. This antibody is a procoagulant and is associated with accelerated clotting, not abnormal bleeding. In a large series of patients with this finding who underwent major surgery, there were two minor complications (wound hematoma), neither of which required re-exploration [38]. Thus, the further testing, physical trauma and complications to which the patient in the case presentation was subjected were entirely unnecessary.

Table 2.2 Factors that identify risk for increased perioperative bleeding

Patients generally at risk for increased bleeding can generally be ruled out by the following five questions; in the absence of a positive response to at least one of the questions, the patient should be considered low risk for bleeding
1. Do you personally have a diagnosed bleeding disorder?
2. Does anyone in your family have a diagnosed bleeding disorder?
3. Do you bleed or bruise easily (e.g., bruising with minimal or no trauma, bleeding from the gums for a full 5 min after stopping brushing teeth, history of transfusion for minor trauma or surgery, very heavy menses requiring intervention, heavy bleeding after prior surgery or vaginal delivery)
4. Do you take a blood thinning medication such as coumadin, lovenox, heparin, Plavix or Pradaxa?
5. Do you have a medical condition that predisposes to bleeding such as advanced liver or kidney disease?

Medical Tests with Special Ethical Significance

Many blood tests have few social implications. But while the negative impact of most unnecessary blood tests may therefore be restricted to cost, patient discomfort and the risks that they will lead to further tests, costs and potential complications, some tests carry serious social risks for patients –up to and including their very safety. Examples of such tests are HIV, hepatitis, and mandatory pregnancy testing.

HIV and Hepatitis

Screening testing for the presence of HIV and hepatitis infection may be advisable in some limited patient populations. For example, screening in pregnant women may increase the probability that an infant born to an HIV-positive mother can receive early therapy and avoid chronic HIV infection. But screening in the routine preoperative population is impossible to justify.

It has been shown that the incidence of positive findings on routine preoperative screening for HIV and hepatitis B and C prior to elective orthopedic surgery is low (0.4% in a large population) [39]. Weber and colleagues concluded that the costs of testing are not warranted by the results [39]. Prevalence of hepatitis C in elective orthopedic surgery patients is about 0.6% [40]. A similar prevalence for hepatitis B and C (0.41%) was found in an elective orthopedic surgical population with a much higher prevalence of abnormal liver function tests (LFTs) (13%). The most common cause of elevated transaminases by far was nonalcoholic steatohepatitis and not infectious agents [41].

The prevalence of asymptomatic HIV infection in elective orthopedic surgery patients has been shown to be low (0.15%) and testing in this low-prevalence population is associated with an equal rate of false positive to true positive tests (0.11% versus 0.15%) [42]. Thus for every patient correctly identified as being HIV positive, one will be falsely labeled as such.

There are two arguments for carrying out routine testing for infectious agents in the perioperative period. The first is that the patient may suffer from a disease that substantially increases their risks in the perioperative period. However, asymptomatic HIV and hepatitis patients are NOT at substantially increased risk for perioperative complications during elective surgery and anesthesia. The second is that provider injury during surgical care of patients with the infectious agent may expose the provider to increased risks, and early intervention after such an injury, prior to the patient's recovery from anesthesia, will reduce the provider's risks. But early intervention in the postanesthesia care unit (PACU) is not necessary in the first steps after hollow needle stick or other blood borne pathogen exposure in the operating room.

Some providers may order such tests so that they can identify positive patients and single them out for "extra precautions." However, this belief lies in a misunderstanding of infectious disease. A true negative antibody test can occur in patients who do not have infection, and also occur in those who have very early infection and have not yet developed the antibodies that turn the test positive. Both test results are true negatives and correctly identify patients without antibodies. But early in infection before antibody development, viral load is often at its greatest and the patient most infectious. Thus, the Centers for Disease Control (CDC) recommends "universal precautions," rather than precautions only directed at test-positive patients.

Testing for HIV and hepatitis without consent may violate patient privacy rights, is unnecessary, and may lead to further unnecessary cost and stress in patients when intraoperative provider injury is uncommon. Most hospitals have established procedures for when such provider injuries occur, including approaching the patient to obtain consent for testing, protection of patient privacy rights, and providing often legally required counseling to patients who find out in this way that they have a serious chronic infectious disease.

Adverse social consequences for HIV positive patients include employment discrimination, loss of insurance, and social isolation. Mandatory HIV testing prevents some patients from seeking medical care. HIV seropositivity is associated with marital breakup, abandonment, and verbal and physical violence against women whose HIV status is disclosed [43]. The U.S. thus includes acquired immune deficiency syndrome (AIDS) patients in the protections afforded under the Americans with Disabilities Act, and legislation specifically protects the privacy of a patient's HIV status.

Pregnancy Testing

Routine preoperative pregnancy testing has ethical ramifications analogous to HIV testing. Preoperative pregnancy testing is most logical early in pregnancy, when it is not obvious to either the patient or her provider that she is pregnant. But during early pregnancy, maternal rights are generally recognized to supersede fetal interests in most of the United States.

In many states, an adult female's right to privacy regarding reproduction issues is absolute, up to and including a decision to terminate pregnancy. In many states, those rights are awarded without restriction to minor females as well. Minor females are often awarded rights to seek reproductive care without parental permission because there is concern that without such privacy rights, many pregnant minors would forgo prenatal or other pregnancy care. But a more serious and sinister reason is also argued: childhood pregnancies may be the result of child abuse, incest or rape within the child's home. Informing the parents of a minor of her positive pregnancy test can place the child in jeopardy of further physical harm, since it may be evidence of criminal behavior on the part of a family member, or family friend or acquaintance. Many states have statutory requirements for physicians to report evidence of child abuse, and some authorities recommend reporting pregnant minors to Child Protective Services for investigation of possible sexual abuse. Such repercussions lead to fears of physical violence and even death on the part of vulnerable girls in social environments where their pregnancy is not accepted [44].

Against such potentially great harm, what are the potentially beneficial outcomes of pregnancy testing? Evidence of harm from elective anesthesia and surgery in early pregnancy is surprisingly scant. Several specific factors are of concern with regard to elective surgery in early pregnancy: radiation, manipulation of the uterus or pelvis, and exposure to anesthetic drugs and agents.

Fetal radiation exposure above 5Gy is known to cause increased rates of cancer, although malformations are not generally reported [45]. Thus, procedures exposing the fetus to either direct radiation in utero (as might happen with lower spine surgeries, for example) or indirect scatter radiation from intraoperative procedures involving fluoroscopy or other radiation devices are of particular concern. But the fetal radiation exposure in even orthopedic procedures is generally below 5Gy [46].

Large scale studies of pregnancy outcomes following pelvic or abdominal surgery on a pregnant patient have not been done, however, small series and case reports are increasingly reporting that laparoscopic surgery in the pregnant woman can be safely done. A recent review demonstrates increased fetal loss that may be partially mitigated by selection of surgical approach (open vs. laparoscopic) [47].

Well-designed population studies do not demonstrate that anesthetics lead to early fetal loss or increased fetal malformation [48–50]. In fact the ASA Task Force on Perioperative Testing judged the literature to be "inadequate" to support concerns about fetal exposure to anesthetics [23]. Fewer than one-third of US anesthesiology practices demand pregnancy testing prior to surgery [51].

Many patients may choose not to undergo elective surgery if they know they are pregnant. However, coercing a female patient to have a test against her wishes explicitly violates patient autonomy. Physician self-interest (defensive medicine) is not a sufficient justification for disregarding patient autonomy or violating a patient's privacy. It is the joint recommendation of the ASA Task Force on Preoperative Testing and the ASA Committee on Ethics that anesthesiologists offer the choice of preoperative pregnancy testing to any female patient who might desire one, explain the potential risks and benefits, and obtain informed consent for the test [25].

Informed Consent for Preoperative Testing

Consent for preoperative testing of any kind is the same as informed consent for any other aspect of medical care. Risks and benefits of the tests should be explained to the patient, including the risks of not being tested. Respect for patient autonomy requires us in general to respect patient choice about preoperative testing.

Targeted tests are much easier to justify to patients, because there is a specific reason that makes the test important in this patient. It may be difficult to justify to a patient that the only reason for a test is "because we always do it." In fact, if the test has a low probability of yielding a meaningful, management-altering result, it is tough to justify the test on either ethical or medical grounds. Even with minimal justification, however, patients may respond positively to the desire to do a test to avoid the inconvenience of an unexpected cancellation. That, however, should be their choice. It is not appropriate to routinely do medical tests that have potential economic, social and medical harms, to prevent inconvenience to the operating room schedule, surgeon or anesthesiologist.

What If the Patient Refuses Preoperative Testing?

Patients, when given accurate information on the likelihood that medical tests will benefit them, may be unwilling to undergo routine preoperative tests.

Physicians are never required to provide futile, bizarre or substandard care. If the lack of testing would lead to such a situation, it may be at the physician's discretion to refuse to proceed with surgery if the patient refuses testing. However, the fact that many if not most physicians thoughtlessly order unnecessary tests before surgery does not make such testing "standard," or the lack of it "substandard." The "standard of care" depends increasingly on the medical evidence and guidelines of professional organizations, and less and less on individual practices. If there are no or little demonstrable benefits to having the test done, it is unlikely that it can be labeled substandard to forgo it, even if it is a common test. Furthermore, most guidelines and standards now no longer endorse most preoperative screening examinations: it is not therefore likely that failure to do a screening examination would be considered substandard from a medico-legal standpoint.

If the physician feels there is a specific reason for a preoperative test, this obviously should be disclosed to the patient, particularly if failure to test or a particular test result could result in cancellation of the surgery.

In a recent case in the author's practice, for example, a woman presented for hysterectomy due to a genetic disorder that not only caused spontaneous miscarriages early in pregnancy, but also life-threatening bleeding with menses and with her miscarriages. After becoming pregnant several times and experiencing life-threatening hemorrhage, she elected to undergo prophylactic hysterectomy. The hospital she chose was a Catholic organization who did not inform her that a pregnancy test was required by hospital policy prior to surgery in women of child-bearing years on religious grounds. She did not want a pregnancy test, since it was painful to her to think that she might be causing the end of another pregnancy during her surgery, even though it had no hope of being carried to completion. When the nursing staff insisted that she undergo the test, she began to cry and told the author that, had she known of the requirement, she would have scheduled her surgery at a competing hospital down the street that had no such policy.

When test results carry very important relevance to patients, anesthesiologists and surgeons have an ethical obligation to respect that fully informed patients may make choices in order to manage their own health care goals, including seeking another provider–and that they have an absolute right to do so.

References

1. Bryson GL, Wyand A, Bragg PR. Preoperative testing is inconsistent with published guidelines and rarely changes management. Can J Anaesth. 2006;53:236–41.
2. Carrier ER, Resschovsky JD, Katz DA, Mello MM. High physician concern about malpractice risk predicts more aggressive diagnostic testing in office-based practice. Health Aff (Millwood). 2013;32:1383–91.
3. DeKay ML, Asch DA. Is the defensive use of diagnostic tests good for patients, or bad? Med Decis Making. 1998;18:19–28.
4. Kumar A, Srivastava U. Role of routine laboratory investigations in preoperative evaluation. J Anaesthesiol Clin Pharmacol. 2011;27:174–9.
5. Kalantri SP. Ethics, evidence and anaesthesiology. Ind J Anaesth. 2004;48:108–10.
6. Polaris JJ, Katz JN. "Appropriate" diagnostic testing: supporting diagnostics with evidence-based medicine and shared decision-making. BMC Res Notes. 2014;7:922.
7. Burger IM, Kass NE. Screening in the dark: ethical considerations of providing screening tests to individuals when evidence is insufficient to support screening populations. Am J Bioeth. 2009;9:3–14.
8. Alderson P, Bunn F, Lefebvre C, Li WP, Li L, Roberts I, et al. Human albumin solution for resuscitation and volume expansion in critically ill patients. Cochrane Database Syst Rev. 2004;18:CD001208.
9. Gotzsche PC, Nielsen M. Screening for breast cancer with mammography. Cochrane Database Syst Rev. 2013;1:CD001877.
10. Ubel PA, Asch DA. Creating value in health by understanding and overcoming resistance to de-innovation. Health Aff (Millwood). 2015;34:239–44.
11. Hoffmann TC, Del Mar C. Patients' expectations of the benefits and harms of treatments, screening and tests: a systematic review. JAMA Intern Med. 2015;175:274–86.
12. Gaspoz JM. Smarter medicine: do physicians need political pressure to eliminate useless interventions? Swiss Med Wkly. 2015;145:w13125.
13. Onuoha OC, Arkoosh VA, Fleisher LA. Choosing wisely in anesthesiology: the gap between evidence and practice. JAMA Intern Med. 2014;174:13991–5.
14. Nash GF, Cunnick GH, Allen S, Cook C, Turner LF. Preoperative electrocardiograph examination. Ann R Coll Surg Engl. 2001;83(6):381–2.
15. Atkins RF, Roizen MF. Predicting the utility of the preoperative electrocardiogram: ageism and its economic impact. J Clin Monit. 1994;10:70–2.
16. Noordzij PG, Boersma E, Bax JJ, Feringa HH, Schreiner F, Schouten O, et al. Prognostic value of routine preoperative electrocardiography in patients undergoing noncardiac surgery. Am J Cardiol. 2006;97:1103–6.
17. Fleisher LA. The preoperative electrocardiogram: what is the role in 2007? Ann Surg. 2007;246:171–2.
18. Munro J, Booth A, Nicholl J. Routine preoperative testing: a systematic review of the evidence. Health Technol Assess. 1997;1:i–iv,1–62.
19. Correll DJ, Hepner DL, Chang C, Tsen L, Hevelone ND, Bader AM. Preoperative electrocardiograms: patient factors predictive of abnormalities. Anesthesiology. 2009;110:1205–6.
20. Liu LL, Dzankic S, Leung JM. Preoperative electrocardiogram abnormalities do not predict postoperative cardiac complications in geriatric surgical patients. J Am Geriatr Soc. 2002;50:1186–91.
21. Tait AR, Parr HG, Tremper KK. Evaluation of the efficacy of routine preoperative electrocardiograms. J Cardiothorac Vasc Anesth. 1997;11:752–5.
22. Fleisher LA, Beckman JA, Brown KA, et al. ACC/AHA 2007 guidelines on perioperative cardiovascular evaluation and care for noncardiac surgery. Anesth Analg. 2007;104:15–26.
23. American Society of Anesthesiologists Task Force on Preanesthesia Evaluation. Practice advisory for preanesthesia evaluation: a report by the American Society of Anesthesiologists Task Force on Preanesthesia Evaluation. Anesthesiology. 2002;96:485–96.

24. de Sousa S, Brandao RR, Mourao MR, Azevedo VL, Figueiredo AV, Trindade ES. Relevance of routine testing in low-risk patients undergoing minor and medium surgical procedures. Braz J Anestesiol. 2013;63:197–201.
25. Czoski-Murray C, Lloyd Jones M, McCabe C, Claxton K, Oluboyede Y, Roberts J, et al. What is the value of routinely testing full blood count, electrolytes and urea, and pulmonary function tests before elective surgery in patients with no apparent clinical indication and in subgroups of patients with common comorbidities: a systematic review of the clinical and cost-effective literature. Health Technol Assess. 2012;16:i–xvi, 1–159.
26. Hirsch IA, Tomlinson DL, Slogoff S, Keats AS. The overstated risk of preoperative hypokalemia. Anesth Analg. 1988;67:131–6.
27. Wong KC, Sperry R. What is an acceptable preoperative serum potassium level for surgery? Anesthesiology. 1994;81:269.
28. Fritsch G, Flamm M, Hepner DL, Panisch S, Seer J, Soennichsen A. Abnormal pre-operative tests, pathological findings of medical history, and their predictive value for perioperative complications. Acta Anaesthesiol Scand. 2012;56:339–50.
29. Johnson RK, Mortimer AJ. Routine pre-operative blood testing: is it necessary? Anaesthesia. 2002;57:914–7.
30. Kaplan EB, Sheiner LB, Boeckmann AJ, Roizen MF, Beal SL, Cohen SN, et al. The usefulness of preoperative laboratory screening. JAMA. 1985;253:3576–81.
31. Dützmann S, Gessler F, Marquardt G, Seifert V, Senft C. On the value of routine prothrombin time screening in elective neurosurgical procedures. Neurosurg Focus. 2012;33:E9.
32. Townsend JC, Heard R, Powers ER, Rueben A. Usefulness of international normalized ratio to predict bleeding complications in patients with end-stage liver disease who undergo cardiac catheterization. Am J Cardiol. 2012;110(7):1062–5.
33. Seicean A, Schiltz NK, Seicean S, Alan N, Neuhauser D, Weil RJ. Use and utility of preoperative hemostatic screening and patient history in adult neurosurgical patients. J Neurosurg. 2012;116(5):1097–105.
34. Samkova A, Blatny J, Fiamoli V, Dulicek P, Parizkova E. Significance and causes of abnormal preoperative coagulation test results in children. Haemophilia. 2012;18:e297–301.
35. van Veen JJ, Spahn DR, Makris M. Routine preoperative coagulation tests: an outdated practice? Br J Anaesth. 2011;106:1–3.
36. Eckman MH, Erban JK, Singh SK, Kao GS. Screening for the risk for bleeding or thrombosis. Ann Intern Med. 2003;138:W15–24.
37. Chee YL, Crawford JC, Watson HG, Greaves M. BJH guidelines on the assessment of bleeding risk prior to surgery or invasive procedures. British Committee for Standards in Haematology. Br J Haematol. 2007;140:496–504.
38. Chng WJ, Sum C, Kuperan P. Causes of isolated prolonged activated partial thromboplastin time in an acute care general hospital. Singapore Med J. 2005;46(9):450–6.
39. Weber P, Eberle J, Bogner JR, Schrimpf F, Jansson V, Huber-Wagner S. Is there benefit to routine screening of infectivity for HIV, hepatitis B and C virus before elective orthopedic operations? Infection. 2013;41(2):479–83.
40. Wiegand J, Kaiser T, Lobstein S. Low prevalence of chronic hepatitis C, but high prevalence of elevated transaminases in a cohort of 2026 patients referred for orthopedic surgery in the eastern part of Germany. Z Gastroenterol. 2006;44:11–4.
41. Lobstein S, Kaiser T, Liebert U, Wojan M, Leichtle A, Mossner J, et al. Prevalence, aetiology and associated co-morbidities of elevated aminotransferases in a German cohort of orthopedic surgery patients. Z Gastroenterol. 2008;46:415–20.
42. LaPorte DM, Mont MA, Jones LC, Padden DA, Hungerford DS. Human immunodeficiency virus testing for elective orthopedic procedures: results in a community-based hospital. Orthopedics. 2001;24(1):52–5.
43. Lester P, Partridge JC, Cheesny MA, Cooke M. The consequences of a positive prenatal HIV antibody test for women. J Acquir Immune Defic Syndr Hum Retrovirol. 1995;10:341–9.

44. Henshaw SK, Kost K. Parental involvement in minors' abortion decisions. Fam Plann Perspect. 1992;24:196–207.
45. Williams PM, Fletcher S. Health effects of prenatal radiation exposure. Am Fam Physician. 2010;82:488–93.
46. Gaymer CE, Achten J, Auckett R, Cooper L, Griffin D. Fluoroscopic radiation exposure during hip arthroscopy. Arthroscopy. 2013;29:870–3.
47. Juhasz-Boss I, Solomayer E, Strik M, Raspe C. Abdominal surgery in pregnancy–an interdisciplinary challenge. Dtsch Arztebl Int. 2014;111:465–72.
48. Brodsky JB. Anesthesia and surgery during early pregnancy and fetal outcome. Clin Obstet Gynecol. 1983;26:449–57.
49. Mazze RI, Kallen B. Reproductive outcome after anesthesia and operation during pregnancy: a registry study of 5405 cases. Am J Obstet Gynecol. 1989;161:1178–85.
50. Mazze RI, Kallen B. Appendectomy during pregnancy: a Swedish registry study of 778 cases. Obstet Gynecol. 1991;77:835–40.
51. Kempen PM. Preoperative pregnancy testing: a survey of current practice. J Clin Anesth. 1997;9:546–50.

Chapter 3
Informed Consent and the Disclosure of Surgeon Experience

Logan K. Chastain and Sabha Ganai

Abstract This chapter provides an overview of ethical issues and legal precedent relevant to informed consent for surgical procedures including the disclosure of the surgeon's experience. The process of informed consent will be examined in a systematic fashion, including methods to improve physician-patient communication and important considerations for documentation of the consent process. Ethical principles including respect for patient autonomy, beneficence, nonmaleficience, distributive justice, and duty to tell the truth will be explored as relevant to the doctrine of informed consent.

Keywords Ethics • Informed Consent • Autonomy • Surgical Decision Making • Disclosure

Case Presentation

Ms. B. is a 38-year-old obese female with a body mass index of 47 kg/m^2. Despite numerous attempts at weight reduction with dietary interventions and exercise, she has failed to maintain her weight loss. She complains of chronic lower back pain and has been recently diagnosed with hypertension, diabetes,

L.K. Chastain, MD (✉)
Department of Radiology, Southern Illinois University School of Medicine, 315 W. Carpenter St., PO Box 19638, Springfield, IL 62794, USA
e-mail: lchastain@siumed.edu

S. Ganai, MD, PhD
Department of Surgery, Southern Illinois University School of Medicine, Simmons Cancer Institute at Southern Illinois University, 315 W. Carpenter St., PO Box 19638, Springfield, IL 62794, USA
e-mail: sganai@siumed.edu

B.G. Jericho (ed.), *Ethical Issues in Anesthesiology and Surgery*,
DOI 10.1007/978-3-319-15949-2_3

and obstructive sleep apnea, all of which her primary care physician attributes to the patient's morbid obesity. Her primary care physician advised her that weight loss is essential to improve her health and longevity.

Ms. B. meets with a bariatric surgeon to discuss the options of different surgical approaches to address her morbid obesity, including laparoscopic sleeve gastrectomy and Roux-en-Y gastric bypass. She learns about the risks, benefits, and alternatives of the different surgical procedures, and their relative probabilities of weight regain. She is instructed that she will be required to participate in a yearlong process of psychological and nutritional counseling prior to surgery, will meet with others who have undergone the procedure, and will join a support group of patients who plan to undergo bariatric surgery. As the surgical date approaches, the patient will also meet with the anesthesiologist in the anesthesia clinic. Her surgeon advises her that she can change her mind about having surgery at any time, even the day of surgery. Her surgeon then asks her if she has any questions. The patient asks for the disclosure of the surgeon's prior surgical experience in bariatric surgery.

Introduction

Informed consent is an essential component in the daily practice of surgeons and anesthesiologists. While the process of informed consent is meant to expand and protect patient autonomy, it gives patients the opportunity to decide what is truly in their best interests and make a decision on whether or not to receive a specific treatment based on their own perception of benefit. The ethical principle of autonomy becomes a fundamental part of discourse relevant to informed consent, and recognizes that patients have an intrinsic right to decide what happens to their body, regardless if others believe they are making the "correct" choice. However, one may still question how many patients are truly informed; understand the risks, benefits, and alternatives of the procedure; and are informed of the surgeon's experience for a specific procedure. This chapter will explore some of the nuances and complexities relevant to the obtaining of informed consent and the disclosure of surgeon experience.

Informed Consent Principles: Disclosure and Understanding

Informed consent may be incorrectly perceived to be just a signature and just one more task to get marked off on a preoperative checklist. Furthermore, while the disclosure of the indications, risks, benefits, and alternatives of a procedure is given in the process of obtaining informed consent from a competent patient with decision making capacity, it does not assure a patient's true understanding of the information received by that patient to make an autonomous decision. Moreover, the patient's signature on a consent form is hardly sufficient as legal protection against litigation regarding informed consent issues. Informed consent should ultimately be a conversation between the patient and physician within the framework of shared decision making with the document only being a record that this discussion took place.

Disclosure of the Risks, Benefits, Alternatives

Canterbury v. Spence established the legal standard of informed consent as an "objective" duty to disclose, otherwise known as the reasonable patient test [1]. In *Canterbury v. Spence*, Jerry Canterbury sued his physician for negligence after complications ensued, alleging that he was not properly informed of the risks involved with an elective laminectomy performed for back pain [1]. The content of the disclosure of the risks of a procedure to the patient has been approached in terms of subjective, community, and reasonable person standards. "*Subjective*" standards require the disclosure of what a specific patient would need to know pertinent to the patient's particular circumstances; "*community practice*" standards require disclosure of information that other local practitioners in a local community deem appropriate for disclosure; and "*reasonable person*" standards require the disclosure of what a reasonable patient would want to know under the given circumstances. In *Canterbury v. Spence*, the court ultimately stated that "full" disclosure was a norm that was prohibitive and unrealistic to demand from physicians, so it was favored to require disclosure of risk as "material when a reasonable person, in what the physician knows or should know to be the patient's position, would be likely to attach significance to the risk or cluster of risks in deciding whether or not to forego the proposed therapy" [1]. Current legal precedent thus requires the disclosure of information that would be relevant to the ability of a patient to make a decision under given circumstances. This information includes discussion of the risks and benefits, potential alternatives, and expected postoperative course relevant to a procedure or disease process in order for it to be a truly informed decision. Unfortunately, the "objective" legal standard focusing on information that a reasonable person would want to know can still be considered ambiguous and subjective as the content can vary widely among different patients.

Patient Understanding

Once the physician discloses information to the patient, it is essential to confirm that the patient understands this information and the risks, benefits, and alternatives of the procedure. In *The Nichomachean Ethics,* Aristotle discusses *nous* (comprehension) as not based only on the acquisition of *episteme* (knowledge), *techne* (craft), or *phronesis* (practical wisdom), but as exercising an opinion in order to render a decision or judgment [2, 3]. Using the framework of Aristotlean virtue ethics, informed consent requires the provision of sufficient information and the confirmation of the patient's understanding of the provided information that will allow for judgment at a personal level [4]. The process of disclosure of relevant information can be extensive, as this discourse may not only be procedure-specific and disease-specific, but also patient-specific. However, the patient's understanding of this information is critical to the informed consent process.

In the discussion between Ms. B. and her bariatric surgeon, the surgeon asks if the patient has any questions and thus begins to explore the patient's level of comprehension and what additional information is relevant for her as a person. While the informed consent process for bariatric surgery may take over a year and may be assisted and supplemented by support groups and teams to ensure that adequate disclosure and understanding has taken place, it can be argued that the majority of surgical procedures and anesthetics cannot be practically undertaken with such liberty to educate the patient.

Despite physicians presenting information to patients in the obtaining of informed consent, the patients' recall and understanding of this information can be limited. In a study of patients undergoing an open inguinal hernia repair, patient understanding and recall were poor only 4–5 days after informed consent was obtained [5]. In fact, only two-thirds of patients understood that they would have mesh in their groin, and less than 3% of patients were aware of the potential to develop chronic pain [5]. Furthermore, a study of patients with rectal cancer on a multidisciplinary clinical pathway including neoadjuvant therapy followed by a surgical procedure with multiple preoperative visits by the surgical team showed that patients still retained very little of informed consent discussions, and most still did not perceive these decisions surrounding surgery as being reflective of a true choice [6]. However, even with elective surgery, up to 13% of patients did not know the major risks of the procedure or even the procedure being performed (major deficits), and another 33% of patients did not have their values, preferences, or goals assessed [7].

Moreover, it is challenging to know when a patient truly does understand all of the relevant information, even if a patient verbalizes understanding. A recent study showed that while two-thirds of patients felt that they were extremely to moderately well-informed about their procedure, there was no relationship between perceptions of being informed and actual knowledge scores [8]. While these findings may lead to the conclusion that we are doing a poor job of informing our patients, these findings also highlight challenges in the process of the disclosure of information to patients. Interestingly, while surgeons and anesthesiologists are considered important sources of information for the consent process, the majority of patients seeking elective surgery may have already decided on whether they want the procedure done prior to even meeting their surgeon [9].

Informed Consent

The content and methods of informed consent have led both patients and physicians to be dissatisfied with the process of consent [10, 11]. It has been argued that the eras of paternalism and patient autonomy have led to a general dissatisfaction of the physician-patient relationship by both stakeholders, and that the current era of "bureaucratic parsimony", or "shared decision making," is appealing because it fosters both autonomy and collegiality in the decision making process [12]. This new paradigm effectively requires clinicians to relinquish their role as a sole authority, but rather than give up their expertise, they must train to become more effective coaches [13]. To further explore the process of informed consent in the context of a shared decision making framework, we will divide this section into two parts: (1) informing the patient, and (2) obtaining consent [11].

Informing the Patient

Informing the patient can be the more challenging of the components of informing the patient and obtaining consent. Informing the patient can be divided into three requirements to be met during the informed consent process: (1) physician disclosure, (2) assessing patient understanding, and (3) shared decision making [14]. In clinical practice, these stages are less distinct, and can happen over time and over multiple patient encounters, but we will examine each of them individually.

Physician Disclosure

Physician disclosure is performed before the informed consent document is actually signed by the physician and patient or patient's surrogate decision maker. Ideally, the act of disclosing information to the patient or surrogate decision maker should take place as early as possible in the clinical setting. This early disclosure of information to the patient will allow the patient time to reflect on the given information and to formulate and ask pertinent questions. Certainly, this ability to disclose information to the patient may be influenced by the emergent nature of the procedure and the patient's decision making capacity and competence.

The act of physician disclosure can be challenging, partly because of the breadth and complexity of the information. Whether in an elective or acute setting, it may be impossible to discuss every facet of the procedure and anesthetic with the patient, so the physician should focus on the most important values and interests as determined by the patient and the physician together and what a reasonable patient would want to know under the given circumstances. The discussion should include the diagnosis, an explanation of the procedure and anesthetic, risks and benefits of the procedure and anesthetic, and alternatives including nonsurgical management or non-intervention. Disclosure can also include other topics that could be relevant to the patient, such as prognosis depending on treatment choice, change in functional status after the procedure, side effects, and the expected postoperative course.

The language used during disclosure is important, and if the physician is not thoughtful the physician can unintentionally coerce the patient into making a decision initially not wanted by the patient. The goal is to be as objective as possible while delivering information to the patient, and to try to avoid personal opinions until after disclosure is complete unless the patient specifically asks for recommendations. For example, a physician may only tell a patient "there are risks from this surgery, but your quality of life will be much worse if you don't have this procedure." This statement can be construed as manipulative and coercive and can negatively impact the decision making process. However, when the physician states "about a third of people who undergo this procedure have complications, however choosing this surgery ultimately leads to a cure in more patients compared to observation," this statement may be preferable as it provides information relevant to making an autonomous decision. It is also beneficial to the patient to counteract framing bias by presenting the data in both directions: "one out of five people develop a recurrence after this procedure; that means that four out of five do not." A physician can make recommendations to the patient, yet must not coerce the patient or manipulate the patient into making a decision. Furthermore, a patient's decision to not accept a physician's recommendation for a procedure should be respected in accordance with the ethical principle of patient autonomy.

The word "doctor" is derived from the Greek *docere*, meaning 'to teach.' An essential component of disclosure requires that physicians teach their patient as much as practical about their disease process, how surgery and other therapies may influence their disease course, including the provision of anesthesia as appropriate. During discussions with the patient, the physician should use simple and easy to understand language to aid the patient's comprehension, especially since patients do not typically ask for clarification. Drawings and illustrations may facilitate the description of medical procedures and the education of the patient. Decision making tools, videos, and pamphlets may also assist with the provision of relevant information to help patients make an informed choice about their anesthesia and surgery. Moreover, the use of an official interpreter is necessary when there is a language barrier between the patient and physician.

Patient Understanding

A second component of informing the patient is assessing patient understanding. One method of assessing patient comprehension is for the physician to consider the type and content of questions patients are asking the physician. When patients ask questions suggesting an incorrect understanding of the information or are reluctant to ask questions, the physician should ask probing questions to clarify the patient's misunderstanding and attempt to address the confusion. The goal is to encourage patient participation in an open dialogue about the current situation and the choices available. Another method to assess patient understanding is the repeat-back method. This requires the patient to use their own words to tell you what they understand about the procedure and can simply be performed by asking the patient to explain the procedure and its risks, benefits, and alternatives back to the physician. Of interest, a multicenter, randomized controlled trial showed that adding the repeat-back method significantly improved patient comprehension with no differences in patient anxiety or satisfaction, and it only added about 2.5 min to the time spent by the provider [15]. This was substantiated by another study that found that total consent time and use of the repeat-back method were both strong predictors of patient comprehension [16]. The use of these methods and unbiased, easy to understand language in the patient's spoken language will allow the patient to understand the information presented by their physician. At this point the patient should ideally be ready to make a decision about his or her treatment or procedure with the help of the physician.

Shared Decision Making

A third component in informing the patient is shared decision making which involves the patient analyzing the information presented by the physician and discussing their goals with the physician in accordance with the patient's stated preferences and values. There are three main components of shared decision making: (1) the sharing of information between parties, (2) the clinician offering options then describing their risks and benefits, and (3) the patient expressing his or her preferences and values [13]. Shared decision making is best facilitated when the physician acts less like a paternalistic authority and more like a coach or partner in making the decision. It is also important to note that patients often need time to reflect, process information, and make an informed choice, and that they may also value the opinion of their primary care doctor and family in addition to the perspective of the surgeon and anesthesiologist. While this is certainly not realistic in emergencies or cases in which urgent care is required, physicians should ideally limit having extensive discussions on the same day that the consent document is being signed in order to allow adequate time for the patient to process the information.

We expect that when providers use the advice provided above in a systematic fashion, it will allow the physician and patient to discuss and make decisions about complex issues effectively, with respect to underlying duties to protect patient autonomy and avoid undo harm to the patient.

Obtaining Informed Consent

The consent form can be signed by the patient (authorization of the patient) only after the following components of obtaining informed consent are addressed: competence and decision making capacity, disclosure, understanding, voluntariness, and the decision of the patient to proceed with a procedure/treatment or not. While others can assist with the task of documentation, the primary physician should personally confirm consent on the day of the procedure, as the patient's understanding may have changed or the patient may have additional questions.

There are several essential components that must be included in the informed consent document [14]. The documentation of obtaining informed consent must include the name and description of the planned and possible alternative procedures and their risks and benefits; describe the anticipated outcomes both positive and negative, in the near and distant future; and provide the options of non-intervention or observation with their corresponding risks and benefits [14]. Furthermore, there should be accompanying documentation that the patient had the opportunity to ask any further questions and that the physician answered these questions satisfactorily. These components of the informed consent discussion between patient and physician should also be documented in the patient's medical record. The physician and the patient or surrogate decision maker subsequently sign the consent form(s) for surgery and anesthesia if the patient so agrees. In situations in which there is a language barrier between the physician and the patient, informed consent must be obtained with a trained medical interpreter with documentation of the interpreter on the informed consent.

The process of informed consent promotes and respects patient autonomy while fostering the physician-patient relationship. Physicians will not only fulfill the important ethical and legal requirements for obtaining informed consent by putting the above recommendations into practice, but also patients will have a better understanding of their procedures to be able to make decisions regarding their health care voluntarily.

Other Considerations

The Patient Decides Not to Proceed with the Surgical Procedure

There are still many situations in which the process of obtaining consent remains challenging. For instance, a previously consented patient may decide that he or she no longer wants a procedure. This can be perceived as a frustrating situation, and care must be taken in how we respond to the patient in such circumstances. The patient has the right to refuse a procedure, even if he or she has previously given consent to treatment. The physician should explore the reasons behind the patient changing their decision as it can offer insight into the patient's thought process. Furthermore, it is important to articulate that refusing treatment does not imply that the patient will lose the care and support of the physician, but efforts should be made to inform the patient of the further health implications of treatment refusal. Depending on the circumstance, the physician should also make sure that the patient understands that refusing treatment now may not necessarily preclude having the procedure done at a later time.

Decision Making Capacity

Physicians can determine if patients have the capacity to participate in shared decision making, but the determination of competency is a legal issue that is determined by a court of law. Decision making capacity involves the patient being able to (1) understand the relevant information, (2) appreciate the medical consequences of the situation, (3) reason about the treatment options, and (4) communicate a choice [17]. All of these criteria must be met for a patient to be considered to have decision making capacity.

There are situations when it is unclear if a patient has the decision making capacity to consent to treatment. As physicians, we often assess decision making capacity of our patients on a moment-to-moment basis, yet a change in a patient's medical condition can suddenly or gradually result in a loss of decision making capacity. Of interest, a study of medical inpatients with acute conditions revealed that the clinical team responsible only identified one quarter of this group as having impaired decision making capabilities [18]. If there is ambiguity as to whether the patient has decision making capacity, a psychiatry evaluation may be obtained. If a patient lacks decision making capacity after reversible causes have been addressed, the physician should review the patient's advance directive to review the patient's treatment goals and to identify the patient's surrogate decision maker. If a surrogate decision maker is not identified with the advance directive, then the physician should consult their state law and/or their institutional ethics committee for local rules on determining surrogacy. In a situation where there is a disagreement or dispute on which treatment decision is in the best interest of the patient and which treatment would respect a patient's wishes, an ethics committee consult can be obtained. Moreover, if a physician believes the surrogate decision maker is not making a decision in the best interest of the patient or is not making a decision that the patient would have clearly wanted based on prior discussion, an ethics committee consultation should be requested prior to considering the intervention of the courts. There is evidence that ethics consultation services can effectively build consensus in disagreements regarding perceived nonbeneficial treatments and are a valuable resource [19]. Unfortunately, in a survey study, physicians with the least training in ethics were also the least likely to have access to an ethics consultation service [20].

Disclosure of Surgeon Experience

Whether surgeons are legally required to disclose their experience for certain procedures is unclear, as legal precedent on this issue remains unsettled. Currently, there have been two state Supreme Court cases that examined this issue, with both courts coming to opposite conclusions [21, 22]. In *Johnson v. Kokemoor* (1996), the legal standards of informed consent were expanded to include providing a surgeon's performance data if considered material to the decision making process [21]. However, Duttry *v. Patterson* (2001) indicated that a physician's prior experience is outside the scope of an informed consent claim [22].

The disclosure of surgeon-specific performance data to aid patients in making a decision regarding their choice of a surgeon has been controversial and criticized. While the ultimate goal of reporting surgeon-specific performance ratings is to improve the quality of surgical care and enhance patient autonomy, it is questionable whether the reporting of these ratings actually enhances autonomous decision making [23]. While sharing of data within peer groups to improve performance rates is currently justifiable from a quality and process improvement perspective, it is unclear of the benefit unadjusted surgeon-specific outcomes data provides to patients. Schwarze argues that disclosure of performance ratings would be similar to mandated disclosure of flight disasters faced by individual pilots, provide an excess burden on the consumer to make a decision that may not be feasible or even relevant to their future, and certainly question the ability of the airline industry to self-police [23]. Furthermore, the application of prediction models developed at a population level cannot reliably be applied to individual surgeons – this is otherwise known as an ecological fallacy. Of interest, patients may not even be influenced by performance data if available, but instead may be influenced more by the opinion of their referring physician [24].

The disclosure of surgeon-specific performance ratings has been criticized for being complex and difficult to understand for potential patients [25]. Disparate outcomes from surgeons may not be controlled for patient comorbidities, surgical volume, referral patterns, and team characteristics, and may not be reflective of the expertise and technical skill of an individual surgeon [4]. At this time, some experts believe that since surgeon-specific performance data are currently inaccurate and misleading, there may be no ethical obligation to disclose this data as part of the informed consent process [23, 24]. Using comparative data in an unadjusted fashion, it becomes unclear if a heart surgeon has a high complication rate because of poor technique, because he or she performs surgery on moribund patients, or because he or she is readily available as backup to salvage complications from a particularly aggressive interventional cardiology group. Furthermore, an expert pancreas surgeon may have a higher complication rate than a novice surgeon who has performed only a few cases without any morbidity. Individual statistics unadjusted for volume or comorbidity may not tell the whole story of a surgeon's performance in a straightforward manner. If the accuracy and applicability of these statistics improve in the future, then a case may be made that physicians do have an ethical duty to disclose surgeon-specific performance ratings in order to minimize patient harm.

Competing with the patient's autonomous choice of selecting a surgeon is the ethical principle of justice. A patient still may have to weigh the relative degree of importance of a surgeon's skill with issues related to access to care and the distance to travel to receive the surgeon's care, as well as the importance of containing the cost of the patient's deductible by staying within "in-provider" insurance networks.

For the disclosure of surgeon experience to be beneficial to the patient, it is essential that there is a potential for a patient to be able to make an autonomous decision [23]. The disclosure of a surgeon's experience and surgeon-specific data is probably most relevant for rare or unusual disease processes and highly complex procedures with greater associated risks in which the surgeon has limited experience. For example, there is data supporting the relationships of hospital and surgeon volume and in-hospital mortality for pancreatectomy and esophagectomy [26, 27].

However, as an example, a socioeconomically disadvantaged patient in a rural location may not be able to be medically evaluated by a high-volume esophageal surgeon with excellent patient outcome data. This situation exemplifies the ethical issue of justice as well as the patient's inability to exercise his or her autonomous choice secondary to travel distance and financial concerns. Furthermore, there may be regions of the country with only one surgeon available within a several hour radius that does perform such complex procedures. Under this circumstance, it is essential for the rural surgeon to disclose to the patient the surgeon's level of training, case experience, and outcomes (if they are known), and allow the patient to decide if he or she wishes to travel to another center or stay closer to home. While it remains unclear whether there is an ethical or legal obligation of full disclosure of surgical experience, it is fundamental to uphold professional standards to patients with respect to truth-telling [4]. It is essential to honestly disclose surgeon experience to the patient, respect the patient's right to decide on their treatment, and offer the patient a referral to a more experienced surgeon if requested by the patient.

Conclusion

The process of informed consent promotes and respects patient autonomy while fostering the physician-patient relationship. Both anesthesiologists and surgeons will not only fulfill the important ethical and legal requirements for obtaining informed consent by putting the above recommendations into practice, but also patients will have a better understanding of their procedures to be able to make decisions regarding their health care voluntarily.

During the process of informed consent, "it may be appropriate to not only disclose risk, but to articulate the level of uncertainty around risk estimates, especially when there is greater system complexity surrounding both disease process and technique" [4]. We feel that humility and intellectual honesty in the process of the disclosure of surgeon experience will help engender trust in the surgeon and will strengthen the surgeon-patient relationship.

References

1. Canterbury v. Spence, 464 F.2d 772 (D.C. Cir. 1972).
2. Aristotle. The Nichomachean ethics. 2nd ed (trans: Irwin T). Indianapolis: Hackett Publishing Co.; 984.
3. Aristotle. Aristotle's Nichomachean ethics (trans: Bartlett RC, Collins SD). Chicago: The University of Chicago Press; 2011.
4. Ganai S. Disclosure of surgeon experience. World J Surg. 2014;38:1622–5.
5. Uzzaman MM, Sinha S, Shaygi B, Vitish-sharma P, Loizides S, Myint F. Evaluation of patient's understanding and recall of the consent process after open inguinal hernia repairs. Int J Surg. 2012;10:5–10.

6. Scheer AS, O'Connor AM, Chan BP, Moloo H, Poulin EC, Mamazza J, Auer RC, Boushey RP. The myth of informed consent in rectal cancer surgery: what do patients retain? Dis Colon Rectum. 2012;55:970–5.
7. Ankuda CK, Block SD, Cooper Z, Correll DJ, Hepner DL, Lasic M, Gawande AA, Bader AM. Measuring critical deficits in shared decision making before elective surgery. Patient Educ Couns. 2014;94:328–33.
8. Sepucha KR, Fagerlin A, Couper MP, Levin CA, Singer E, Zikmund-Fisher BJ. How does feeling informed relate to being informed? The DECISIONS survey. Med Decis Making. 2010;30(5 suppl):77S–84.
9. Hall DE, Morrison P, Nikolajski C, Fine M, Arnold R, Zickmund SL. Informed consent for inguinal herniorrhaphy and cholecystectomy: describing how patients make decisions to have surgery. Am J Surg. 2012;204:619–25.
10. Faden RR, Becker C, Lewis C, Freeman J, Faden AI. Disclosure of information to patients in medical care. Med Care. 1981;19:718–33.
11. Katz J. Reflections on informed consent: 40 years after its birth. J Am Coll Surg. 1998;186:466–74.
12. Siegler M. The progression of medicine: from physician paternalism to patient autonomy to bureaucratic parsimony. Arch Int Med. 1985;145:713–5.
13. Barry MJ, Edgman-Levitan S. Shared decision making—the pinnacle of patient-centered care. N Engl J Med. 2012;366:780–1.
14. Childers R, Lipsett PA, Pawlik TM. Informed consent and the surgeon. J Am Coll Surg. 2009;208:627–34.
15. Fink AS, Prochazka AV, Henderson WG, Bartenfeld D, Nyirenda C, Webb A, et al. Enhancement of surgical informed consent by addition of repeat back: a multicenter, randomized controlled clinical trial. Ann Surg. 2010;252:27–36.
16. Fink AS, Prochazka AV, Henderson WG, Bartenfeld D, Nyirenda C, Webb A, et al. Predictors of comprehension during surgical informed consent. J Am Coll Surg. 2010;210:919–26.
17. Appelbaum PS. Assessment of patients' competence to consent to treatment. N Engl J Med. 2007;357:1834–40.
18. Raymont V, Bingley W, Buchanan A, David AS, Hayward P, Wessely S, Hotopf M. Prevalence of mental incapacity in medical inpatients and associated risk factors: cross-sectional study. Lancet. 2004;364:1421–7.
19. Nelson R. Nonbeneficial treatment and conflict resolution: building consensus. Perm J. 2013;17:23–7.
20. DuVal G, Clarridge B, Gensler G, Danis M. A national survey of U.S. internists' experiences with ethical dilemmas and ethics consultation. J Gen Intern Med. 2004;19:251–8.
21. Johnson v. Kokemoor, 545 NW 2d 495 (Wis. Supreme Court 1996).
22. Duttry v. Patterson, 771 A.2d 1255 (Pa. Super. 2001).
23. Schwarze ML. The process of informed consent: neither the time nor the place for disclosure of surgeon-specific outcomes. Ann Surg. 2007;245:514–5.
24. Burger I, Schill K, Goodman S. Diclosure of individual surgeon's performance rates during informed consent: ethical and epistemological considerations. Ann Surg. 2007;245:507–13.
25. Schneider EC, Lieberman T. Publicly disclosed information about the quality of health care: response of the US public. Qual Health Care. 2001;10:96–103.
26. Birkmeyer JD, Siewers AE, Finlayson EV, Stukel TA, Lucas FL, Batista I, et al. Hospital volume and surgical mortality in the United States. N Engl J Med. 2002;346:1128–37.
27. Birkmeyer JD, Stukel TA, Siewers AE, Goodney PP, Wennberg DE, Lucas FL. Surgeon volume and operative mortality in the United States. N Engl J Med. 2003;349:2117–27.

Chapter 4
Perioperative Considerations of Do Not Resuscitate and Do Not Intubate Orders in Adult Patients

Joseph F. Kras

Abstract The vast majority of medical orders are for the purpose of some action being taken; for example, orders to admit patients to the hospital and orders to administer medications. DNR (Do Not Resuscitate) and DNI (Do Not Intubate) orders, however, are exceptions to these medical orders that initiate an action. DNR and DNI orders in the perioperative period may pit patients' rights to decide which actions are (or are not) performed on their bodies against the surgeon and anesthesiologist's duties to do their best to treat patients and to do no harm.

Autonomy figures prominently in Western medical ethics and, especially, in the United States (US). Patients should be able to directly (or through their surrogate) express their wishes for what type(s) of care they wish provided to them. Automatic suspension of DNR orders compromises patients' abilities to decide their own fate.

Surgeons may feel duty-bound by the principle of beneficence to only perform actions that will physically benefit patients and feel, that by requesting surgery, patients implicitly want their surgeon to "get them through" the surgery, no matter what. Such an attitude would preclude letting patients die on the operating room table if they could be saved by cardiopulmonary resuscitation. Anesthesiologists often feel guided by nonmaleficence, going so far as to say that they "don't want to be a patient's executioner." Like many of their surgical colleagues, they view standing by while patients die from potentially totally reversible events as being totally antithetical to their calling.

Keywords Perioperative Do Not Resuscitate • Do Not Resuscitate • Suspending Do Not Resuscitate Perioperatively • Surgery and Do Not Resuscitate

---

J.F. Kras, MD, DDS, MA
Department of Anesthesiology, Washington University School of Medicine, 660 S. Euclid Avenue, Campus Box 8054, St. Louis, MO 63110, USA
e-mail: krasj@wustl.edu

B.G. Jericho (ed.), *Ethical Issues in Anesthesiology and Surgery*,
DOI 10.1007/978-3-319-15949-2_4

Case Presentation

The patient is a 66-year-old male who is a retired Chief Executive Officer of a large manufacturing firm. Four years ago, he was treated for Stage III colorectal cancer with a right hemicolectomy with primary anastomosis, chemotherapy and targeted therapy. Seven months ago, the patient presented with multiple lung and liver metastases from his colorectal cancer. The patient has been receiving chemotherapy and targeted therapy in an attempt to slow the progression of his disease. Recognizing that he has terminal cancer, the patient signed an advance directive 2 months ago. The advance directive states that while the patient does wish to receive all treatment that will relieve his pain and prolong his life with him in a conscious state, the patient does not want to be resuscitated.

He is referred to you for treatment of an intestinal obstruction of the descending colon, after an unsuccessful attempt at stenting the blockage by the gastrointestinal laboratory.

Notes on Abbreviations

DNR (Do Not Resuscitate) and DNI (Do Not Intubate) are currently the two most common forms of orders written to limit resuscitation in US institutions. In some locales and institutions, these orders have different names such as DNAR (Do Not Attempt Resuscitation) or DNACPR (Do Not Attempt Cardiopulmonary Resuscitation). One more recent nomenclature for such orders is AND (Allow Natural Death). As the nomenclature "DNR" is probably the most uniformly recognized, it will be used throughout this chapter when referring to the ethical conflicts surrounding all such orders.

The History of Do Not Resuscitate Orders

Before considering the above case regarding perioperative DNR orders, it is helpful to consider briefly the history of cardiopulmonary resuscitation and the institution of DNR orders in general.

Cardiac arrest is the final common occurrence of all natural death, absent intensive interventions such as mechanical ventilation and cardiac assist devices. Prior to the middle of the twentieth century, there were few invasive technologies available for artificially sustaining life, and there were no commonly available methods of reversing cardiac arrest. The period from the 1950s to the 1970s witnessed a large increase in the number and intensity of treatments that could stave off physiologic demise at the end of life. Furthermore, in the post-World War II period, endotracheal intubation and positive pressure ventilation became much more common during surgery with the discovery of the medical uses of curare and other nondepolarizing muscle relaxants [1]. Yet, some patients ventilated during surgery could not successfully undergo tracheal extubation at the end of the surgical case. The need to provide care for these postoperative patients and other seriously ill patients requiring ventilator support lead to the development of recovery rooms and intensive care units (ICUs). In fact, Bjorn Ibsen, an anesthesiologist, opened what was most likely the first ICU in Copenhagen, Denmark in 1953 [2].

The development of improved methods of resuscitation began in the late 1950s. Safer and colleagues demonstrated the superiority of mouth-to-mouth ventilation over back pressure/arm lift or chest pressure methods of ventilation [3]. Furthermore, Gurvich, Kouwenhoven, and Zoll all contributed significantly to proving that electrical countershocks could restart a fibrillating heart [4]. One of Kouwenhoven's students, Knickerbocker made the serendipitous discovery that pressure on the chest produced an arterial waveform [5]. Closed chest massage was subsequently combined with ventilation to resuscitate pulseless patients in the operating room [6]. Cardiopulmonary resuscitation (CPR) and advanced cardiac life support (ACLS) were first used primarily in the operating room and recovery areas, but soon spread throughout the hospital. In a country that had conquered polio and was sending men to the moon, anything seemed possible. The ability to prolong life was assumed to be a good thing. So, CPR training soon expanded to include the general public and paramedics who provided prehospital care.

By the early 1970s, the practice of resuscitation was universal and most always provided when the heart stopped. Even if a patient's family expressed their wish not to have their loved one resuscitated, physicians and hospitals felt that they might become liable for performing "passive euthanasia" if they did not attempt resuscitation. Patients and their families came to feel, at times, trapped by the very measures designed to help them. Western medical practice and law had evolved to require informed consent for medical interventions, yet what patients and their families now wanted was informed refusal.

Since the 1970s, there has been a trend of increasing patient autonomy in the medical arena. In 1976, the New Jersey Supreme Court decided that life-sustaining ventilation could be removed from Karen Quinlan who was in a persistent vegetative state (PVS). The US Supreme Court decided a similar case in 1990 when Nancy Cruzan's guardian successfully argued that her feeding tube should be removed after several years of being in a PVS [7]. Subsequently, the US Congress passed the Patient Self-Determination Act that required all hospitals, nursing homes, and surgicenters to determine on admission whether patients had signed advance directives regarding their preferences for future care, should patients become unable to communicate their preferences at that time. All patients who did not have directives were to be offered education on advance directives. Although advance directives may be far from being perfectly utilized or followed, patients and their surrogates, for the most part, have been afforded the opportunity to refuse care (including resuscitation) that was not felt to be consistent with their goals. The current standard within US hospitals is that CPR is routinely provided unless patients or their surrogates have consented to a written DNR order.

Although DNR orders have been a mainstay in American institutions for decades, the one area of the hospital that has resisted embracing these orders is the surgical arena. The surgical arena includes both the operating rooms and the surgical ICUs. For many years, health care professionals practicing medicine in the surgical arena have assumed that if patients presented to an acute care area then all DNR orders were to be automatically suspended. Surgeons have either assumed that patients wanted everything done to save them or had conversations with patients preoperatively in which the surgeons believed they had obtained implicit buy-in from the patient to the operation and any measures the surgeon felt necessary to perform postoperatively [8, 9]. Anesthesiologists have also been slow to embrace the possibility of a valid DNR order in the perioperative period. In one study done in 1993, 60% of anesthesiologists surveyed assumed that DNR orders would be automatically suspended when a patient came to the operating room [10]. The American Society of Anesthesiologists (ASA) issued guidelines in 1993 stating that when patients presenting for surgery had existing DNR orders there should be "required reconsideration" of such orders. Subsequently in the 1990s, the American College of Surgeons issued guidelines regarding DNR orders similar to the ASA's guidelines [11]. A more recent study of patient and doctor attitudes suggests that thinking has evolved, as 38% of surgeons and only 18% of anesthesiologists believed that DNR orders should be automatically suspended when patients come to the operating room [12].

Do Not Resuscitate Orders Outside of the United States

The process of deciding to provide CPR to patients or to withhold CPR and other resuscitation efforts from patients is not the same around the world. In the United States, unless there is a specific order approved by patients or their surrogates not to perform resuscitation, it is almost exclusively expected that patients in cardiac arrest will receive resuscitative measures. This is certainly not the case in most other countries around the world.

In the United Kingdom (UK), the General Medical Council (GMC) licenses and regulates all physicians. The GMC publishes a guidance for physicians, including "Treatment and care towards the end of life: good practice in decision making" [13]. The portion of the guidance that addresses resuscitation decisions for patients without decision-making capacity begins in a way familiar to a US audience, stating "If a patient lacks capacity to make a decision about future CPR, you should consult any legal proxy who has authority to make the decision for the patient. If there is no legal proxy with relevant authority, you must discuss the issue with those close to the patient and with the healthcare team" [13]. The document further prescribes how a physician should proceed if a patient's proxy disagrees with the physician's judgment, stating "If the legal proxy requests that CPR with a small chance of success is attempted in the future, in spite of the burdens and risks, or they are sure that this is what the patient wanted, and it is your considered judgement that CPR would not be clinically appropriate and not of overall benefit for the patient, you should explore the reasons for the proxy's request" [13]. However, it quickly becomes apparent that the ultimate decision on whether or not to attempt CPR rests with the medical practitioner and not the patient or their proxy. "If after further discussion you still consider that attempting CPR would not be of overall benefit for the patient, you are not obliged to offer to attempt CPR in the circumstances envisaged. You should explain your reasons and any other options that may be available to the legal proxy, including their right to seek a second opinion" [13]. Resuscitation is viewed alongside all other treatments as something that may or may NOT be beneficial and medically indicated for a particular patient. Similar to other medical treatments, resuscitation decisions are viewed primarily as medical decisions to be made by physicians. Thus, it is not surprising that perioperative DNR orders in the UK were formerly routinely suspended, just as they were in the US for similar reasons as described previously. Legal decisions and common practice over the last several years have granted greater autonomy to patients refusing interventions in the UK, and thus there are a greater number of surgeries being performed with some form of a DNR order in place [14].

Across the rest of Europe, the involvement of patients and their surrogates in end-of-life decisions and resuscitation varies somewhat from country to country. All available evidence points to a common denominator of physicians making the final decision to resuscitate patients. However, patient autonomy is increasing on the continent, as it is elsewhere. In Austria, a 2006 law created a formal process for advance directives for the first time. If notarized, these forms and the patient's preferences are binding on physicians; however, "Patients document their personal views regarding extension of treatment, e.g. mechanical ventilation, resuscitation or nutrition and they can express their wishes, e.g. concerning pain therapy *but only in accordance with best clinical practice* (emphasis added)" [15]. In France, there has been a shift towards sharing end-of-life decisions by having physicians consult with patients and family members; yet, all resuscitation decisions are made by physicians [16].

In Asia, there is a high degree of paternalism embedded in Asian medical practice. In Japan, if physicians believe that CPR is unjustified and futile, physicians are not even required to inform their patients that they have entered a DNR order [16]. In Hong Kong, many physicians routinely ask patients to suspend their DNR orders during surgery, and patients are expected to comply with the physician's request. There are no specific rules regarding CPR, either in or out of the operating theater, as again all aspects of resuscitation are considered medical decisions. That being said, the Hospital Authority tells physicians that it is desirable to involve patients and family members in DNR decisions, and operations under a DNR order have occurred [17].

The majority of Middle Eastern countries are Muslim. Islamic law allows DNR orders for those who are terminally ill and allows unilateral decisions by three physicians to enter such an order without patient or family involvement. One survey showed that only about 66% of Muslim physicians were aware that a DNR order was allowed in Islam [18]. However, in Israel, a largely Jewish population (although it is composed of a sizable minority of "secular Jews") follows traditional Jewish practices when nearing end of life. Traditional Jewish law considers dying a natural progression from life to death [16]. Unless a person is one who is considered to be very close to death (a *gosess*), Jewish law prescribes that all measures should be taken to preserve life, including CPR [19]. Thus, in the Middle East, there appears to be a variation in practice concerning DNR orders.

Now that we have considered the past and current state of DNR orders, it is time to consider the arguments for and against suspending such orders in the perioperative period.

Anesthetic Arguments for Suspending Do Not Resuscitate Orders Perioperatively

One of the primary reasons anesthesiologists give to justify suspending perioperative DNR orders is that the performance of a well-administered anesthetic shares many components with the procedures undertaken when resuscitating patients who have had a cardiac arrest. When a cardiac arrest occurs, resuscitation typically consists of multiple different elements including not only chest compressions and shocking the heart, but also endotracheal intubation and ventilating the patient, starting an intravenous (IV) line and administering fluids, and giving a patient vasoactive medications intravenously that affect both heart rhythm as well as contractility. Depending on how a DNR order is written or interpreted, most such orders would prohibit the normal administration of an anesthetic.

As stated, a typical general anesthetic involves many of the same interventions performed during a cardiac arrest. Confusion may ensue if an anesthesiologist is performing tasks during a typical general anesthetic that are "forbidden" in a DNR order. These tasks may include placing an IV line, administering IV fluids, administering oxygen, endotracheal intubation, ventilating the patient, and administering vasoactive medications. Even some of the language used while treating a patient with a cardiac arrest and one being cared for during a major operation are the same. In the operating room, when a patient is losing blood or has an abnormally low blood pressure due to another medical condition such as sepsis, the anesthesiologist speaks of "resuscitating" the patient, even though the heart has not yet stopped.

A second reason for suspending DNR orders perioperatively is that CPR and other resuscitative interventions were originally designed to rescue those who arrested in the operating room secondary to anesthetic medications given, surgical interventions, or trauma. Resuscitative measures (CPR, electroshocks, and powerful vasoactive medications) soon spread to be used outside of the operating room, but remain today more effective when applied in the operating room than when performed on a regular medical floor. This is probably due to the fact that a patient has a physician at the bedside in the operating room when an event occurs, IV access is already present, and a defibrillator is immediately at hand. Suspending resuscitation in the operating room may seem to be the last place one would want to restrict it, since it is most efficacious there.

Patients may suffer an arrest due to iatrogenic causes, such as a relative overdose of anesthetic medications. When such events occur, it is usually a relatively simple and quick process to resuscitate a patient, as compared to arrests caused by other causes such as shock and massive trauma. It is certainly understandable, though, that anesthesiologists would believe that they, themselves, are personally responsible if a patient dies following an action they performed that could have been reversed except for the patient's DNR order. This situation differs from a patient spontaneously arresting on the medical floor, the awareness that a patient is DNR, and no action is taken to resuscitate the patient as per the patient's wishes.

Finally, most anesthesiologists believe that the operating room is a place where patients come to GET treated, and not to have treatment withheld or withdrawn. The thrust of all anesthesiology training is in maintaining and saving patients, not in allowing patients to die in the operating room. Anesthesiologists may believe that their talents and the resources of the operating room should only be used to treat patients to the best of their ability. Patients dying in the operating room is certainly a possibility, but it is viewed as a bad outcome, and never an acceptable one.

Surgical Arguments for Suspending Do Not Resuscitate Orders Perioperatively

Surgeons are often said to form a covenantal relationship with their patients [20]. If patients trust their surgeons to take them on this (surgical) journey, then surgeons will do everything in their power to safely guide their patients to a successful outcome. Attempting to rescue patients utilizing every means at one's disposal is part of such a covenant. Not to do so might constitute abandoning patients in the eyes of their surgeons.

A variation of the above argument, and a reason shared with anesthesiologists is the "surgeon as causative agent" of the precipitating event leading to the arrest. Surgery, by its very nature, is very cause and effect, and generally occurs over a relatively short timeline. A patient presents with a potentially surgically correctable problem, a surgeon presents a plan to fix the problem, and the patient either does or does not get better. Although many patients proceed with their surgeries exactly as planned, it is accepted that some patients will undergo complications. Some of these complications may be due to factors inherent to the patient, while other complications may be due directly to surgical causes (for example, unanticipated excess hemorrhage). As much as a surgeon feels bound to rescue the patient from any adverse event while under the surgeon's care, this imperative is especially felt when the surgeon perceives himself or herself as contributing to the patient's demise. Surgeons who were asked to consider whether they would agree to remove postoperative life support from a patient they had performed an operation on were significantly less likely to agree if they believed that the patient had suffered a complication that they had caused [21].

Surgeons often believe that they have achieved "buy-in" from patients preoperatively, whether or not they have specifically discussed patient preferences for resuscitative efforts [8, 9]. Especially in the situation of "big" operations, surgeons expect that if patients are willing to commit to the operation itself, then patients should also be willing to commit to all necessary postoperative care, including extreme measures. Surgeons describe getting this "buy-in" from patients in their preoperative discussions with the patients. Yet, regardless of the fact that the majority of surgeons have such discussions with their patients the majority of the time, it is also true that such discussions don't usually include any explicit talk of when or how to limit treatment if events don't go as planned [9].

Surgeons are selected and trained to be bold, decisive, and indefatigable. To let a patient die when he or she might still be saved through intensive measures would traditionally be perceived by colleagues as a sign of weakness, as well as perhaps abandonment of the patient. In the perceived battle against disease, surgeons are taught to win, whatever the cost. Two often heard aphorisms are "Do it. Do it right. Do it right now!" and "A chance to cut is a chance to cure." The not so subtle underlying message is that "standing by idly" while a patient is allowed to die is completely unacceptable.

In addition to peers looking over one's shoulder, there is the very real aspect of surgical practice whereby society constantly watches you (or at least your results). In a world where the public demands increased quality and accountability, the American College of Surgeons (ACS) has responded by setting up the ACS NSQIP (National Surgical Quality Improvement Program). This program tracks rates of complications and death for thirty days postoperatively for hospitals and individual surgeons [22]. This data is utilized both by national certifying agencies and for publicity by individual hospitals [23]. Thus, there is a distinct incentive for surgeons to keep their patients alive until day 31, in order to look better on paper. It is easy to see how surgical temperament, training, tradition, and tracking information all work together to favor the suspension of DNR orders in the perioperative arena.

Arguments for Not Suspending Do Not Resuscitate Orders Perioperatively

Many people and other players have an ethical stake in what happens in an operation. These include the patient, surgeon, anesthesiologist, nurses and technicians, hospital, and society as a whole. Except for the patient experiencing a "life event", everyone in the operating room is "coming to work". It is the patient who has the most to gain or lose from the procedure, and who may have to live a lifetime with the results. Therefore, it is only right that concerns of the patient should be primary (though not exclusive) when making decisions regarding the patient's care. The primary ethical principle underlying the patient's ability to direct their care is autonomy.

In regard to our case mentioned previously, the state of the art in cancer therapy and treatment of other serious diseases has improved greatly in the last few decades. Some patients are cured, some patients have their lives significantly prolonged, and some patients experience failure of their treatment. Still, in those patients whose life can be prolonged, there may be medical problems that need to be addressed surgically. Surgery may be performed either as an adjunct to other treatment (for example, placing a percutaneous feeding tube) or for palliation (for example, relieving a colon obstruction) as in our case mentioned previously. Patients who have previously chosen not to be resuscitated because of their overall physical condition and underlying values (as in our clinical case) should not be forced to undergo resuscitation because others (surgeons and anesthesiologists) would feel uncomfortable watching patients die. Indeed, a patient may believe that dying under anesthesia is far preferable than experiencing pain and air hunger while conscious and dying. Although there are unique aspects of the operating room environment and anesthetic practice, in essence there is still the interaction of patients and physicians. If taking away a patient's autonomy is wrong in other doctor-patient interactions, then it is also wrong here in the operating room and the perioperative period.

Although some surgeons and anesthesiologists may believe that DNR orders should be automatically suspended in the perioperative period, patients do not necessarily agree. In one study, 92% of patients expected doctors to discuss their requests not to be resuscitated [12]. In this same study, 79% of patients stated that if DNR orders were suspended perioperatively, then the DNR orders should be reinstituted at a predetermined time postoperatively.

Furthermore, patients and their surrogates can be educated regarding the differences between resuscitation in the operating room and other locations in the hospital. It may take some time to explain these differences, but it is certainly no more difficult to explain such differences than it is to explain some of the more complex treatments in medicine (for example, ventricular assist devices) or esoteric concepts such as brain death.

Finally, surgeon and anesthesiologist mortality tracking should not be a reason to override a patient's right to make his or her own resuscitation decisions. Laws and policies can be easily amended such that a separate category of deaths (those with preexisting DNR orders) is counted separately in a practitioner's statistics. Patients and their families should not be expected (or forced) to undergo more suffering because policies and laws were poorly written.

Options for Resuscitation Orders in the Operating Room and Perioperative Period

Ethical options for resuscitation orders in the perioperative period for patients or their surrogates include the following:

1. **Suspending DNR orders for a specified period of time**

   Perhaps the primary reason that the default position in most institutions has been (and in some cases, still remains) for DNR orders to be routinely suspended in the perioperative period is that it is often clearly the right thing to do. When a patient pursues an operation or procedure, there is often at least a temporary change of goals on the patient's part. Because of this, as well as the other reasons stated above, suspending DNR orders in the perioperative period is often a rational choice. As long as there is an open and frank discussion of options between the medical team and the patient and the patient freely agrees to this option, it can be a very good option for the patient. The time when DNR orders are to be reinstituted needs to be mutually agreed upon by the patient and his or her team preoperatively.

2. **Continuing DNR orders, as written, to the operating room and beyond**
   In some situations, DNR orders are continued through the perioperative period. If a patient is having minimal sedation for a procedure that will not change his or her overall goals, then he or she may choose to continue his or her DNR status without modification. The medical team must accept that even if the "cause" of the patient's heart stopping is something that was done as part of the procedure, they will not resuscitate the patient.
3. **Modifying DNR orders for a specified period of time, specifying which procedures would be allowed**
   In some circumstances, a patient may choose to continue their DNR status through the perioperative period with modification of the DNR orders. Patients who want to exert the most control possible in the situation may wish to specify exactly which procedures are allowed and which are forbidden. For example, a patient may agree to endotracheal intubation and the use of vasopressor medications, but may refuse chest compressions and defibrillation.
4. **Modifying DNR orders for a specified period of time, with resuscitative discretion left up to the treating team, based on mutually agreed upon goals of care**
   Because all causes and presentations of cardiac and respiratory failure are somewhat different, patients may wish to allow their physicians to decide for them during the critical situation whether to resuscitate, as well as which procedures to employ. For instance, if the event is perceived at the time to be most likely easily reversible, with treatment most likely returning the patient to his or her preoperative state, then the patient and team may agree ahead of time to proceed with resuscitation. On the other hand, if an event is perceived to be major, with little hope of quickly returning the patient to his or her preoperative state, then he or she may wish to have the team "let him or her go" by not providing resuscitation. Allowing the physicians to make judgment calls at the time a critical incident occurs may lead to the patient's values and wishes being more closely adhered to. The downside of proceeding in this manner is that it depends on a high level of mutual understanding on the part of the patient and his or her physicians, as well as a high level of trust on the patient's part that the physicians will follow through when the event occurs. This option also depends on extremely good communication between all of the physicians on the perioperative team, and most importantly, between the physicians on the perioperative team and those physicians who will assume care for the patient after the operation.

What Constitutes the "Perioperative Period"?

Assuming a patient is to suspend or modify the DNR orders for the perioperative period, exactly how long does this last? Most people would agree that it starts when the patient is taken to the operating room, but when does it end? When the patient leaves the operating room, when the patient leaves the recovery area, a few days postoperatively, or longer? The answer is that it depends, and everything is negotiable.

If a patient is having a feeding tube placed surgically, the perioperative period might be logically said to have ended when the patient leaves the recovery area. By that time, the major effects of the anesthetic should have worn off, and there should have been no major blood loss from the surgery to compromise the patient's state. On the other hand, if a patient were to decide to have an aortic valve replacement (which usually involves several days of care postoperatively in an ICU), then it would make more sense to consider the perioperative period to extend longer. The patient might agree to have his or her DNR orders suspended for 3 days postoperatively, for as long as he or she is in the ICU, or perhaps time-limited to "no longer than 7 days, even if still in the ICU". Surgeons may want to extend the concept of the perioperative period even longer, especially if the patient is agreeing to undergo major surgery. Yet, these decisions need to be mutually agreed upon and documented in the medical record.

Addressing Conflicts Between Physicians and the Patient's Goals and Wishes

When discussing if, when, and how long to suspend or modify a DNR order, a patient needs to listen to the physician's explanations of the medical reasons for why certain actions are done, and doctors need to listen to a patient's goals and desires for their care and treatment. In most cases, such discussions will lead to a mutually agreeable plan. But ultimately, a physician does not have to operate on or provide anesthesia to a patient if the physician does not believe he or she can provide care consistent with the patient's goals and wishes. Furthermore, patients can consult with another physician if the patient does not believe their treatment goals and desires are being met. In the rare instance when a patient needs to undergo urgent or emergent surgery, and their assigned physician cannot agree with the

Case Resolution

In our clinical case, the patient's wishes for the perioperative period were clarified and documented in the medical record. The patient wanted to have the surgical procedure to relieve the obstruction of the descending colon. The patient accepted endotracheal intubation for the surgery and the use of vasopressor medications, but with the stipulation that these modalities were not to continue for more than 7 days postoperatively. During the surgery and postoperative period, the patient did not want CPR or defibrillation to be performed on him. The surgery was successful and the patient underwent tracheal extubation the next morning.

patient's wishes, then the physician may withdraw from caring for the patient, as long as there is another physician willing to care for the patient. If no other physician can be identified or is available to care for the patient, then the assigned physician is obliged to care for the patient, reasonably honoring the patient's goals and wishes.

References

1. Raghavendra T. Neuromuscular blocking drugs: discovery and development. J R Soc Med. 2002;95:363–7.
2. Berthelsen P, Cronqvist M. The first intensive care unit in the world: Copenhagen 1953. Acta Anaesthesiol Scand. 2003;47:1190–5.
3. Safar P, Escarraga L, Elam J. A comparison of the mouth-to-mouth and mouth-to-airway methods of artificial respiration with the chest-pressure arm-lift methods. New Engl J Med. 1958;258:671–7.
4. Safer P. From control of airway and breathing to cardiopulmonary-cerebral resuscitation. Anesthesiology. 2001;95:789–91.
5. Kouwenhoven W, Jude J, Knickerbocker G. Closed-chest cardiac massage. JAMA. 1960;173:1064–7.
6. Safar P, Brown T, Holtey W, Wilder R. Ventilation and circulation with closed chest cardiac massage in man. JAMA. 1961;176:574–6.
7. Monahan J, Lawhorn E. Life-sustaining treatment and the law: the evolution of informed consent, advance directives and surrogate decision making. Ann Health Law. 2010;19:107–13. Art 23.
8. Schwarze M, Redmann A, Alexander G, Brasel K. Surgeons expect patients to buy-in to postoperative life support preoperatively: results of a national survey. Crit Care Med. 2013;41(1):1–8.
9. Pecanac K, Kehler J, Brasel K, Cooper Z, Steffens N, McKneally M, Schwarze M. It's big surgery: preoperative expressions of risk, responsibility, and commitment to treatment after high-risk operations. Ann Surg. 2014;259:458–63.
10. Clemency M, Thompson N. "Do Not Resuscitate" (DNR) orders in the perioperative period-a comparison of the perspectives of anesthesiologists, internists, and surgeons. Anesth Anal. 1994;78(4):651–8.
11. Burns J, Edwards J, Johnson J, Cassem N, Truog R. Do-Not-Resuscitate order after 25 years. Crit Care Med. 2003;31(5):1543–50.
12. Burkle C, Swetz K, Armstrong M, Keegan M. Patient and doctor attitudes and beliefs concerning perioperative Do Not Resuscitate orders: anesthesiologists' growing compliance with patient autonomy and self determination guidelines. BMC Anesthesiol. 2013;13:2. http://www.biomedcentral.com/1471-2253/13/2. Accessed 26 Feb 2015.
13. General Medical Council. Treatment and care towards the end of life: good practice in decision making. 2010. http://www.gmc-uk.org/static/documents/content/Treatment_and_care_towards_the_end_of_life_-_English_0914.pdf. Accessed 12 Apr 2015.
14. Knipe M, Hardman J. Past, present, and future of 'Do Not Attempt Resuscitation' orders in the perioperative period. Br J Anaesth. 2013;111(6):861–3.
15. Schaden E, Herczeg P, Hacker S, Schopper A, Krenn C. The role of advance directives in end-of-life decisions in Austria: survey of intensive care physicians. BMC Med Ethics. 2010;11:19. http://www.biomedcentral.com/1472-6939/11/19. Accessed 21 Feb 2015.
16. Santonocito C, Ristagno G, Gullo A, Weil M. Do-Not-Resuscitate order: a view throughout the world. J Crit Care. 2013;28:14–21.

17. Chan WL. The "Do-Not-Resuscitate" order in palliative surgery: ethical issues and a review on policy in Hong Kong. Palliat Support Care. 2015. doi:10.1017/S1478951514001370.
18. Saeed F, Kousar N, Aleem S, Khawaja O, Javaid A, Siddiqui M, Holley J. End-of-life care beliefsamongMuslimphysicians.AmJHospPalliatCare.2014.doi:10.1177/1049909114522687.
19. Gordon M. Cardiopulmonary resuscitation in the frail elderly: clinical, ethical and halakhic Issues. Isr Med Assoc J. 2007;9:177–9.
20. Buchman T, Cassell J, Ray S, Wax M. Who should manage the dying patient?: rescue, shame, and the surgical ICU dilemma. J Am Coll Surg. 2002;194(5):665–73.
21. Schwarze M, Redmann A, Brasel K, Alexander G. The role of surgeon error in withdrawal of postoperative life support. Ann Surg. 2012;256(1):10–5.
22. ACS NSQIP Program Specifics, Inclusion/Exclusion Criteria. http://site.acsnsqip.org/program-specifics/inclusionexclusion-criteria-4/. Accessed 2 Mar 2015.
23. Northwestern Medicine. Death within 30 days following vascular or general surgery. http://www.nmh.org/nm/quality-30-day-mortality-vascular-and-general-surgery. Accessed 2 Mar 2015.

Chapter 5
Pediatric Patients: Do Not Resuscitate Decisions

Rose J. Campise-Luther and Christina D. Diaz

Abstract The ethical challenges surrounding do not resuscitate (DNR) decisions in pediatric patients differ significantly from those in adult patients. Pediatric patients are in an ethical class of their own, and rely, in most cases, on their parents to make decisions for them, albeit with the pediatric patient's assent when appropriate. Both the initial decision to enter a DNR order and then the reevaluation of that order in the perioperative setting require timely, open, and compassionate communication on the part of the healthcare providers with the involved parties. The physician's primary obligation in these cases is to the patient with thoughtful awareness of the needs of the family. It is the family that will have to cope with the death of their child and the decisions they have made for the rest of their lives.

Keywords Do Not Resuscitate Orders • Pediatric Patients • Anesthesia • Surgery • End-of-Life Decisions

Case Presentations

Case Presentation 1

A 3-year-old girl presents to the operating room for an exploratory laparotomy secondary to a small bowel obstruction. The patient is experiencing septic shock and requires an epinephrine infusion to support her blood pressure. The patient has acute lymphocytic leukemia, which despite extensive chemotherapy and a bone marrow transplant has not gone into remission. The parents have decided on palliative care for their child at this point in time. The surgeon and anesthesiologist contact the oncologist to clarify if the patient has a DNR order. The oncologist answers, "We touched on the subject and the

R.J. Campise-Luther, MD, FAAP (✉) • C.D. Diaz, MD
Department of Anesthesiology, Medical College of Wisconsin-Children's Hospital of Wisconsin, 9200 W. Wisconsin Ave, P.O. Box 1997, MS 735, Milwaukee, WI 53226, USA
e-mail: rcampise@mcw.edu; cdiaz@mcw.edu

B.G. Jericho (ed.), *Ethical Issues in Anesthesiology and Surgery*,
DOI 10.1007/978-3-319-15949-2_5

parents would like to be contacted should the child suffer a cardiac arrest intraoperatively to discuss the options and make the decision at that time."

Case Presentation 2
A 6-year-old boy is scheduled for an emergency ventriculoperitoneal (VP) shunt revision. He has a brainstem glioma for which he previously received chemotherapy and the placement of a VP shunt for the ensuing hydrocephalus. The patient has intractable headaches and nausea/vomiting secondary to the malfunction of the VP shunt. The patient's prognosis is grave and the parents, the child, and the oncology team agreed on a DNR order, which they would like to maintain throughout the perioperative period. The neurosurgeon and anesthesiologist told the family that the DNR order would be upheld in the perioperative period, but now the neurosurgeon takes the anesthesiologist aside and states "under no circumstances will I let this child die in the operating room."

Introduction

Shortly after the advent and propagation of cardiopulmonary resuscitation in the 1960s, the enthusiasm of reviving every cardiac arrest patient was hampered by the unintended consequences that patients and healthcare providers had to face. It quickly became clear that not every patient could or should be resuscitated. The weighing of the benefit of prolonging a patient's life versus the burden of the patient suffering and postponing the inevitable had to be addressed. In 1974, the American Medical Association published the "Standards for Cardiopulmonary Resuscitation (CPR) and Emergency Cardiac Care (ECC)", which stated "CPR is not indicated in certain situations, such as in cases of terminal irreversible illness where death is not unexpected" and also proposed that Do Not Resuscitate (DNR) orders be written in the chart [1]. About the same time, the modern medical ethics movement gained traction, including the upholding of the principle of patient autonomy. In 1990, the Patient Self-Determination Act was passed mandating"…that, in those healthcare institutions which receive Medicare or Medicaid funding, patients must be informed in writing upon admission of (1) their right to accept or refuse treatment, (2) their right under existing state laws regarding advance directives, and (3) any policies which the institution has regarding the withholding or withdrawing of life-sustaining treatments" [2]. Yet, the acceptance of DNR orders in the perioperative setting was slow (see Chapter 4 for a more detailed discussion on this topic). Finally in 1993, The American Society of Anesthesiologists established the "Ethical Guidelines for the Anesthesia Care of Patients with Do-Not-Resuscitate Orders or Other Directives that Limit Treatment" that recommended that DNR orders be reevaluated for the perioperative period to reflect the patient's wishes [3]. Subsequently the American College of Surgeons released the "Statement on Advance Directives by Patients:

"Do Not Resuscitate" in the Operating Room", which also recommended the reevaluation of existing DNR orders prior to surgery [4].

The ethical challenges surrounding perioperative DNR decisions in pediatric patients can differ from those in the adult patient. In fact, some would consider pediatric patients an ethical class of their own [5]. Pediatric patients are at the beginning of their life, whereas the elderly patient has often lived a long and fulfilled life by the time end-of-life issues have to be addressed. Also, pediatric patients include multiple age groups unlike adults, ranging from neonates to adolescents. Moreover, adults with decision-making capacity can make their own decisions regarding perioperative DNR orders unlike most pediatric patients. With medical-decision making in most pediatric cases, informed permission from the parent or guardian is obtained with assent of the patient if the child is of a particular developmental age. The evaluation of a child's ability to assent has to be done in the context of their developmental age and decision-making abilities, and not necessarily based on their chronological age alone. See Chap. 1 for a more detailed discussion on informed consent for pediatric patients, adolescents, and emancipated minors.

This chapter addresses perioperative do not resuscitate decisions in pediatric patients, the reluctance of physicians to address do not resuscitate decisions, potential obstacles to honoring perioperative do not resuscitate orders, and futile cardiopulmonary resuscitation in pediatric patients.

Reluctance to Address Do Not Resuscitate Decisions

The reluctance and delay of physicians in addressing DNR decisions in critically or terminally ill children can unnecessarily prolong a child's suffering and the child's exposure to ineffective therapy instead of focusing efforts on the comfort of the child and the preservation of the child's dignity [6, 7]. Also, entering a DNR order when death is imminent may not allow the parents and other relatives enough time to prepare emotionally for the child's death. From a parent's perspective, the decision to agree to a DNR order may be perceived as betraying their child. Moreover, the time immediately prior to the death of their child as well as how their child dies, will probably remain forever in the parents' minds and influence the rest of their lives [8].

Because of the potential parental guilt and long-term emotional after effects, it may be challenging for some physicians to initiate these end-of-life discussions. Some physicians feel uncomfortable presenting bad news and causing sadness to patients and their families, lack the knowledge and experience on how to present unpleasant news, anticipate conflict with the patient and/or family, have medical-legal concerns, are in denial that the death in unavoidable, or have limited knowledge of advance directives [9]. In fact, in a study by Connors et al., only 41% of patients engaged in a discussion with their physicians about CPR, and in 80% of the cases the physicians misunderstood the patient's preferences [10]. In a study by Hilden et al. the attitudes, practices, and challenges of pediatric oncologists involving end-of-life care were assessed [11]. This study identified physician communication and the lack of formal training as barriers in addressing end-of-life issues [11]. In fact, 47% of the pediatric oncologists did not initiate a discussion of advance directives and, thus, the burden of initiating this discussion was placed on the family [11]. Furthermore, only 10% of the pediatric oncologists had formal courses in pediatric end-of-life care in medical school and only 2.2% had a clinical rotation in hospice or palliative care [11]. Despite the gravity of the situation, parents are able to participate in discussions with the physicians [12]. In fact, in a recent study from the Netherlands addressing communication between physicians and parents concerning end-of-life decisions for their children, the study in most cases indicated that "parents' intense emotions of anxiety, grief, and distress did not hinder them from asking relevant questions and from clearly explaining their considerations and preferences" [12].

Potential Obstacles to Honoring Perioperative Do Not Resuscitate Orders

Surgeons and anesthesiologists have a mutual goal of taking the patient through an anesthetic and surgery with no patient mortality or morbidity. Because of this mutual goal and the uniqueness of the operating room environment, at times these physicians may be reluctant to continue DNR orders in the perioperative period.

The perioperative environment is unlike any other environment in the hospital. Patients enter the operating room to receive very specific interventions usually aimed to improve or even cure an underlying problem. During the anesthetic and surgery, patients may experience hemodynamic perturbations, which are usually transient and routinely treated with measures that may be perceived as resuscitation measures in areas outside of the operating room. Moreover, in the event of an anesthesia-related cardiopulmonary arrest, patient outcomes are more favorable in the operating room than in other areas of the hospital most likely because of the ability of physicians to respond immediately to the patient and the controlled nature of the environment. In fact, in a survey of more than 250,000 patients, 92% of patients were successfully resuscitated in the operating room [13]. With some DNR orders, physicians may not be able to treat these iatrogenic perturbations or cardiopulmonary arrests, leaving them feeling personally responsible for the demise of their patient [14]. Furthermore, a physician may be reluctant to have documentation of a potentially avoidable adverse patient event logged in their patient outcome records.

Perioperative Do Not Resuscitate Orders

Despite guidelines from the American Society of Anesthesiologists, American College of Surgeons, and the Association of Perioperative Nurses to respect a patient's preferences for perioperative DNR orders [3, 4, 15], not all physicians practice required reconsideration of perioperative DNR orders and not all physicians honor a patient's preferences. Furthermore, not all hospitals appear to have a policy addressing pediatric DNR orders. A survey of surgeons and anesthesiologists showed that 75.3% of surgeons and 69.2% of anesthesiologists would uphold a DNR order for palliative procedures. For elective procedures, though, only 49.6% of surgeons and 46.7% of anesthesiologists were willing to uphold such orders [6]. For those children with existing DNR orders, the majority of anesthesiologists and surgeons discuss resuscitation concerns with parents prior to surgery. Although the majority of surgeons and anesthesiologists agree that there should be a hospital policy addressing pediatric DNR orders, only 50.5% of anesthesiologists and 27.5% of surgeons worked in a hospital that had such a policy [6].

As presented in the guidelines of the American Society of Anesthesiologists and American College of Surgeons, the perioperative reevaluation/reconsideration of DNR orders occurs prior to beginning a procedure [3, 4]. DNR orders for children are often discussed when the resuscitation of the pediatric patient would not be beneficial to the child but instead would only prolong their suffering and delay death. As early as possible, the primary care physician, surgeon, and anesthesiologist should talk with the family and, when appropriate, the child concerning perioperative DNR orders. This discussion is not intended to convince the parent or guardian to suspend the DNR order for the perioperative period, but to determine the course of action to preserve the patient's best interests. The conversations should be aimed at understanding the patient's and family's wishes and goals, since often times neither the surgeon nor the anesthesiologist had a prior relationship with the patient or the parents or the guardian. Moreover, pediatric patients should participate in decision-making consistent with their developmental age.

After obtaining informed consent and delineating the perioperative DNR decision, the surgeon and anesthesiologist must communicate the decision concerning the patient's DNR status with the perioperative team and document the decision in the medical record. If at any time either the surgeon or anesthesiologist cannot abide to the agreed upon perioperative DNR decision, the physician should withdraw from the care of the patient, while identifying in a timely manner another physician willing to abide to the DNR decision.

Options regarding the consideration of a perioperative DNR order include the following:

1. **The unaltered maintenance of a preoperative DNR order**.
2. **The suspension of the DNR order** may be considered by some anesthesiologists and surgeons to allow more flexibility concerning actions that can be taken during the course of a procedure [16]. The time of reinstatement of the DNR order must be discussed and communicated to the patient's primary physician so that the time and date of the reinstated DNR order can be recorded in the patient's medical record and medical orders. A study by Fallat et al. showed that 55.1% of anesthesiologists and only 38.2% of surgeons believed the perioperative period ended when the patient left the recovery room [6]. Yet, 39.5% of surgeons believed that this period should continue until 24 h after the surgery was completed [6]. Thus, it is essential to clarify with the parent or guardian and patient, if appropriate, when the perioperative period ends and when the DNR order is to be reinstated.

3. **The goal-directed approach** focuses on the goals and preferences of the parent or guardian and patient [17]. With the goal-directed approach, there is a strong trust and mutual understanding among the anesthesiologist, surgeon, patient as applicable, and parent or guardian. During the procedure, the physicians will make clinical judgments to resuscitate the patient or not, based on discussed and mutually understood goals, values, and preferences.
4. **The procedure-directed approach** discusses a series of procedures that are likely to be used during the procedure. For example, the patient, if applicable, and parent or guardian may accept tracheal intubation, chest compression, and the administration of vasoactive medications but not defibrillation.

Futile Cardiopulmonary Resuscitation

In his article, "Is It Always Wrong to Perform Futile CPR," Truog alludes to situations in which a parent's interest may supersede the pediatric patient's interests [18]. Performing futile cardiopulmonary resuscitation on a child may be what the parents need to find appropriate closure, being reassured that they did everything they could for their child as opposed to questioning if they neglected their parental duties and abandoned their child at the child's time of greatest need. Physicians should not participate in nonbeneficial care to patients if it causes suffering to the patient and diverts healthcare resources away from another patient with resulting harm [18]. Yet, Truog also states "…actions surrounding the moment of death are highly symbolic and often of great significance to the surviving family. By sometimes agreeing to provide futile CPR, we send a message to our communities not that clinicians can be bullied into performing procedures that good medical judgment would oppose, but our hospitals are invested in treating patients and families with respect and concern for their individual needs" [18].

Conclusion

The ethical challenges surrounding DNR decisions in pediatric patients significantly differ from those in adult patients. Pediatric patients are in an ethical class of their own, and rely, in most cases, on their parents to make decisions for them, albeit with the pediatric patient's assent when appropriate. Both the initial decision to enter a DNR order and then the reevaluation of that order in the perioperative setting require timely, open, and compassionate communication on the part of the healthcare providers with the involved parties. The physician's primary obligation in these cases is to the patient with thoughtful awareness of the needs of the family. It is the family that will have to cope with the death of their child and the decisions they have made after their loved one has passed on.

Case Resolution

Case Presentation 1

The lack of clarification concerning the DNR status of the child was most likely secondary to the reluctance of the oncologist to broach the topic. A provider that has an established relationship with the patient and family should initiate discussions regarding the DNR status of the child and allow ample time for the family to discuss the care of the child, ask questions, and make a decision. The lack of timely end-of-life discussions can lead to prolongation of the suffering of the patient. Additionally, the lack of a preemptive discussion of the patient's DNR status puts the healthcare providers in the operating room, including the anesthesiologist and surgeon, in a difficult position of discussing the patient's DNR status "at the operating room door."

In this case, the oncologist, surgeon, and anesthesiologist met with the family and discussed the prognosis of the child; the risks, benefits, and alternatives of the treatment and anesthesia; and the potential for an intraoperative cardiopulmonary event. The family decided to proceed with the surgery to relieve their child's bowel obstruction with full resuscitation measures being employed regardless of the cause. The child underwent a colon resection and the creation of a colostomy, was admitted to the intensive care unit, and passed away 10 days later.

Case Presentation 2

The remarks of the surgeon are not respectful of the wishes of the family, despite the surgeon informing the family that the DNR order would be honored in the perioperative period. The anesthesiologist is obliged to inform the neurosurgeon that the neurosurgeon will need to honor the patient's and family's wishes. Should the surgeon not be able to honor the DNR order in perioperative period, the surgeon should withdraw from the care of the patient in accordance with ACS and ASA guidelines [3, 4] and find an alternative surgeon in a timely manner. If necessary, the institutional ethics committee should be consulted. If another surgeon is not readily available to perform the emergency VP shunt revision, the original scheduled surgeon should proceed with the emergency surgery with adherence to the family's and patient's wishes and goals.

References

1. American Heart Association. National Academy of Sciences-National Research Council: standards for cardiopulmonary resuscitation (CPR) and emergency cardiac care (ECC). JAMA. 1974;227(7 Suppl):833–68.
2. Ulrich L. The patient self-determination act: meeting the challenges in patient care. Washington, DC: Georgetown University Press; 2001.

3. American Society of Anesthesiologists Committee on Ethics. Ethical guidelines for the anesthesia care of patients with do-not-resuscitate orders or other directives that limit treatment. Approved by the American Society of Anesthesiologists House of Delegates on October 17, 2001, and last amended on October 16. 2013. http://www.asahq.org/quality-and-practice-management/standards-and-guidelines. Accessed 27 June 2015.
4. American College of Surgeons Committee on Ethics. Statement on advance directives by patients: "do not resuscitate" in the operating room. Revised Oct 2013. http://bulletin.facs.org/2014/01/statement-on-advance-directives-by-patients-do-not-resuscitate-in-the-operating-room/. Accessed 28 June 2015.
5. Goldberg DS. The ethics of DNR orders as to neonatal & pediatric patients: the ethical dimension of communication. Houst J Health Law Policy. 2007;7(1):57–83.
6. Fallat ME, Deshpande JK. Do-not-resuscitate orders for pediatric patients who require anesthesia and surgery. Pediatrics. 2004;114:1686–92.
7. Truog RD, Campbell ML, Curtis JR, Haas CE, Luce JM, Rubenfeld GD, et al. Recommendations for end-of-life care in the intensive care unit: a consensus statement by the American Academy of Critical Care Medicine. Crit Care Med. 2008;36:953–63.
8. Sayeed SA. The marginally viable newborn: legal challenges, conceptual inadequacies, and reasonableness. J Law Med Ethics. 2006;34(3):600–10.
9. Morrison MF. Obstacles to doctor-patient communication at the end of life. In: Steinberg MD, Youngner SJ, editors. End-of-life decisions: a psychosocial perspective. Washington, DC: American Psychiatric Press; 1998. p. 123–8.
10. Connors AF, Dawson NV, Desbiens NA, Fulkerson WJ, Goldman L, Knaus WA, et al. A controlled trial to improve care for seriously ill hospitalized patients: the study to understand prognoses and preferences for outcomes and risks of treatments (support). JAMA. 1995;274:1591–8.
11. Hilden JM, Emanuel EJ, Fairclough DL, Link MP, Foley KM, Clarridge BC, et al. Attitudes and practices among pediatric oncologists regarding end-of-life care: results of the 1998 American Society of Clinical Oncology Survey. J Clin Oncol. 2001;19(1):205–12.
12. de Vos MA, Bos AP, Plotz FB, van Heerde M, de Graaff BM, Tates K, et al. Talking with parents about end-of-life decisions for their children. Pediatrics. 2015;135(2):e465–76.
13. Olsson GI, Hallen B. Cardiac arrest during anesthesia: a computeraided study of 250,543 anesthetics. Acta Anaesthesiol Scand. 1988;32:653–4.
14. Bosk CL. Forgive and remember: managing medical failure. Chicago: University of Chicago Press; 1979.
15. Association for Perioperative Nurses (AORN). AORN position statement on perioperative care of patients with do-not-resuscitate or allow-natural-death orders. Approved 1995. Reaffirmed 2014. http://www.google.com/search?q=+aorn+staement+of+perioperative+dnr&hl=en&gbv=2&oq=+aorn+staement+of+perioperative+dnr&gs_l=heirloom-serp.3..30i10.331848.331848.0.332164.1.1.0.0.0.0.117.117.0j1.1.0....0...1ac.1.34.heirloom-serp..0.1.117.Oh_SsWhsGh0. Accessed 28 June 2015.
16. Fine PG, Jackson SH. Do not resuscitate in the operating room: more rights and wrongs. Am J Anesthsiol. 1995;22:46–51.
17. Truog RD, Waisel DB, Burns JP. DNR in the OR: a goal-directed approach. Anesthesiology. 1999;90:289–95.
18. Truog R. Is it always wrong to perform futile CPR? N Engl J Med. 2010;362(6):477–9.

Chapter 6
Ethical Care of the Children of Jehovah's Witnesses

Liza-Marie Johnson and James M. West

Abstract The right of adults with full decision-making capacity to refuse specific treatments such as a blood transfusion is well-established in the legal and ethical realms. In adults who have lost their decision-making capacity, the principle of substituted judgment has also been well-defined. However, in the case of parents or guardians who refuse a child's recommended medical treatments for religious or other reasons, conflicts may arise. In this chapter, we examine the clinical case of an adolescent with a malignancy requiring surgery and, quite likely, a blood transfusion whose parents are some of Jehovah's Witnesses (JW). We also discuss the ethical, legal and medical ramifications of this clinical situation.

Keywords Capacity • Consent • Assent • Jehovah's Witness • (Refusal of) Transfusion • Decision-Making • Pediatric

Case Presentation

A 16-year-old African-American female presents to the emergency room with complaints of flank pain and hematuria. Medical evaluation reveals a large mass in her left kidney. The patient subsequently undergoes a transcutaneous biopsy of her kidney which reveals that the patient has renal medullary carcinoma. The patient is then referred to a pediatric oncologist who, after consulting with the pediatric surgeon, recommends a radical left nephrectomy with

L.-M. Johnson, MD, MPH, MSB (✉)
Department of Pediatric Medicine, St. Jude Children's Research Hospital,
262 Danny Thomas Place, MS #260, Memphis, TN 38112, USA
e-mail: Liza.johnson@stjude.org

J.M. West, MD, MA
Department of Anesthesiology, Methodist-LeBonheur Healthcare, 5229 Cosgrove Cove,
Memphis, TN 38117, USA
e-mail: Jwest@comcast.net

B.G. Jericho (ed.), *Ethical Issues in Anesthesiology and Surgery*,
DOI 10.1007/978-3-319-15949-2_6

intraoperative lymph node evaluation. The medical team, adolescent patient, and her parents agree that surgery is in her best interest and offers the only reasonable chance of cure. The family understands that refusal of surgery would result in spread of the cancer and ultimately death. As practicing Jehovah's Witness (JW) followers, the patient and her parents desire "no blood" and do not provide consent to allow the receipt of blood products during surgery. An ethics consultation is requested after the surgeon and anesthesiologist state that they could not "in good conscience" allow a pediatric surgical patient to hemorrhage in the operating room should complications develop during the nephrectomy.

Introduction

Jehovah's Witnesses are an international religious organization and comprise approximately 0.6–0.8% of the adult population in the United States with the greatest percentage residing in the South (36%) or West (29%) [1]. Interestingly, the majority of Jehovah's Witnesses (63%) have no children [1]. However, Jehovah's Witnesses have the lowest retention rate of any religious group with only 37% of individuals raised in the faith as children keeping this religious affiliation into adulthood [2].

JWs began as a sect of Christianity in 1870, as a bible study group formed by C. T. Russell in Allegheny, Pennsylvania. Among other things, JW's have their own translation of the bible and believe that it is inspired by Jehovah and is scientifically and historically correct. The global headquarters of Jehovah's Witnesses is located in Brooklyn, New York where a governing body has ultimate authority over all issues of doctrine.

Though JWs started in 1870, it was not until 1945 that a ban on blood transfusions was placed for JW's [3]. This ban on blood transfusions was based on quotes from the Bible, especially the following: (*New World Translation of the Holy Scriptures – 2013 Revision*) [4].

> Genesis 9:3 - …. Only flesh with its life – with its blood – you must not eat
>
> Leviticus 17:10–12 - 'If any man of the house of Israel or any foreigner who is residing in your midst eats any sort of blood, I will certainly set my face against the one who is eating the blood, and I will cut him off from among his people (Leviticus 17:10). For the life of the flesh is in the blood, and I myself have given it on the altar for you to make atonement for yourselves, because it is the blood that makes atonement by means of the life in it (Leviticus 17:11). That is why I have said to the Israelites: "None of you should eat blood, and no foreigner who is residing in your midst should eat blood" (Leviticus 17:12).
>
> Acts 15:28–29 - …to keep abstaining from things sacrificed to idols and from blood…

A 1951 *Watchtower* article explained the reasoning that led to this ban on blood transfusion: "…when sugar solutions are given intravenously, it is called intravenous feeding. …The transfusion is feeding the patient blood and …(the patient) is **eating it (blood)** through his veins" [bold type added] [5].

It is a common misconception that if you give a JW blood against his or her will, then the JW is still subject to eternal damnation. Another misconception is that if a JW accepts blood then he or she, too, would be subject to eternal damnation with no chance of repentance. Neither of these is true. According to an e-mail communication with the JW lead office:

> "A forced blood transfusion would not be viewed as a sin. Also, if under extreme pressure & while experiencing undue stress a JW was to compromise their belief and accept blood transfusions, in other words, if they caved in at a moment of spiritual weakness yet still held to their beliefs, that individual would not be ostracized by the JW community, rather, kindness would be shown and pastoral help offered. Nevertheless, a forced transfusion or a compromise with one's conscience may leave the patient with deep emotional scars."

In fact, since 2000 JWs are not "disfellowshipped" for accepting blood. JWs are considered to have voluntarily "disassociated" from the Church. This means that if a JW does repent he or she can remain in the fold.

In order to keep up with advances in medicine (for example, renal dialysis; cardiopulmonary bypass; blood harvesting including cell saver (cell salvage), acute normovolemic hemodilution and autologous blood donation; and organ transplant), new guidelines for JWs have been developed to aid members in addressing these clinical situations [6]. Table 6.1 shows a timeline of significant events in the Jehovah's Witness faith and transfusion medicine.

Alternatives to Blood Transfusion and What a Practicing Jehovah's Witness Will Accept

There are few if any true substitutes for a blood transfusion if one is truly needed and an exhaustive discussion of these is beyond the scope of this chapter. However, there are some measures that can be taken to decrease the need for a blood transfusion. It is important to define which, if any of these, will be acceptable to an individual JW patient.

Just as in any organized religion, there can be a difference between official doctrine and personal belief. Therefore, it is not always the case that a patient

Table 6.1 Events in the history of the Jehovah's Witness Church and transfusion

1870	Study group formed
1879	First issue of Watchtower published
1901	Discovery of ABO blood groups
1914	First blood bank transfusion
1931	Changed name to Jehovah's Witnesses
1945	Ban placed on transfusions
1961	Transfusions become a "disassociating" offense
2013	7.9 million members worldwide and 1.2 million members in U.S.

professing to be a JW will not accept any blood products. In a study of pregnant JW patients, up to 10% of these patients stated that they would accept blood products in an emergency situation; however, it was not confirmed whether these patients were baptized [7]. Furthermore, there is a sect known as "Advocates for Jehovah's Witness Reform on Blood" formerly called "Associated Jehovah's Witnesses for Reform on Blood" whose members will accept blood and blood products in many circumstances [8, 9]. They have also worked to reform the Church from the inside [9]. Despite the fact that some JWs accept blood products, in general, few practicing Jehovah's Witnesses will accept whole blood, packed red blood cells, plasma, platelet concentrates, or white blood cell transfusions [6]. Few practicing JWs will accept pre-donated autologous blood since the blood is out of contact with their body for a significant period of time, yet acute normovolemic hemodilution is acceptable to many of the faithful. With cell saver, acute normovolemic hemodilution (ANH), cardiopulmonary bypass, and renal dialysis, *The Watchtower* states that it is an individual JWs decision to receive these treatments if the blood is kept in a continuous circuit with their body and is not stored for any period of time. Cardiopulmonary bypass and dialysis would always involve a continuous circuit. Of course with cell saver and ANH a continuous circuit is not routinely used, but a continuous circuit can easily be created. Other products and procedures are also left to the "discretion of the practicing Christian" including albumin, cryoprecipitate, cryo-poor plasma, individual factors, as well as organ and bone marrow transplantation (Table 6.2).

When faced with major surgery, it is imperative that the anesthesiologist and surgeon determine, in as much detail as possible, what if any of the "optional" products the patient will accept. In addition, it will often become necessary to educate the patient not only on what each of these products and techniques entails, but also on the fact that they are indeed optional.

Ethical and Legal Issues in the Care of Pediatric Jehovah's Witness Patients

The ethical and legal right of capacitated adults to make medical decisions for themselves is well-established [10]. Autonomous decision making provides adults with the leeway to make authentic choices consistent with their beliefs and values [11]. If an adult patient makes a "bad decision," the clinician may confirm capacity and attempt to use gentle persuasion to redirect the patient, but little precedent exists to override their refusal. It may even be considered battery if consent is not obtained from a capacitated adult patient and his or her known preferences are overridden.

When adult patients are unable to make medical decisions on their own behalf, clinicians try to identify a person to act as the patient's "surrogate" and make decisions as his or her proxy. In other words, clinicians ask the surrogate to make decisions based on the patient's previously expressed wishes (if known), or to make decisions consistent with the patient's known values and interests. In pediatrics, children have developing and evolving decisional capacity as well as beliefs and

Table 6.2 Blood product guidelines for Jehovah's Witness patients

Type of blood product or procedure	Accept/refuse/personal decision (PD)[a]	Specific concerns
Whole blood	Refuse	
PRBC's	Refuse	
Plasma	Refuse	
Platelets Platelet gel	Refuse PD	
White cells	Refuse	
Cryoprecipitate	PD	
Cryo-poor plasma (cryosupernatant)	PD	
Fractionated factors	PD	
Albumin	PD	
Erythropoetin	PD	Most erythropoietin is albumin coated and is a PD. Darbepoetin contains no albumin
Recombinant factors VII and IX	Accept	Not made from blood, though some may still object
Cell saver	PD	If kept in continuous circuit
Acute normovolemic hemodilution	PD	If kept in continuous circuit
Cardiopulmonary or veno-venous bypass	PD	Continuous circuit rule
Renal dialysis	PD	Continuous circuit rule
Stored autologous blood	Refuse	Not in continuous circuit
Organ and bone marrow transplant	PD	

The worksheet that many JW's have does not include all of these products and/or techniques, but those not on the worksheet have been verified by The Watchtower.

[a]The term "personal decision" is used here to denote actions that the Watchtower has said are optional. In reality these are all personal decisions for each patient

values. Parental authority and familial autonomy over their developing, vulnerable child creates a unique dynamic that is different from the moral space in which surrogates make medical decisions [12].

Infants and children lack the ability to make autonomous medical decisions and therefore parents (or legal guardians) are presumed to have a liberty interest in the "care, custody, and management" of their children [13]. Furthermore, as children age and mature they are able to play an increasing role in the medical decision making process creating a triangle of decision making between patient, parent, and provider, which may raise additional complexities [14]. While parents are allowed broad discretion in medical decision making, this right is not absolute. As was noted in the case of *Prince v Massachusetts*, "…Parents may be free to become martyrs themselves. But it does not follow they are free, in identical circumstances, to make martyrs of their children before they have reached the age of full and legal discretion when they can make that choice for themselves" [15]. Responding to parents who are refusing a recommended medical intervention is often challenging to clinicians. It is the fiduciary responsibility of the clinician to advocate for the interests of his or her patient (the child) in a manner that promotes the child's interests while minimizing infringements on familial autonomy and parental authority as a whole.

When a child has a reasonable prognosis, the parental refusal of a recommended therapy obliges physicians to (1) analyze the risks and benefits of the parental request versus the recommended intervention and (2) consider if other alternative interventions may be reasonable. It is generally helpful to engage in shared decision making with the family, involving colleagues skilled in communication if necessary, to reach a mutually agreeable decision. If persistent conflict cannot be resolved with referral to another clinician or through involvement with clinical ethics consultation, state intervention may be required. This is most often indicated when parental decision making is perceived to significantly violate a child's best interest or put the child at risk of serious harm.

Evaluation of Medical Decision Making Involving Minors

Child's Best Interest and the Harm Principle

The "best interest of the child" standard is based on the ethical principles of beneficence, or the "moral obligation to contribute to the good of others" [16]. In the context of medical decision making, it aspires to identify the medical care (decision) that is in the best interest of the child. When parental decision making aligns with a proposed medical therapy, the care is often delivered without deliberate consideration of this ethical standard. When differences of opinion exist, the standard may be invoked to substitute the views of a third party (the physician, the courts) over the views of the parents [17]. One expects that most parents do not seek to make decisions they perceive as harmful, so why do clinicians and families sometimes collide over what interventions are best for the pediatric patient?

The best interest standard and the evaluation of the benefits and harms of alternative medical pathways are inherently subjective, value-laden judgments. Consider a patient with osteosarcoma – based on tumor location and the response to chemotherapy, the oncologist and surgeon may recommend amputation rather than a limb-sparing technique, but after evaluation of the information and consideration of their personal preferences and beliefs, the family may still elect to pursue limb-sparing. The teenager may feel that it is in his long-term best interest to not have a prosthesis and is willing to accept any increased risks associated with declining amputation (amputation being what the physicians consider to be his present day best interest). Finally, children are highly dependent on their parents who bear the burden of their care. Parents are likely to consider familial needs – this is the balancing and rank ordering of the interests of the parents, siblings, and their child who is the patient in order to reach a determination of what is the best medical decision [18].

Because of the difficulty using best interest alone, it is helpful to consider what risk of increased harm can be tolerated before a threshold is crossed and the potential risks of harm becoming so great that it becomes necessary to pursue legal action and request that the state order a parent to comply with the medical recommendation. The pursuit of a child protective services referral for medical neglect or a court order may irreversibly damage a provider's relationship with a family and negatively color future interactions with medical professionals. Therefore, the decision to request that a state agency overtake medical decision making should not be taken lightly. If there is significant prognostic uncertainty or low risk of benefit even with the recommended intervention (i.e. chemotherapy for high risk cancer), state agencies are generally adverse to overriding parental decision making. In this context, it is helpful to consider the answers to eight basic questions, as proposed by Diekema, when considering whether to seek state intervention [19]:

1. "By refusing to consent, are the parents placing their child at significant risk of serious harm?
2. Is the harm imminent, requiring immediate action to prevent it?
3. Is the intervention that has been refused necessary to prevent the serious harm?
4. Is the intervention that has been refused of proven efficacy and, therefore, likely to prevent the harm?
5. Does the intervention that has been refused by the parents also place the child at significant risk of serious harm and do its projected benefits outweigh its projected burdens significantly more favorably than the option chosen by the parents?
6. Would any other option prevent serious harm to the child in a way that is less intrusive to parental autonomy and more acceptable to the parents?
7. Can the state intervention be generalized to all other similar situations?
8. Would most people familiar with the situation agree that the state intervention was reasonable?"

Assent and Children's Role in Medical Decision Making

As children mature, they develop an increasing ability to evaluate proposed medical interventions and consider the risks and benefits of the alternatives. Children are not treated as rational, autonomous adults but allowed to participate in decisions in a manner consistent with their developing capacity. Meaningful pediatric assent, which is less stringent than consent, allows children the opportunity to state their preferences within the context of their developmental abilities and desire to participate [20]. The "rule of sevens" can provide general guidance for clinicians assessing developmental capacity in pediatrics. Children under the age of 7 are presumed to lack capacity, children 7–13 years of age have an evolving sense of capacity and should be evaluated on a case-by-case basis, and children over 14 are presumed to have capacity unless evidence exists to the contrary [21]. It may be helpful to consider the practical example of a common pediatric intervention, vaccination. A 4-year-old is unlikely to want to receive a shot, but most all 4-year-old children will be unable to articulate a meaningful decline, and may actively cry or hide in anticipation of the intervention. A 10-year-old is unlikely to want a shot, and may protest against it because it may hurt, but will usually sit cooperatively for administration of the immunization. A teenager may not want the shot, but realize that it is beneficial and not protest, or they may articulate a reasonable response for declining the immunization.

It is important to remember that there will be older children who lack developmental maturity to participate meaningfully and younger children who have significant illness experience prompting greater consideration of their opinion. If the child does not have a true choice in the final medical decision, then they should not be offered a false choice.

Evaluating Transfusion Refusals in Pediatric Jehovah's Witness Patients

Refusals of transfusion should be evaluated in a manner similar to other refusals. Providers should consider if alternative interventions (or nonintervention) exist and evaluate the risks and benefits of the treatment being refused against other proposed alternatives. It may be helpful to solicit the reason for the refusal and engage in an open discussion to see if the refusing party can be gently persuaded through assuasion of fears or misperceptions. In our local experience, families have sometimes presented with inaccurate information, such as vastly overestimating infection risks associated with transfusion or expecting more immediate (within days) benefit from the use of erythropoietin. If the intervention refused is not essential or can be deferred without substantial risk, the refusual may be binding. In considering adolescent refusals, it is important to note the low retention rate in the religious tradition and consider that the 16-year-old refusing transfusion today, may be unlikely to hold the same beliefs as an adult. This may be a consideration when there are high risks of harm to the adolescent if the declination of transfusion is honored.

Families often understand that physicians have a fiduciary responsibility to their patient, the child. Some families may be willing to sign an "acknowledgement statement" which documents that the parents have been informed that emergency transfusion will not be withheld regardless of parental refusal to sign official transfusion consent. Acknowledgement statements may allow for the avoidance of state intervention. Due to variability in legal precedent between states, we recommend conferring with institutional legal counsel for appropriate language. In some circumstances it may not be possible to avoid state intervention. Also, in some circumstances it may be impractical to override refusal – for example an adolescent patient strongly opposed to transfusion who has been offered a myeloablative bone marrow transplant. In this case, the child would require multiple tranfusions over time as an iatrogenic consequence of therapy and the logistics of overriding a resistant patient on multiple occasions may alter the risk-benefit assessment. Obtaining a clinical ethics consultation is advisable for complex or challenging cases. Figure 6.1 is a proposed model for clinicians evaluating familial refusal of transfusion for a pediatric patient.

If a pediatric patient ultimately requires transfusion, it is important to solicit familial preferences about receiving transfusion-related information and to deliver the transfusion in the most respectful manner. Consider transfusing the child when other visitors who may be Witnesses are not present, covering the blood product with an opaque bag, or transfuse while the child is sleeping if viewing the transfusion will be upsetting.

What Are the Surgeon's and Anesthesiologist's Rights and Obligations in Regard to These Patients?

Some physicians believe that caring for a patient who refuses standard care in the operating room (for example, blood transfusion) puts them in a situation of not being able to fully carry out their professional responsibilities. The American Society of Anesthesiologists has developed Guidelines for the Anesthesia Care of Patients with Do- Not-Resuscitate Orders or Other Directives that Limit Treatment [22]. These guidelines should be applicable to surgeons as well. These guidelines state [22]:

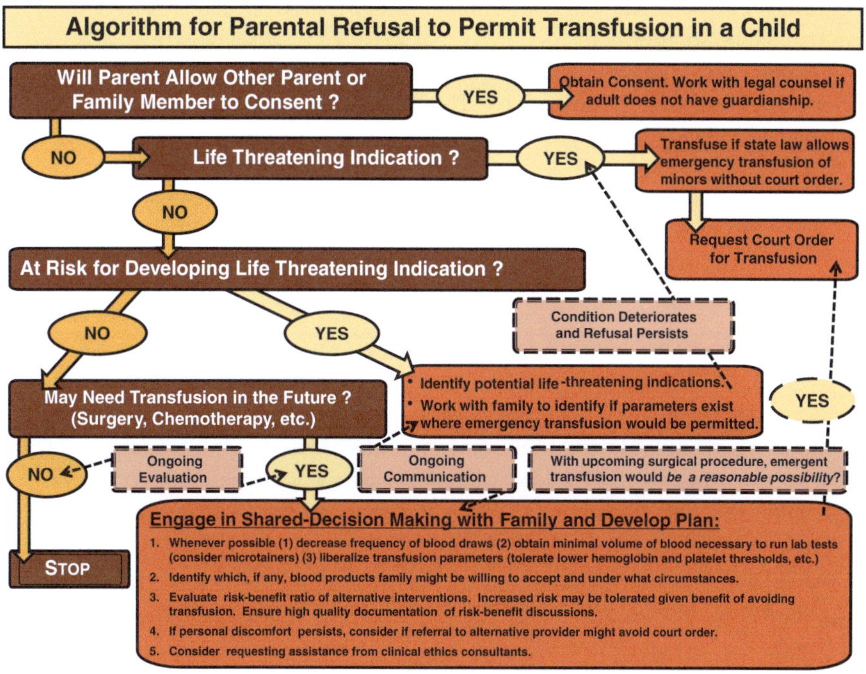

Fig. 6.1 Proposed model for clinicians evaluating familial refusal of transfusion for a pediatric patient

> When an anesthesiologist finds the patient's or surgeon's limitations of intervention decisions to be irreconcilable with one's own moral views, then the anesthesiologist should withdraw in a nonjudgmental fashion, providing an alternative for care in a timely fashion.
>
> If such alternatives are not feasible within the time frame necessary to prevent further morbidity or suffering, then in accordance with the AMA's Principles of Medical Ethics, care should proceed with reasonable adherence to the patient's directives, being mindful of the patient's goals and values.

However, it is important that physicians ensure that by objecting they are not inappropriately applying their own personal moral convictions and beliefs to the physician-patient relationship.

In reality, most ethical dilemmas raised by conscientious refusal can be prevented by forethought, communication, planning and accommodation. However, when push comes to shove, in nonemergent situations, anesthesiologists and surgeons have the right to withdraw themselves from a patient's care, as long as they refer the patient to another health care provider. Not only can the referral be to another physician, but the patient can be referred to another medical center that has expertise in caring for JW patients which may be the best way for these patients to receive optimum care.

If the situation is a life-or-death emergency with no time to make a referral, then the physician is obligated to care for the patient, trying as much as possible to adhere to the patient's and his or her parents' wishes. However, if the physician is concerned that he or she will not be able to comply, then the patient and/or the parents should be so informed.

Of note, these guidelines are similar to the Management of Anaesthesia for Jehovah's Witnesses, published by The Association of Anaesthetists of Great Britain and Ireland in 2005 [23].

Case Resolution

The patient and her mother were active members of their church and were assisted in articulating the grounds for their refusal by a member of the local Jehovah's Witness Hospital Liaison Committee. During a family care conference the surgeon and anesthesiologist shared measures they commonly employ with any patient to reduce the likelihood of transfusion. Furthermore they outlined additional preoperative measures (such as hypervolemic hemodilution) that could be employed to reduce loss of blood cells during surgery. The anesthesiologist led the mother through a checklist of interventions that she would and would not accept for her daughter [24]. The patient and mother made a personal decision to decline whole blood and its components (packed red cells, leukocytes, platelets, and plasma), immune globulin, or autotransfusion of previously banked blood/blood components. The patient and her family were willing to grant permission for use of a cell saver intra-operatively and albumin or other volume expanders. Case consultation involved the office of legal services and the general counsel was able to draft an acknowledgement statement as outlined above.

In a similar case involving a younger child needing a nephrectomy, the family was unwilling to sign an acknowledgement agreement. In this second case, the hospital pursued a court order seeking permission to transfuse if necessary to preserve life and the request was granted. In the end, both children underwent an uncomplicated nephrectomy and neither child required the use of blood or blood products.

References

1. http://religions.pewforum.org/reports. Accessed 12 June 2015.
2. http://www.pewforum.org/2008/02/01/chapter-2-changes-in-americans-religious-affiliation/. Accessed 12 June 2015.
3. How can blood save your life? http://www.jw.org/en/publications/books/blood/how-can-blood-save-your-life/. Accessed 12 June 2015.
4. New World Translation of the Holy Scriptures – 2013 Revision.
5. Anonymous. Questions from readers. The Watchtower. 1 July 1951. p. 415.
6. Jehovah's Witnesses—religious and ethical position on medical therapy, child care, and related matters. Watchtower Bible and Tract Society of Pennsylvania; 2001.
7. Gyamfi C, Berkowitz RL. Responses by pregnant Jehovah's Witnesses on health care proxies. Obstet Gynecol. 2004;104(3):541–4.
8. Elder L. Why some Jehovah's Witnesses accept blood and conscientiously reject official Watchtower Society blood policy. J Med Ethics. 2000;26(5):375–80.
9. Associated Jehovah's Witnesses for reform on blood. www.ajwrb.org. Accessed 12 June 2015.
10. Berg JW, Appelbaum PS, Lidz CW, Parker LS. Informed consent: legal theory and clinical practice. 2nd ed. New York: Oxford University Press; 2001.
11. Brudney, D. Patients, doctors and the good life (for the patient). J Med Ethics. 2015: medethics-2014.
12. Hester DM. Consultation: ethical issues in pediatrics. In: Hester DM, Schonfeld T, editors. Guidance for Healthcare Ethics Committees. New York: Cambridge University Press; 2012. p. 114–21.
13. Santosky v. Kramer, 455 US 745. 1982.
14. Antommaria AHM, Weise KL, Fallat ME, Katz AL, Mercurio MR, Moon MR, et al. Conflicts between religious or spiritual beliefs and pediatric care: informed refusal, exemptions, and public funding. Pediatrics. 2013;132(5):962–5.
15. Prince v. Massachusetts, 321 US 158, 166, 177. 1944.
16. Diekema D. Parental refusals of recommended medical interventions. In: Diekema DS, Mercurio MR, Adam MB, editors. Clinical ethics in pediatrics: a case-based textbook. New York: Cambridge University Press; 2011. p. 14–7.
17. Carbone J. Legal applications of the "best interest of the child" standard: judicial rationalization or a measure of institutional competence? Pediatrics. 2014;134 Suppl 2:S111–20.
18. Ross LF. Children, families, and health care decision-making. New York: Oxford University Press; 1998.

19. Diekema DS. Parental refusals of medical treatments: the harm principle as threshold for state intervention. Theor Med Bioeth. 2004;24:243–64.
20. Bartholome WG. Informed consent, parental permission, and assent in pediatric practice. Pediatrics. 1995;96(5):981–2.
21. Ungaru Y. Pediatric decision-making: informed consent, parental permission, and child assent. In: Diekema DS, Mercurio MR, Adam MB, editors. Clinical ethics in pediatrics: a case-based textbook. New York: Cambridge University Press; 2011. p. 1–6.
22. Ethical guidelines for the anesthesia care of patients with do not resuscitate orders or other directives that limit treatment. American Society of Anesthesiologists; 2009 (updated 2013). Available from: https://www.asahq.org/For-Members/Standards-Guidelines-and-Statements.aspx. Accessed 12 June 2015.
23. Management of anaesthesia for Jehovah's Witnesses. 2nd ed. London: The Association of Anaesthetists of Great Britain and Ireland; 2005. http://www.aagbi.org/sites/default/files/Jehovah's%20Witnesses_0.pdf. Accessed 12 June 2015.
24. http://aggelia.be/km_nov2006.pdf. Accessed 12 June 2015.

Chapter 7
Fatigue and the Care of Patients

Richard J. Kelly and Chen Nisynboim

Abstract This chapter examines the ethical questions that are raised by fatigued medical professionals in the care of their patients. The chapter starts with a review of the science of sleep deprivation and explains why fatigued physicians are at high risk for medical errors. The chapter then provides an ethical analysis of fatigue in the context of physicians' duties to their patients and arrives at the conclusion that physicians who treat patients while impaired by fatigue violate certain ethical responsibilities to their patients. The chapter finishes up with a review of the current regulation of physician work hours in the United States and shows that, while progress has been made, there may be a need to establish coherent and enforceable limitations on work hours for all practicing physicians.

Keywords Fatigue • Ethics • Sleep Deprivation • Physician Work Hours

---

R.J. Kelly, MD, JD, MPH, FCLM (✉)
Department of Anesthesiology and Perioperative Medicine, Health Policy Research Institute, University of California Irvine School of Medicine, 101 The City South Drive, Route 81A, Building 53, Room 203, Orange, CA 92868, USA
e-mail: r.kelly@uci.edu

C. Nisynboim, LLB, JD
University of California Irvine School of Law, 401 E. Peltason Dr., Irvine, CA 92697, USA
e-mail: cnisinbo@lawnet.uci.edu

B.G. Jericho (ed.), *Ethical Issues in Anesthesiology and Surgery*,
DOI 10.1007/978-3-319-15949-2_7

Case Presentation
You've been very busy over the past week performing surgeries and taking multiple night calls. It's now 5 pm on a Friday and you've just completed your week when your office calls to tell you that there has been a scheduling error and you must take an additional night of call for your private group practice. You try to rest but at 10 pm you receive a call that a patient with a ruptured abdominal aortic aneurysm will be coming emergently to the operating room. You begin the surgical procedure, but as the surgery progresses, you become acutely aware that you are severely impaired by fatigue. You begin to wonder whether you will be able to stay awake and alert for the duration of the surgery.

Introduction

Since the time of William Osler, physicians in training have spent long days and sleepless nights working in hospitals to learn from their sick patients and sage professors. While the work was arduous and the hours long, both the professors and their young apprentices, who, more often than not, were unmarried and lived in the hospital, believed that the innumerable hours spent caring for patients was a necessary component of a quality medical education [1].

Over the years, however, evidence has been accumulating that fatigue caused by sleep deprivation may be harmful not only to the health of physicians but to their patients as well. The fact that physicians at all levels, from the intern to the highly experienced clinician, are at risk for fatigue has important ethical and legal implications in the care and treatment of patients.

This chapter starts with a review of the three different types of sleep deprivation and their effects on neurocognitive performance. The second section examines the moral and ethical principles supporting a duty by the medical profession to ensure a practice environment where physicians are not impaired by fatigue. The third section reviews the current regulation of work hours for physicians in the United States.

Effects of Sleep Deprivation on Physician Performance

The purpose of sleep remains elusive, but no matter how hard we try, sleep cannot be eliminated from our daily lives without important biological and neurological consequences [2, 3]. Although the precise amount of sleep modern humans need on a daily basis is unknown, sustained periods of sleep deprivation can cause substantial problems at both a personal and a societal level.

For individuals, sleep deprivation causes excessive daytime sleepiness, declines in neurocognitive and motor function, decreased libido, and depressed mood, all of which can not only interfere with personal and professional relationships but also put individuals at risk for errors in judgment, accidents, and even death [4–6].

On a societal level, sleep deprivation has been implicated in a substantial number of motor vehicle accidents in the United States. According to a study commissioned by the United States (US) National Highway Traffic Safety Administration, over a 5-year period of time, it was estimated that approximately 1.35 million drivers may have been involved in traffic accidents attributable to some form of fatigue [7].

Sleep Deprivation Physiology

Three different but overlapping types of sleep deprivation cause the mental and physical impairments one normally sees in response to periods of restricted sleep. They are classified as acute sleep deprivation, chronic partial sleep deprivation, and sleep inertia.

Acute Sleep Deprivation

Acute sleep deprivation, defined as no sleep or a reduction in the usual total sleep time over a period of 1–2 days, is commonly seen in physicians and others who work shifts of 24 hours or more. Acute sleep deprivation is characterized not only by a significant decline in cognitive function, but also self-assessment and decision-making ability, memory, motor skills, and attention [5, 8–10]. The decline of cognitive function is similar to the effect of a blood alcohol concentration that is above the legal limit for driving (about 0.1%) [11].

Chronic Partial Sleep Deprivation

Chronic partial sleep deprivation, defined as several successive nights of sleep for less than 5–6 hours, causes a similar decline of cognitive function, decision-making, performance, and vigilance [12]. Subjects in a study who slept only 6 hours each night over a period of 2 weeks had similar declines in neurocognitive performance as study subjects who had been awake continuously for 24 hours [4]. Acute sleep deprivation synergistically worsens chronic partial sleep deprivation to the extent that alertness and performance are impaired more than either type of sleep deprivation by itself [13].

Sleep Inertia

Sleep inertia, the third physiological consequence of sleep deprivation, is defined as a state of reduced alertness and performance upon awakening [14]. Sleep inertia is most pronounced for the initial 10–15 minutes after awakening but, in some individuals, may take hours to resolve entirely [15]. The magnitude of the neurocognitive impairment can be similar to the effects of 26 hours of continuous sleep deprivation [16].

These three types of sleep deprivation processes work synergistically such that a physician working at night for one week who is disturbed from sleep in the middle of the night will suffer not only from acute sleep loss but also suffer from chronic partial sleep deprivation and sleep inertia. Such a physician in this sleep-deprived state is at very high risk for making medical errors that compromise the safety of patients.

Strategies to Reduce the Effects of Sleep Deprivation

It has been difficult to address the problem of sleep deprivation because of the degree to which people suffer neurocognitive decline after periods of sleeplessness varies dramatically from individual to individual. Intrinsic factors, such as age and gender, as well as factors that can be modified, such as motivation and training, all interact to determine the degree to which an individual may be affected by sleep deprivation [16, 17].

In individuals, a nap for 30 minutes during a night shift can substantially improve overall cognitive performance and diminish feelings of fatigue [18]. For some, however, the sleep inertia that occurs after awakening can impair cognitive performance for variable periods of time following the nap [19]. In one study, a group of emergency room physicians took 40 minute naps during their night shifts. While they had memory impairment immediately upon awakening, they later showed improved attention and driving performance [20].

Cognitive enhancers such as caffeine and modafinil have been shown to improve neurocognitive function during episodes of acute sleep deprivation and fatigue [21]. Caffeine can make individuals feel more alert and allow them to stay awake for extended periods of time. In a study of novices receiving simulation-based training in laparoscopic procedures, 150 mg of caffeine (equivalent to about one cup of coffee) [22] reversed some of the neurocognitive effects of sleep deprivation [23] but higher doses, equivalent to about four cups of coffee, were needed to have any lasting improvement in cognitive function [24].

Modafinil is a pharmaceutical drug that, similar to caffeine, temporarily mitigates cognitive decline and the subjective sense of fatigue by improving attention, working memory, and cognitive flexibility [24]. Unlike amphetamines, however, modafinil is not known to cause behavioral excitation [25–27] or rebound hypersomnolence [27–29].

Shift pattern manipulation has been the primary means by which the medical profession has sought to ameliorate the effects of sleep deprivation. The Accreditation Council for Graduate Medical Education (ACGME) in the United States mandates that all residents in their first postgraduate year work maximum shift durations of 16 hours and have at least 8 hours each day free of clinical duties when working for extended periods of time. Currently, attending physicians do not have restrictions on the number of hours they may work.

Ethics of Physician Fatigue: The Physician Charter

In 2002, The American Board of Internal Medicine Foundation, the American College of Physicians Foundation, and the European Federation of Internal Medicine collaborated to author *Medical Professionalism in the New Millennium: A Physician Charter,* a document that was subsequently endorsed by more than 130 medical organizations around the world. The charter is based on three fundamental principles operative in the practice of medicine: (1) patient welfare; (2) patient autonomy; and (3) social justice. Revolving around these fundamental principles, the *Physician Charter* has "commitments" that include patient confidentiality, honesty in our interactions with patients, professional competence, quality of patient care, maintenance of appropriate relations with patients, and professional responsibility [30].

Primacy of Patient Welfare

The *Principle of the Primacy of Patient Welfare* is the ethical precept that requires physicians to provide patient care that primarily upholds the best interests of their patients and cannot be compromised by market forces, societal pressures, autonomy interests, or administrative exigencies [30]. A few of the Physician Charter "commitments" that correspond with this fundamental principle are relevant to the ethics of physician fatigue.

First, the Physician Charter declares a commitment to "professional competence," which, among other things, mandates that the medical profession as a whole work towards "improving quality of care" and "strive to see that all of its members are competent" by "ensur[ing] that appropriate mechanisms are available for physicians to accomplish this goal" [30]. Second, the Charter not only mandates that physicians maintain clinical competence but also requires physicians to work with other professionals "to reduce medical error, and increase patient safety" [30]. Moreover, "[p]hysicians … must take responsibility for assisting in the creation and implementation of mechanisms designed to encourage continuous improvement in the quality of care" [30]. And finally, the Physician Charter declares a third commitment to "maintaining appropriate relations with patients," that includes avoiding the exploitation of patients for private purposes [30].

As discussed previously, sleep deprivation leads to substantially decreased neurocognitive performance that, in turn, may lead to considerably increased risks for patients. A fatigued physician who suffers from severe sleep deprivation – whether acute, chronic, or both – may display neurocognitive performance that is so impaired as to render the physician incompetent to treat patients [11, 31]. Physicians in such a state will necessarily provide a lower quality care to their patients. Thus, the *Principle of the Primacy of Patient Welfare* along with the commitments to professional competence and quality of care mandates that physicians should be properly rested in order to maintain levels of neurocognitive performance that would ensure the delivery of an adequate quality of care to patients.

Some ethicists, however, may argue that mandating physicians to be well-rested is unethical. Physicians, after all, have their own autonomy interests including the right to decide their own work hours [32]. Such a position is valid provided the physicians' own autonomy interests do not lead to fatigue and the possibility of providing lower quality of care to patients. If physicians choose to work in a manner that causes their own fatigue, they are subordinating their patients' best interests to their own autonomy interests that, in turn, violates their commitment to maintain appropriate relations with their patients and infringes on their ethical commitment to increase patient safety [32].

The second argument against any mandate relates to cost. Limiting physician work hours to ensure they are rested increases costs for hospitals, medical centers, and private practices [32]. In order to cover for the lost work hours of current physicians on staff, such institutions may find it necessary to hire more physicians at an additional expense. The *Principle of the Primacy of Patient Welfare* requires physicians to dedicate themselves to serving the best interests of patients in a manner that must not be compromised by market forces or administrative exigencies [30]. An interest in costs, therefore, cannot be superior to concerns for patient safety.

Finally, some ethicists may argue that, for the sake of continuity of care [32], physicians should not be required to be well-rested. They may assert that patients' best interests are better served by the attention of the same physician over many continuous hours rather than by a series of physicians who provide fragmented observations and treatment [32]. Shorter working hours inevitably lead to more frequent transfers of patient information from one physician to the next that, in turn, increases the probability of errors in communication [32]. Under this patient's best interest argument, the continuity of care may promote the *Primacy of Patient Welfare* by longer rather than shorter physician work hours. For this argument to succeed, however, the benefits to the patient must outweigh the increased risk of fatigue-related medical errors. Indeed, there may be cases in which continuity of care may benefit the patient more than being cared for by well-rested physicians but, at a certain point, the treating physician's fatigue will become so severe and debilitating that the probability of harm from continued treatment would clearly outweigh the benefits of continuity of care. Thus, continuity of care arguments cannot justify allowing physicians to work in an unlimited capacity.

Patient Autonomy

The *Principle of Patient Autonomy* of the Physician Charter has a more recent history. Events in history, such as the abuse of Nazi prisoners of war and the Tuskegee Syphilis Study, gave rise to the ethical concept that patients themselves have the right to determine what should be done to their bodies.

According to the *Principle of Patient Autonomy*, "physicians must be honest with their patients and empower them to make informed decisions about their treatment" [30]. Within the parameters of ethical and professional constraints, "patients' decisions about their care must be paramount" [30]. The Physician Charter commitment that corresponds with this principle is the commitment to "honesty with patients" [30]. This commitment mandates physicians to "ensure that patients are completely and honestly informed …." [30]. Furthermore, patients must be "empowered to decide on the course of therapy" [30]. For the patient's consent to be validly informed, the physician must provide the patient with the information needed to understand the procedure, including the nature and purpose of the treatment, as well as its risks, potential benefits, and available alternatives [30].

As explained previously, physicians who are severely sleep deprived present substantially increased risks for their patients. Patients, in fact, are interested to know whether their physicians are sleep deprived. A study in the United States showed that the vast majority of patients feel anxious about their safety when they learn that the doctor who is about to perform surgery on them has been on duty for 24 consecutive hours [33]. Furthermore, another study reported that 80 percent of patients would want to be treated by a different physician if they discover their assigned physician has been on duty continuously for 24 hours [34]. Considering that physician fatigue presents a substantial added risk of injury to patients and is something patients consider to be an important factor in deciding about their treatment, the *Principle of Patient Autonomy* and the commitment to honesty with patients mandate disclosure of this added risk.

Those who oppose the disclosure to patients of a physician's degree of fatigue argue along two lines. First, they argue that physicians should assess their own physical or mental preparedness to perform their clinical responsibilities in particular clinical situations. A fatigued surgeon, for example, may want to perform a simple surgical procedure but decide that he or she is not sufficiently rested to perform a more complex surgery. Second, they argue that if sleep deprivation requires disclosure to patients then issues such as family conflict, stress at work, financial difficulties, or other factors that may affect the physician's clinical ability to focus and make medical decisions in the care of patients should also be disclosed [35].

To argue, however, that physicians should assess their own physical or mental preparedness to fulfill their clinical responsibilities in a particular clinical situation presents a false dichotomy. Varying degrees of fatigue and of treatment complexity present differing degrees of added risks to patients. If the fatigue-related risk is large, physicians should be ethically obligated to refrain from the treatment of patients in accordance with the *Principle of the Primacy of Patient Welfare* and its corresponding commitments. Conversely, if the fatigue-related risk is trivial, the physician need not disclose their fatigue. In between these two extremes are circumstances in which the added risk is such that the physician's work is permissible provided the patient has been advised of the risk and has provided consent.

The second argument posited is that if sleep deprivation requires disclosure to patients then other factors such as family strife, financial concerns, and the like should be similarly disclosed. Whether the physician should disclose these personal factors, however, depends not on the intrinsic nature of the phenomenon but rather on whether the personal factors will put the patient's safety at risk. Thus, where other factors, such as family conflict or financial concerns, do give rise to a high degree of added risk to patients, then these factors may require disclosure as well.

Thus, the *Principle of Patient Autonomy* and the corresponding commitment to honesty with patients mandate that physicians disclose their own fatigue when such degrees of fatigue may give rise to substantial additional risk to their patients.

Social Justice

The third of the three fundamental principles is that of *Social Justice* which requires the medical profession to promote a "fair distribution of health care resources" and to "work actively to eliminate discrimination in health care, whether based on race, gender, socioeconomic status, ethnicity, religion, or any other social category" [30]. A relevant Physician Charter commitment that corresponds with this principle is the commitment to "improving access to care." According to this commitment, "medical professionalism demands that the objective of all health care systems be the availability of a uniform and adequate standard of care" [30]. Thus, physicians should "work to eliminate barriers to access [to health care] based on education, laws, finances, geography, and social discrimination" [30].

Fatigued physicians violate the *Principle of Social Justice* because they do not provide the same quality of medical care to their patients as when they are not impaired by fatigue. Some ethicists may reasonably argue that limiting physicians to work only when they are not fatigued is also a violation of the *Principle of Social Justice*. In geographical areas with shortages of qualified physicians, limiting physician work hours will exacerbate any physician shortage and may actually reduce access to medical services for certain patients. While limiting physician work hours to prevent fatigue may not be practical in some settings, this does not imply that limiting physician work hours in all settings is justified [32]. Instead, the work hours of physicians must be structured in a manner that accommodates settings where medical services are in short supply. Flexible physician work hour limitations that are sensitive to different practice settings do not violate the *Principle of Social Justice* and the commitment to improving access to care but actually promote them.

Ethical Duty to Limit Physician Fatigue

The principle of *Primacy of Patient Welfare* and the related commitments to professional competence, improving quality of care, and maintaining appropriate relations with patients provide strong justifications for requiring physicians not to work while impaired by fatigue. Indeed, consideration of patients' welfare must trump all other interests, including the physicians' own autonomy interests and the financial considerations of medical institutions. Although the desire for continuity of care may counsel against providing fragmented treatment in some circumstances, consistent with the *Primacy of Patient Welfare*, this interest does not support the notion that physician work hours should be structured in a manner that allows physicians to work while fatigued.

Similarly, the *Principle of Social Justice* and the related commitment to improving access to care would be well served by structuring physician work hours that are flexible and sensitive to settings that suffer from workforce shortages.

While the *Principle of Patient Autonomy* and the related commitment to honesty with patients do not directly call for limitations on physician work hours, they suggest that fatigued physicians have a duty to inform patients of their status when their fatigue is severe enough to carry a substantial added risk to their patients.

Duty Hour Limitations for Physicians in the United States

When graduating medical students begin their residencies, they embark on an intense course of training that involves long hours, challenging patient care situations, regular shifts of overnight call, and increasing levels of responsibility. In the past, these resident physicians worked in hospitals without any regulation of their work hours. Some in the medical profession defended these long working hours as necessary to expose residents to diverse populations of patients, to develop skills in triaging patients, to learn multitasking skills, and have the opportunity to be actively involved in the care of their patients. Studies have shown, however, that residents working these long hours experienced high rates of depression and burnout [36–38].

Despite emerging concerns about the long working hours of residents, some thought shorter working hours would compromise residents' professional development, interrupt continuity of care, and diminish residents' dedication and commitment to their patients [39]. In addition, the reduction of resident work hours would increase the number of patient transfers of care that, in turn, would increase the potential for medical errors [40].

As evidence of the deleterious effects of sleep deprivation was more widely reported [41], many residency programs in the United States responded by reducing resident call responsibilities but, in many cases, residents continued to work more than 100 hours per week.

New York State Regulations for Duty Hours

In 1989, in the wake of the famous *Libby Zion* case in which a young woman died while under the care of under-supervised fatigued residents [42], New York became the first state to limit the working hours of physicians in training. New York Health

Code section 405 now limits the work of residents to 24 consecutive hours and an average of 80 hours per week over a 4-week period [43]. Interestingly, the statute imposes a special limitation of 12 consecutive work hours per shift not only for residents but also for attending physicians working in the emergency departments of hospitals [43]. The New York State regulations have been plagued by limited compliance and problematic enforcement. Over the years, some New York hospitals have been found to schedule residents beyond the prescribed limits, casting doubt on the effectiveness of the statute [44].

Accreditation Council for Graduate Medical Education Duty Hour Guidelines

Since 2003, the Accreditation Council for Graduate Medical Education (ACGME) has required all accredited medical training programs to implement a policy that limits resident work hours. The ACGME work hour restrictions followed the Institute of Medicine's (IOM) landmark report *To Err is Human* in which resident fatigue was identified as one of the primary causes of medical errors [45], and was a response to society's demand to reduce medical errors resulting from physician sleep deprivation. The implementation of the ACGME duty hour policy was the first attempt to limit resident work hours throughout the United States.

As a follow-up to the ACGME work hour restrictions, the Institute of Medicine reviewed, at the request of the United States Congress, existing data addressing the relationship between resident work hours and the safety of patients. In 2008, the IOM reported a scarcity of research on the topic, but recommended further reductions in resident duty hours [46].

Currently, the ACGME guidelines (revised in 2011) consist of the following for residents in all specialties:

- 80-hour work week averaged over 4 weeks
- maximum of 28 continuous hours
- not more than every third night call on average
- 10 hours off after each long shift
- at least 1 day off per week averaged over 4 weeks
- 16-hour work hour limits for interns.

Despite the ACGME guidelines and duty hour restrictions, subsequent studies showed no change in the rate of patient morbidity or mortality, resident board examination pass rates, or voluntary withdrawal of residents from residency programs [47–49]. Interns, however, did report fewer errors in the care of patients and subjectively felt less sleep deprived [50].

In order to implement the most recent ACGME guidelines, many medical training programs have scheduled residents to work a week of nights. One shift at night, however, causes disrupted sleep and results in significant sleepiness at work [51–53].

Furthermore, consecutive night shifts cumulatively increase sleep loss, sleep deficit, and fatigue [54]. Thus, changing from a traditional call schedule (one call every fourth night) to a week of night shifts does not reduce resident fatigue [55].

The changes in the duty hour requirements for residents are in need of further development to further reduce sleep deprivation and its effects on patient safety. Members of the medical profession should look to other industries to investigate staffing models that optimize continuity-of-care of patients, minimize sleep disruption, and reduce fatigue [56].

Conclusion

Physician fatigue presents a significant risk to patient safety and will continue to do so as long as sleep-deprived and overworked physicians continue to work inordinately long hours. Until we have a better understanding of sleep deprivation and its effects on neurocognitive performance, process improvements must be implemented to protect patients and physicians from being harmed from sleep deprivation. Although regulation of attending and resident physician work-hours must be done thoughtfully and must consider the potential implications for patient safety and access to healthcare, there is little justification for the current state of affairs in which many physicians continue to work long hours in varying states of fatigue.

Future studies that elucidate the causal link between fatigue and clinical performance will guide us in the establishment of duty hour requirements that enhance patient safety and maximize physician performance.

References

1. William Osler BM. A life in medicine. Oxford: Oxford University Press; 1999.
2. Dinges DF, Kribbs NB. Performing while sleepy: effects of experimentally-induced sleepiness. In: Monk TH, editor. Sleep, sleepiness and performance. Chichester: Wiley; 1991. p. 97–128.
3. Bonnet MH. Sleep deprivation. Princ Pract Sleep Med. 2000;2:50–67.
4. Van Dongen HP, Maislin G, Mullington JM, Dinges DF. The cumulative cost of additional wakefulness: dose-response effects on neurobehavioral functions and sleep physiology from chronic sleep restriction and total sleep deprivation. Sleep. 2003;26(2):117–26.
5. Pilcher JJ, Huffcutt AI. Effects of sleep deprivation on performance: a meta-analysis. Sleep. 1996;19(4):318–26.
6. Dinges DF, Pack F, Williams K, Gillen KA, Powell JW, Ott GE, et al. Cumulative sleepiness, mood disturbance and psychomotor vigilance performance decrements during a week of sleep restricted to 4–5 hours per night. Sleep: J Sleep Res Sleep Med. 1997;20(4):267–77.
7. NHTSA. National Highway Traffic Safety Administration Report [online]. Available from URL: http://www.nhtsa.gov/people/injury/research/drowsy_driver.html. Accessed 15 May 2015.
8. Alhola P, Polo-Kantola P. Sleep deprivation: impact on cognitive performance. Neuropsychiatr Dis Treat. 2007;3(5):553–67.

9. Dorrian J, Lamond N, Dawson D. The ability to self-monitor performance when fatigued. J Sleep Res. 2000;9(2):137–44.
10. Philibert I. Sleep loss and performance in residents and nonphysicians: a meta-analytic examination. Sleep. 2005;28(11):1392–402.
11. Dawson D, Reid K. Fatigue, alcohol and performance impairment. Nature. 1997;388(6639):235.
12. Carskadon MA, Dement WC. Cumulative effects of sleep restriction on daytime sleepiness. Psychophysiology. 1981;18(2):107–13.
13. Cohen DA, Wang W, Wyatt JK, Kronauer RE, Dijk DJ, Czeisler CA, et al. Uncovering residual effects of chronic sleep loss on human performance. Sci Translat Med. 2010;2(14):14ra3.
14. Downey R, Bonnet MH. Performance during frequent sleep disruption. Sleep. 1987;10(4):354–63.
15. Jewett ME, Wyatt JK, Ritz-De Cecco A, Khalsa SB, Dijk DJ, Czeisler CA. Time course of sleep inertia dissipation in human performance and alertness. J Sleep Res. 1999;8(1):1–8.
16. Van Dongen HP, Baynard MD, Maislin G, Dinges DF. Systematic interindividual differences in neurobehavioral impairment from sleep loss: evidence of trait-like differential vulnerability. Sleep. 2004;27(3):423–33.
17. Van Dongen HP, Vitellaro KM, Dinges DF. Individual differences in adult human sleep and wakefulness: Leitmotif for a research agenda. Sleep. 2005;28(4):479–96.
18. Smith SS, Kilby S, Jorgensen G, Douglas JA. Napping and nightshift work: effects of a short nap on psychomotor vigilance and subjective sleepiness in health workers. Sleep Biol Rhythm. 2007;5(2):117–25.
19. Asaoka S, Fukuda K, Murphy TI, Abe T, Inoue Y. The effects of a nighttime nap on the error-monitoring functions during extended wakefulness. Sleep. 2012;35(6):871–8.
20. Smith-Coggins R, Howard SK, Mac DT, Wang C, Kwan S, Rosekind MR, et al. Improving alertness and performance in emergency department physicians and nurses: the use of planned naps. Ann Emerg Med. 2006;48(5):596–604. e1–3.
21. Sugden C, Aggarwal R, Housden C, Sahakian BJ, Darzi A. Pharmacological enhancement of performance in doctors. BMJ (Clinical Research Ed). 2010;340:c2542.
22. Crozier TW, Stalmach A, Lean ME, Crozier A. Espresso coffees, caffeine and chlorogenic acid intake: potential health implications. Food Funct. 2012;3(1):30–3.
23. Aggarwal R, Mishra A, Crochet P, Sirimanna P, Darzi A. Effect of caffeine and taurine on simulated laparoscopy performed following sleep deprivation. Br J Surg. 2011;98(11):1666–72.
24. Killgore WD, Kahn-Greene ET, Grugle NL, Killgore DB, Balkin TJ. Sustaining executive functions during sleep deprivation: a comparison of caffeine, dextroamphetamine, and modafinil. Sleep. 2009;32(2):205–16.
25. Gallopin T, Luppi P, Rambert F. Effect of the wake-promoting agent Modafinil on sleep-promoting neurons from the ventrolater-al preoptic nucleus: an in vitro pharmacologic study. Sleep. 2004;27(1):19–25.
26. Lagarde D, Milhaud C. Electroencephalographic effects of modafinil, an alpha-1-adrenergic psychostimulant, on the sleep of rhesus monkeys. Sleep: J Sleep Res Sleep Med. 1990;13(5):441–8.
27. Lin J, Gervasoni D, Hou Y, Vanni-Mercier G, Rambert F, Frydman A, et al. Effects of amphetamine and modafinil on the sleep/wake cycle during experimental hypersomnia induced by sleep deprivation in the cat. J Sleep Res. 2000;9(1):89–96.
28. Tourev M, Sallanon-Moulin M, Jouvet M. Awakening properties of modafinil without paradoxical sleep rebound: comparative study with amphetamine in the rat. Neurosci Lett. 1995;189(1):43–6.
29. Edgar DM, Seidel WF. Modafinil induces wakefulness without intensifying motor activity or subsequent rebound hypersomnolence in the rat. J Pharmacol Exp Ther. 1997;283(2):757–69.
30. Medical professionalism in the new millennium: a physician charter. Ann Intern Med. 2002;136(3):243–6.

31. Lamond N, Dawson D. Quantifying the performance impairment associated with fatigue. J Sleep Res. 1999;8(4):255–62.
32. Mercurio MR, Peterec SM. Attending physician work hours: ethical considerations and the last doctor standing. Pediatrics. 2009;124(2):758–62.
33. Czeisler CA, Pellegrini CA, Sade RM. Should sleep-deprived surgeons be prohibited from operating without patients' consent? Ann Thorac Surg. 2013;95(2):757–66.
34. Blum AB, Raiszadeh F, Shea S, Mermin D, Lurie P, Landrigan CP, et al. US public opinion regarding proposed limits on resident physician work hours. BMC Med. 2010;8:33.
35. Pellegrini CA, Britt LD, Hoyt DB. Sleep deprivation and elective surgery. N Engl J Med. 2010;363(27):2672–3.
36. Fahrenkopf AM, Sectish TC, Barger LK, Sharek PJ, Lewin D, Chiang VW, et al. Rates of medication errors among depressed and burnt out residents: prospective cohort study. BMJ (Clin Res Ed). 2008;336(7642):488–91.
37. West CP, Huschka MM, Novotny PJ, Sloan JA, Kolars JC, Habermann TM, et al. Association of perceived medical errors with resident distress and empathy: a prospective longitudinal study. JAMA. 2006;296(9):1071–8.
38. Shanafelt TD, Bradley KA, Wipf JE, Back AL. Burnout and self-reported patient care in an internal medicine residency program. Ann Intern Med. 2002;136(5):358–67.
39. Van Eaton EG, Horvath KD, Pellegrini CA. Professionalism and the shift mentality: how to reconcile patient ownership with limited work hours. Arch Surg. 2005;140(3):230–5.
40. Mukherjee S. A precarious exchange. N Engl J Med. 2004;351(18):1822–4.
41. Friedman RC, Bigger JT, Kornfeld DS. The intern and sleep loss. N Engl J Med. 1971;285(4):201–3.
42. Asch DA, Parker RM. The Libby Zion case. One step forward or two steps backward? N Engl J Med. 1988;318(12):771–5.
43. N.Y. Comp. Codes R. & Regs. tit. 10, § 405.4.
44. Gefell AW. Dying to sleep: using federal legislation and Tort Law to cure the effects of fatigue in medical residency programs. J Law Policy. 2002;11:645.
45. Kohn LT, Corrigan JM, Donaldson MS, editors. To err is human: building a safer health system. Washington, DC: National Academies Press; 2000.
46. Ulmer C, Wolman D, Johns M, editors. Committee on optimizing graduate medical trainee (resident) hours and work schedules to improve patient safety, Institute of Medicine. Resident duty hours: enhancing sleep, supervision, and safety. Washington, DC: National Academies Press; 2008.
47. de Virgilio C, Yaghoubian A, Lewis RJ, Stabile BE, Putnam BA. The 80-hour resident workweek does not adversely affect patient outcomes or resident education. Curr Surg. 2006;63(6):435–9.
48. Volpp KG, Rosen AK, Rosenbaum PR, Romano PS, Even-Shoshan O, Wang Y, et al. Mortality among hospitalized Medicare beneficiaries in the first 2 years following ACGME resident duty hour reform. JAMA. 2007;298(9):975–83.
49. Leibrandt TJ, Pezzi CM, Fassler SA, Reilly EF, Morris JB. Has the 80-hour work week had an impact on voluntary attrition in general surgery residency programs? J Am Coll Surg. 2006;202(2):340–4.
50. McElearney ST, Saalwachter AR, Hedrick TL, Pruett TL, Sanfey HA, Sawyer RG. Effect of the 80-hour work week on cases performed by general surgery residents. Am Surg. 2005;71(7):552–5; discussion 5–6.
51. Åkerstedt T. Shift work and disturbed sleep/wakefulness. Occup Med. 2003;53(2):89–94.
52. Son M, Kong JO, Koh SB, Kim J, Harma M. Effects of long working hours and the night shift on severe sleepiness among workers with 12-hour shift systems for 5 to 7 consecutive days in the automobile factories of Korea. J Sleep Res. 2008;17(4):385–94.
53. Crowley SJ, Lee C, Tseng CY, Fogg LF, Eastman CI. Complete or partial circadian re-entrainment improves performance, alertness, and mood during night-shift work. Sleep. 2004;27:1077–88.

54. Leff DR, Aggarwal R, Rana M, Nakhjavani B, Purkayastha S, Khullar V, et al. Laparoscopic skills suffer on the first shift of sequential night shifts: program directors beware and residents prepare. Ann Surg. 2008;247(3):530–9.
55. Kamine TH, Barron RJ, Lesicka A, Galbraith JD, Millham FH, Larson J. Effects of the new Accreditation Council for Graduate Medical Education work hour rules on surgical interns: a prospective study in a community teaching hospital. Am J Surg. 2013;205(2):163–8.
56. Volpp KG, Landrigan CP. Building physician work hour regulations from first principles and best evidence. JAMA. 2008;300(10):1197–9.

Chapter 8
Conscientious Objection

Ran Cheng and Kenneth R. Abbey

Abstract The phrase "*conscientious objection*" appears to have originated from the military service, but today it can be applied in other fields including education, child immunization, and healthcare. In medicine, conscientious objection refers to the right of providers to refuse to participate in certain types of medical care that they object to on religious or moral grounds. Most commonly, conscientious objection in medicine occurs when providers refuse to participate in abortion. However, conscientious objection is a much broader issue and may also apply to a number of medical and quasi-medical interventions including lethal injection, work with prisoners, futile care, and medical research. Conscientious objection is an issue worthy of consideration by every physician because invoking conscientious objection carries professional responsibilities as well as social, professional, and legal risks. In general, a physician will be better positioned to fulfill their professional responsibilities and minimize their professional risks if they prepare in advance.

Keywords Conscientious Objection • Abortion • Right to Privacy • Lethal Injection • Physician-Assisted Suicide • Prisoners • Roe v. Wade

---

R. Cheng, MD (✉)
Department of Anesthesiology and Perioperative Medicine, Operative Care Division, Oregon Health and Sciences University, 3181 SW Sam Jackson Park Road, Portland, OR 97239, USA
e-mail: Chenra@ohsu.edu

K.R. Abbey, MD, JD
Department of Anesthesiology, Portland Veterans Affairs Medical Center, 3710 SW US Veterans Hospital Road, Portland, OR 97239, USA

Department of Anesthesiology and Perioperative Medicine, Operative Care Division, Oregon Health and Sciences University, Portland, OR, USA
e-mail: Kenneth.Abbey@va.gov; abbeyk@ohsu.edu

B.G. Jericho (ed.), *Ethical Issues in Anesthesiology and Surgery*,
DOI 10.1007/978-3-319-15949-2_8

Case Presentation
You are a young anesthesiologist practicing at a community hospital in Oregon and you are consulted to provide better pain management to a terminally ill patient. The patient is a 67-year-old retired nurse with metastatic lung cancer to his brain. His prognosis is very poor and he has, at most, 6 months to live. While interviewing him, he tells you that he is constantly in agony and cannot bear it anymore. He knows that physician-assisted suicide is legal in Oregon and he asks you to help him end his life. What will you do? If you do not believe in suicide, is it appropriate to decline his request? Do you have an ethical obligation to decline his request? If you decide you cannot in good conscience assist in his suicide, what are your professional obligations to him?

Introduction

Conscientious objection in medicine refers to the right of providers to refuse to participate in certain types of medical care that they object to on religious or moral grounds [1]. Most commonly, conscientious objection in medicine occurs when providers refuse to participate in abortion. Not surprisingly, therefore, the invocation of conscientious objection for legal abortion is controversial and a discussion of conscientious objection is often colored by one's views on abortion [2]. However, conscientious objection is a much broader issue that may apply to a number of medical and quasi-medical interventions including lethal injection, care of prisoners, futile care, and medical research. Moreover, conscientious objection has long held a place in history and applies far beyond medicine to many aspects of society and human interaction. Accordingly, thoughtful discourse about conscientious objection requires consideration of not only its application in the context of abortion but also in many other contexts in which it has been invoked.

The History of Conscientious Objection

The phrase "*conscientious objection*" appears to have originated from the military service and in the modern military refers to a "firm, fixed, and sincere objection to participation in a war in any form or to the bearing of arms, by reason of religious training and or belief" [3].

The oldest known conscientious objector to military service was Saint Maximilian of Tebessa who earned his sainthood for his refusal to serve in the Roman Legions on the basis of his Christian beliefs. He was executed on March 12th, 295 AD, and became a martyr for Christianity [4]. In America, the earliest known conscientious objectors were members of religious sects who refused to bear arms or take part in combat during the American Civil War. During World War I, conscientious objectors were allowed to take non-combatant military roles, but those who refused to serve in *any* position in the military were subjected to imprisonment and even physical abuse [1, 5]. The honorable service received by conscientious objectors, especially during the world wars, has helped to ensure the commitment of the military to the concept of conscientious objection. In fact, the first non-combat conscientious objector to be awarded the Congressional Medal of Honor was Desmond T. Doss, a Seventh Day Adventist who distinguished himself by heroic service as a medic in World War II [6]. Today, the Department of Defense criteria for conscientious objection states that "the belief upon which conscientious objection is based must be the primary controlling force in the applicant's life" [3].

Outside of the military, conscientious objection can be witnessed in education, child immunization, and healthcare. In the United States, compulsory education varies slightly from state to state, but typically begins around the ages of 5–7 and ends between the ages of 16–18 [7]. Home schooling serves as a form of conscientious objection for many parents who would like their children's education to have a certain religious or moral background or who object to some of the classes (e.g. sex education) or topics (e.g. evolution) offered in public schools. Similarly, school immunization laws require parents to vaccinate their children against certain contagious and fatal diseases prior to starting school. However, there are 48 states that allow for religious exemptions and 18 states that allow personal belief exemptions to these immunizations for daycare and school [8]. Many parents elect not to vaccinate their children because of a believed link to autism, although scientific evidence does not support this belief [9]. However, in 2014, an outbreak of measles occurred in the western United States leading to calls for the elimination of conscientious objection exemptions to immunization [10, 11].

The History of Conscientious Objection in Medicine

The history of conscientious objection in medicine is nearly as long as its history in the military. Ironically, given the modern association of conscientious objection to abortion, the original Hippocratic Oath (written in Ionic Greek around the fifth century BC) contained the promise that "I will give no sort of medicine to any pregnant woman, with a view to destroy the child" [12]. Since the Oath was not and is not legally binding, the promise amounted to an assurance that the practitioner would exercise conscientious objection against participation in abortion. But the Oath also called upon physicians to refrain from a number of other interventions: poison, surgery (reserved for surgeons), and broadly to "refrain from injury or wrong from falsehood" [12].

In the United States, the issue of conscientious objection to abortion became acute after the *Roe v. Wade* decision in 1973, in which the Supreme Court found that laws banning abortion were unconstitutional [13]. Congress reacted to *Roe* by passing the Church Amendments that same year, which provide that "receipt of certain federal funds by any individual or entity does not authorize a public authority to require the recipient to perform or assist in the performance of an abortion or sterilization, make its facilities available for an abortion, or provide personnel to perform or assist in the performance of an abortion or sterilization" [14–16]. In 1996, the Public Health Service Act gave more specific guidelines regarding reproductive rights. These guidelines prohibit the "federal government and any state or local agencies receiving federal financial assistance from discriminating against any health care entity on the basis that: the entity refuses to undergo training in the performance of induced abortions, to require or provide such training, to perform such abortions, or to provide referrals for such training or such abortions" [15, 17]. More recently, the Affordable Care Act under Section 1303(b)(4) offers health care providers the right to conscientious objection by stating that "No qualified health plan offered through an Exchange may discriminate against any individual health care provider or health care facility because of its unwillingness to provide, pay for, provide coverage of, or refer for abortions" [18].

At the state level, 49 states provide for at least a limited right of conscientious objection for health care providers [19]. In Michigan, for example, the Conscientious Objector Policy Act allows providers to "decline care if that care compromises the provider's beliefs, except in the event of an emergency" [20]. In Mississippi, the Uniform Health-Care Decisions Act provides that "healthcare providers may decline to comply with healthcare decisions for reasons of conscience" [21]. Vermont is the only state that offers no right of conscientious objection to health care providers [19].

Philosophical Underpinnings of Conscientious Objection in Medicine

Conscientious objection has philosophical support from multiple sources both in the United States and internationally. The Constitution of the United States references both a philosophical and legal basis for conscientious objection in the First Amendment [22].

The First Amendment states "Congress shall make no law respecting an establishment of religion, or prohibiting the free exercise thereof; or abridging the freedom of speech, or of the press; or the right of the people peaceably to assemble, and to petition the Government for a redress of grievances" [22]. The inclusion of religious freedom in the First Amendment was not an arbitrary choice by the founders. Rather, religious freedom was considered essential to American society and distinguished America (at that time) from most other countries reflecting the strong liberal (in the modern vernacular, "libertarian") philosophical beliefs of the founders. Even in modern times, these protections retain a special place in American society and are treated with the greatest respect by American courts and governmental institutions.

Conscientious objection in the United States is supported primarily by the First Amendment. Certainly, it is argued, one cannot be forced to perform acts contrary to one's religious or ethical beliefs any more than one can be forced to, for example, pray to a god one does not believe in. Indeed, with respect to religious freedom, the Supreme Court has been particularly sensitive, applying a "strict scrutiny" test to any failure by the government to accommodate religious beliefs and requiring states to show a "compelling interest" for such failures of accommodation [23].

Outside of the United States, a right of conscientious objection is supported by a number of other countries and international organizations. Article 9 of the European Convention on Human Rights provides an explicit right to freedom of thought, conscience, and religion [24]. Though not absolute, Article 9 does provide support for European physicians to conscientiously object to participation in certain care [24]. The British Medical Association supports a conditional right to conscientious objection, and by statute, British physicians may conscientiously object to participate in abortion and fertility treatments [25].

Current Issues Involving Conscientious Objection in Medicine

Abortion

Perhaps more than any other issue, abortion has sharply divided physicians' views on conscientious objection. At one end of the spectrum, Dr. Julian Savulescu, a bioethicist at Oxford, quoted Shakespeare to say that "[c]onscience is but a word cowards use, devised at first to keep the strong in awe." He went on to say that "[i]f people are not prepared to offer legally permitted, efficient, and beneficial care to a patient because it conflicts with their values, they should not be doctors" [26]. Dr. Savulescu has brought up a number of concerns regarding conscientious objection by physicians. He notes that conscientious objection in medicine may create barriers and inequality in patient care. For example, if obstetricians refuse to perform abortions, or pediatricians refuse to administer rubella vaccines because the vaccine is developed from aborted fetal cells, then these patients are forced to "shop around" for another doctor who is willing to perform these services. This may create a delay in access to care and be burdensome to the patient. He concludes, therefore, that physicians should set aside their moral objections in deference to the wishes of their patients [26]. Furthermore, since the Supreme Court has found a constitutional right to abortion in the United States, Savulescu's analysis would suggest that American physicians are ethically obligated to participate in abortions when called upon or leave the profession.

However, as noted earlier in our discussion of the philosophical basis of conscientious objection, the Constitution also protects the rights of citizens, including doctors, to be accommodated in their religious beliefs and in their freedom to associate (or not associate) with other citizens. To some extent, the same principles of American freedom that the Supreme Court relied upon to support a right to abortion also lend support to a physician's right to conscientious objection.

In 1973, a single pregnant woman challenged the constitutionality of the Texas abortion laws in a class action suit, *Roe v. Wade*. At that time, it was illegal for women to obtain or even attempt to obtain abortions in Texas, except under circumstances where continuation of the pregnancy would jeopardize the mother's life. Roe eventually won the lawsuit as the district court ruled the Texas abortion laws to be vague and to have abridged her rights under the 9th and 14th amendments [13]. In its reasoning, the court reviewed the protection offered by the Constitution for citizens against governmental intrusion into their beliefs and expressions regarding certain "fundamental" areas including: marriage, procreation, contraception, family relationships, child rearing and education. This right to privacy, nowhere specifically mentioned in the Constitution but implied by the "penumbra" of the Bill of Rights, was found by the Court to mean that a person has the right to follow their conscience in these intensely personal areas of life [13, 27, 28].

The reasoning of the Supreme Court in *Roe* was the culmination of academic theory and legal precedent beginning with a law review article written in 1890 by then lawyer and later to be Supreme Court Justice Louis Brandeis entitled, "The Right to Privacy." In "The Right to Privacy" Louis Brandeis advocated for the "right to be let alone" [27]. This concept was developed further in a series of court decisions to encompass the liberty of personal autonomy, belief, and privacy protected by the 1st, 4th, 5th, 9th, and 14th amendments. In Roe's case, this penumbra of rights was deemed broad enough to protect her "decision whether or not to terminate her pregnancy" based upon her consideration, in consultation with her physician, of the many medical, psychological, social, and other factors involved [13, 27]. Thus, the *Roe* court not only honored her decision but also her right to make her decision based on her own ethical principles and practical reasons.

Certainly, physicians, like other citizens, are entitled to their own sphere of privacy just as the Court found applicable to *Roe*. The question, then, is whether that sphere of privacy extends to physicians' decisions about whether to provide certain services to their patients. Savulescu makes the argument that it does not and that physicians, in effect, should leave their personal beliefs at home [26]. However, just as a law criminalizing abortion represents a heavy interference by government into an area of fundamental belief, a prohibition on conscientious objection to abortion would represent a heavy interference by government upon beliefs that carry what the British Medical Association calls great "moral seriousness" [25]. Moreover, while those considering medicine as a career could conscientiously object by not becoming physicians or by choosing specialties where they would not be asked to participate in abortion, most of the same benefit to the patient could be achieved through simple referral to another provider. Concerns about the need to "shop around" for physicians willing to provide abortion services seem anachronistic in modern America where diversity of opinion is prevalent and transportation is relatively cheap. Moreover, in a country that provides for conscientious objection to armed conflict even in an all-volunteer army (on the rationale that a soldier might have a change of beliefs while in service) [1], the notion that those entering medicine should be required to "fish or cut bait" at an early stage of their careers without any tolerance for change in beliefs is draconian and unrealistic.

Prisoners

On December 9, 1946, an "American military tribunal opened criminal proceedings against 23 leading German physicians" [29]. Although formally titled *United States of America v. Karl Brandt, et al.*, the trial became known as the "Doctor's Trial." The doctors were all involved in planning or participating in the "Euthanasia" program in Nazi Germany. In this program, those deemed "unworthy of life" including the mentally retarded, institutionalized mentally ill, and physically impaired were killed. In addition, some of the physicians conducted medical experiments on concentration camp prisoners without the prisoners' consent. The criminal allegations against them included murder and torture [29].

At Guantanamo Bay, the United States has and continues to imprison people designated as "enemy combatants" [30]. It is estimated that at least 780 people have been imprisoned at Guantanamo since 2002 [30]. As of June 2014, 7 prisoners had been convicted of crimes or accepted guilty pleas, approximately 600 had been released without charges, and 149 remained in custody, of whom only 6 had charges of any kind pending [31]. According to the President of the United States, in the course of some Central Intelligence Agency interrogations, "we tortured some folks" [32]. Some of the Guantanamo Bay prisoners were subject to "enhanced interrogations" in which they were exposed to "some beatings", restrained for extended periods in "forced positions", and exposed to "temperature extremes" [33]. Furthermore, some prisoners were subjected to "*waterboarding*", a technique designed to simulate drowning [34]. By report, the basic method of interrogation used was devised by psychologists under contract to the United States government [35]. Also by report, a number of physicians were involved in various aspects of the prisoners' treatment including providing interrogators the medical information of the prisoners which was used to help "break" the prisoner [36]. A number of prisoners participated in hunger strikes, which were broken by placing the prisoners in restraint chairs and force-feeding them via nasogastric tubes [37]. Both the use of confidential medical information to assist interrogators and force-feeding have been criticized as violating medical ethics [36, 37].

One can then imagine the position of military physicians both in Nazi Germany and in Guantanamo Bay. Did these physicians participate in these acts of their own free will, or were they pressured or even forced, into doing so? At what point should the physicians at Guantanamo Bay have conscientiously objected, if at all? Furthermore, while conscientious objection is often viewed as a right held by physicians, in a setting like Guantanamo Bay, where physicians were involved to some extent in activities both harmful to patients and possibly illegal, was conscientious objection in fact an obligation? If so, should that obligation be enforced? Is it the case, for example, that specialty boards, state medical boards, and medical societies have an obligation to investigate questionable actions relating to prisoners by their members? Should they discipline members for failing to conscientiously object to unethical activities?

Lethal Injection

In February 2006, a federal judge in California issued an order requiring an anesthesiologist to be present during all scheduled lethal injections to ensure that the prisoners are adequately anesthetized prior to receiving the lethal injection [38]. The president of the American Society of Anesthesiologists (ASA), Dr. Guidry, reacted and quoted from the American Medical Association's (AMA) Code of Ethics that "an individual's opinion on capital punishment is the personal moral decision of the individual. A physician, as a member of a profession dedicated to preserving life when there is hope of doing so, should not be a participant in a legally authorized execution" [38]. What constitutes involvement in lethal injection is defined as "selecting injection sites; starting intravenous lines as a port for lethal injection device; prescribing, preparing, administering, or supervising injection drugs or their dose or type; testing, or maintaining lethal injection devices; and consulting with or supervising lethal injection personnel" [38]. Dr. Guidry noted that while "ASA does not have a detailed position on anesthesiologist participation in lethal injection," it does support the AMA's "position regarding physician nonparticipation in execution" [38]. Dr. Guidry advised the members to "be well informed on the subject and steer clear" [38]. While the surgical literature is more sparse regarding lethal injection, there are examples of surgeons having participated in the past (for instance, Dr. Alan Doerhoff, a surgeon, supervised 54 executions in Missouri) [39].

While the ethical responsibilities of physicians in regard to lethal injection seem clear at first blush (to "steer clear"), on closer analysis the question is more difficult and good-faith arguments have been advanced supporting participation by anesthesiologists. Savulescu offers a three-part test for what procedures physicians should be prepared to perform: "*(1) legally permitted, (2) efficient, and (3) beneficial care*" [26]. Applying his test demonstrates the challenges presented to physicians by the concept of conscientious objection. By definition, lethal injection is *legal* in much of the United States. Is it *efficient*? Arguments can be advanced on either side. On the one hand, keeping someone prisoner for life is exceedingly expensive, so lethal injection may be less expensive to society. On the other hand, the legal wrangling associated with lethal injection often makes it equally or more expensive than incarceration. It is possible, however, that participation by anesthesiologists would lower the costs of lethal injection by removing many of the legal challenges based on claims of cruelty. Would participation in lethal injection be "*beneficial*"? The obvious answer is no, because participation in the killing of a person can never be beneficial to that person. But what if they are going to die anyway and the anesthesiologist's participation makes their death less painful? Often, physicians treat patients who are dying not to prolong their life, but to make their inevitable death less painful (e.g. hospice). Moreover, some states have made it clear that if they cannot successfully conduct lethal injection due to conscientious objection by physicians or inability to obtain the required drugs, then they will resort to arguably more barbaric methods (e.g., Utah has recently announced a return to the firing squad) [40]. In addition, what if the request for participation of the anesthesiologist comes from the condemned? Does that make it beneficial to participate? As often happens, so-called obvious issues can become much more difficult to resolve upon closer scrutiny. In the end, individual physicians will have to decide for themselves whether to participate in lethal injection and if so, under what conditions.

Physician-Assisted Suicide

Physician-assisted suicide (PAS) is becoming increasingly common. The phrase, physician-assisted suicide, is often used interchangeably with euthanasia, but the two are very different concepts. In the case of euthanasia, the physician is the one that administers the lethal injection to end the patient's life. In PAS, the physician usually prescribes a lethal drug, and the patient uses the drug to end his or her own life [41]. Euthanasia is legal in Belgium, the Netherlands, and Luxembourg. PAS is legal in the Netherlands, Luxembourg, Switzerland, and a few states in the United States [42]. In the United States, Oregon led the way, followed by Washington, Vermont, and New Mexico. The Montana Supreme Court, in the *Baxter v. Montana* case, ruled "although the Constitution did not guarantee a right to PAS, there was nothing in the Montana Supreme Court precedent or Montana statutes indicating PAS is against public policies" [41, 43]. In Oregon, the Oregon Death with Dignity Act states that "in order for a patient to participate, the patient must be 18 years or older, a resident of Oregon, capable of making and communicating healthcare decisions, and diagnosed with a terminal illness that will lead to death within 6 months" [44]. In Washington and Vermont, the restrictions are similar, except that the patient has to be seen by two physicians and both physicians have to agree upon the patient's prognosis [45, 46]. In New Mexico, during the *Morris v. New Mexico* case, a second Judicial Court Judge, Nan Nash, ruled "This court cannot envision a right more fundamental, more private or more integral to the liberty, safety and happiness of a New Mexican than the right of a competent, terminally ill patient to choose aid in dying" [47].

So, would you participate in physician-assisted suicide if it is legal in your jurisdiction and your terminally ill cancer patient asks you to help end his misery? If you are not comfortable doing so and cannot find someone else to take your place, what should you do? If you are willing to prescribe a lethal medication to a dying patient, is that different than participating in lethal injection at the request of the condemned prisoner?

Practical Issues Surrounding the Invocation of Conscientious Objection

Conscientious objection is an issue worthy of consideration by every physician because invoking conscientious objection carries with it professional responsibilities as well as social, professional, and legal risk. In general, physicians will be better positioned to fulfill their professional responsibilities and minimize the risks if they prepare in advance [19].

Invocation of conscientious objection does not absolve physicians of responsibilities to their patient nor does it necessarily end the physician-patient relationship. At a minimum, physicians continue to have a responsibility not to abandon or compromise the care of their patients. Failure to fulfill professional responsibilities carries considerable risk. For example, a fertility clinic that would not inseminate a lesbian patient was sued for discrimination, and a religious hospital was found liable for failing to inform a rape victim about the availability of emergency contraception [48, 49]. In addition to civil liability, a physician who compromises the care of a patient on grounds of conscience may face investigation or discipline by the state board, loss of privileges, or dismissal from their medical practice. Socially, conscientious objection may expose a physician's ethical and religious beliefs to colleagues and associates who find such beliefs either unsophisticated or repugnant.

For all physicians, it is wise to consider in advance situations that might force them to invoke conscientious objection and plan how to fulfill their professional responsibilities while remaining true to their beliefs. To begin with, the physician should consult their institution's policy (if any) on conscientious objection. Most institutions have policies that reflect both the state and federal law on the subject as well as the culture of the institution. At our institution, for example, a physician invoking conscientious objection is required to "refer the patient to other persons who will either provide the intervention or facilitate appropriate referral," and the policy states that "[t]his process must not create undue delay, inconvenience, or impediment to receiving requested services for the patient" [50]. In addition to the hospital policy, the physician should review the relevant state and federal laws as it pertains to their anticipated area of objection.

Once having completed the above research, the physician should attempt to avoid situations that would require conscientious objection. In general, this will require the physician to reveal personal ethical beliefs at least to a limited degree. And while it may be uncomfortable to make even a limited revelation for fear of being ostracized, a limited revelation in advance generally generates less exposure than that created by actual invocation of conscientious objection. The precise method of avoiding patients and cases that may lead to conscientious objection will obviously vary by practice, locale, and situation. However, with some planning, it can usually be accomplished. In the anesthesia department at our institution, for example, we maintain lists of providers who do not wish to be involved in abortion or artificial insemination. Perhaps 10% of our group falls on one or the other list. The lists are available to schedulers (but are not made public) who try not to assign objectionable cases. In the rare instance that a provider is assigned to a case they object to, a simple case swap is carried out before either provider comes into contact with the patient. In this way, the rights of both the patient and the provider are honored without embarrassment.

In most circumstances, referral of a patient to another provider who is willing to provide the requested care will be adequate to fulfill professional responsibilities. However, in situations in which another provider is not available either due to time (i.e. emergency) or skill set, the treating physician will have to be prepared to choose between their professional responsibilities to their patient and their conscience. If possible, involvement of the patient advocate and ethics consult team is advisable, but neither is likely to protect a physician from legal liability or board investigation in the event that a patient's care is compromised.

References

1. Conscientious objection. In: Wikipedia. 2015. http://en.wikipedia.org/wiki/Conscientious_objector (2015). Accessed 7 Jan 2015.
2. Feder J. The history and effect of abortion conscience clause laws. 2015. http://www.law.umaryland.edu/marshall/crsreports/crsdocuments/RS2142801142005.pdf. Accessed 26 Feb 2015.
3. Conscientious objectors. Department of defense instructions. 2007. http://www.dtic.mil/whs/directives/corres/pdf/130006p.pdf (2015). Accessed 27 Mar 2015.
4. Ott M. The Catholic Encyclopedia, vol. 10. New York: Robert Appleton Company; 2013.
5. Yoder AM. Conscientious objection in America. 2007. http://www.swarthmore.edu/library/peace/conscientiousobjection/co%20website/pages/HistoryNew.htm. Accessed 5 Jan 2015.
6. Desmond Doss. In: Wikipedia. 2015. http://en.wikipedia.org/wiki/Desmond_Doss (2015). Accessed 6 Mar 2015.
7. National center for education statistics. 2013. https://nces.ed.gov/programs/statereform/tab5_1.asp. Accessed 30 Apr 2015.
8. Vaccines and immunization. Center for disease control and prevention. 2015. http://www.cdc.gov/vaccines/imz-managers/laws/state-reqs.html (2015). Accessed 24 Feb 2015.
9. Vaccine exemptions. Institute for vaccine safety. 2014. http://www.vaccinesafety.edu/cc-exem.htm (2014). Accessed 11 Feb 2015.
10. Szabo L. California measles outbreak linked to Disneyland. USA Today. 8 Jan 2015. http://www.usatoday.com/story/news/nation/2015/01/07/measles-outbreak-disneyland/21402755. Accessed 6 Feb 2015.
11. Benson L. Measles outbreak sparks call to limit vaccination exemptions. MPR News. 9 Feb 2015. http://www.mprnews.org/story/2015/02/08/measles-outbreak-sparks-call-to-limit-vaccination-exemptions. Accessed 10 Jun 2015.
12. Hippocratic Oath. In: Wikipedia. 2015. http://en.wikipedia.org/wiki/Hippocratic_Oath. Accessed 9 Apr 2015.
13. Roe v. Wade. 401 U.S. 113. 1973.
14. Bradley I. Conscientious objection in medicine: a moral dilemma. Clinical Correlations. 2009. http://www.clinicalcorrelations.org/?p1454. Accessed 15 Jan 2015.
15. Department of Health and Human Services. Ensuring that Department of Health and Human Services funds do not support coercive or discriminatory policies or practices in violation of federal law. Fed Regist. 2008;73(245):78071–101.
16. 42 USC Sec. 300a-7.
17. 42 USC Sec. 2000E[2].
18. Patient protection and affordable care act, 42 U.S.C. § 18001. 2010.
19. Abbey KR, Stepaniak MC. Refusal to do a case on moral or ethical grounds: practical navigation through very troubled waters. In: Marcucci C, Cohen NA, Metro DG, Kirsch JR, editors. Avoiding Common Anesthesia Errors. Philadelphia: Lippincott Williams & Wilkins; 2006. p. 804–8.
20. Michigan conscientious objector policy act. HB-5006. 2004. http://www.legislature.mi.gov/documents/2003-2004/billengrossed/house/htm/2003-HEBH-5006.htm. Accessed on 17 Feb 2015.
21. Miss. Code Ann. Sec. 41-41-215.
22. United States Constitution, Amendment I.

23. Sherbert v. Verner. 374 U.S. 398. 1963.
24. United Nation of Human Rights. Conscientious objection to military service. United nations. 2012. http://www.ohchr.org/Documents/Publications/ConscientiousObjection_en.pdf. Accessed 6 Feb 2015.
25. British Medical Association. Practical support at work, ethics, expressions of doctor's beliefs. 2015. http://bma.org.uk/practical-support-at-work/ethics/expressions-of-doctors-beliefs. Accessed 10 Apr 2015.
26. Savulescu J. Conscientious objection in medicine. Br Med J. 2006;332:294–7.
27. Warren S, Brandeis L. The right to privacy. Harvard LR. 1890;4(5):193.
28. Griswold v. Connecticut. 381 U.S. 479. 1965.
29. United States Holocaust Memorial Museum: The doctors trial: the medical case of the subsequent Nuremberg Proceedings. 2015. http://www.ushmm.org/information/exhibitions/online-features/special-focus/doctors-trial. Accessed 10 Feb 2015.
30. Scheinkman A, et al. The Guantanamo docket. The New York Times. 2015. http://projects.nytimes.com/guantanamo/about (2015). Accessed 13 May 2015.
31. Human Rights Watch. Facts and figures: military commissions v. federal courts. 2015. http://www.hrw.org/features/guantanamo-facts-figures. Accessed 13 May 2015.
32. Hulse C, Mazzetti M. Obama expresses confidence in CIA director. The New York Times. 1 Aug 2014. http://www.nytimes.com/2014/08/02/us/obama-expresses-confidence-in-cia-director-brennan.html?_r=0. Accessed 25 Feb 2015.
33. Lewis NA. Red Cross finds detainee abuse in Guantanamo. The New York Times. 30 Nov 2004. http://www.nytimes.com/2004/11/30/politics/30gitmo.html?pagewanted=all. Accessed 13 May 2015.
34. Lamothe D. Lawyers for 9/11 suspects say interrogation report could help their cases. Washington Post 10 Dec 2014. http://www.washingtonpost.com/news/checkpoint/wp/2014/12/10/lawyers-for-911-suspects-say-cia-interrogation-report-could-help-their-cases. Accessed 16 Feb 2015.
35. ReisnerS.APAfailstosanctionpsychologistinGuantanamotorturecase.Counterpunch.11Feb2014.http://www.counterpunch.org/2014/02/11/apa-fails-to-sanction-psychologist-in-guantanamo-torture-case/.
36. Lewis NA. Interrogators cite doctors' aid at Guantanamo Prison Camp. The New York Times. 24 Jun 2005. http://www.nytimes.com/2005/06/24/politics/24gitmo.html?. Accessed 13 May 2015.
37. Gross M. Force feeding, autonomy, and the public interest. N Engl J Med. 2013;369:103–5.
38. Guidry O. Dr. Orin Guidry on medical ethics and lethal injection. Yes Magazine. 13 Nov 2006. http://www.yesmagazine.org/issues/go-local/1561. Accessed 13 May 2015.
39. Mencimer S. State executions: untrained, incompetent, and "complete idiots". Mother Jones. 7 May 2014. http://www.motherjones.com/politics/2014/05/death-penalty-lethal-injections-untrained-doctors. Accessed 13 May 13 2015.
40. NPR staff. Utah brings back firing squad executions. NPR News. 5 Apr 2015. http://www.npr.org/2015/04/05/397672199/utah-brings-back-firing-squad-executions-witnesses-recall-the-last-one. Accessed 10 Apr 2015.
41. Physician assisted suicide. In: Wikipedia. 2015. http://en.wikipedia.org/wiki/Assisted_suicide. Accessed 16 Feb 2015.
42. Legality of euthanasia. In: Wikipedia. http://en.wikipedia.org/wiki/Legality_of_euthanasia (2015). Accessed 25 May 2015.
43. Baxter v. State. 354 Mont. 234. 2009.
44. The Oregon Death with Dignity Act. ORS 127.800-995. 1994.
45. Patient Choice and Control at End of Life Act. 18 V.S.A. 113. 2013.
46. The Washington Death with Dignity Act. RCW 70.245. 2008.
47. Morris v. New Mexico. 132 S.Ct. 1102. 2012.
48. Stein R. Seeking care and refused. The Washington Post. 16 Jul 2006. http://www.washingtonpost.com/wp-dyn/content/article/2006/07/15/AR2006071500787.html. Accessed 3 Apr 2015.
49. Brownfield v. Daniel Freeman Marina Hospital. 256 Cal. 240. 1989.
50. Personnel & Human Resources, Conscientious Objection Adm. 07.05, Chapter 7. In: Oregon Health and Sciences University Health Care System Administrative Policy Manual. 20 Aug. 2006.

Chapter 9
Ethical Implications of Drug Shortages

Jeffrey S. Jacobs

Abstract Drug shortages have become a ubiquitous occurrence at most perioperative facilities. Dealing with these shortages involves not just administrative challenges, but opens a Pandora's Box of ethical quandaries. This chapter reviews: the causes of medication shortages from manufacturing to distribution, the ethical discussions that arise when dealing with medication shortages from varying perspectives, and the challenges of finding definitive solutions.

Keywords Medication • Drug • Shortages • Group Purchasing Organizations • Drug Manufacturer • Food and Drug Administration • Hoarding

Case Presentation

As a staff anesthesiologist at a community hospital, you have noticed that the supply of propofol has dwindled. The hospital pharmacist informs you that the hospital is unable to obtain any more of this medication from the usual supplier for the foreseeable future. Many questions arise:

1. If there is no more supply of this medication to the hospital, do we need to inform patients of the increased risk of postoperative nausea and vomiting as we switch to etomidate or methohexital for induction?
2. Can we divide some of the 50 cc bottles of propofol into 2 or 3 induction doses for different patients to make the supply last longer?
3. Should we order propofol from some of the other suppliers that are outside of the usual manufacturing and distribution chain?
4. If we are able to get one last shipment of propofol, should we try to order the remaining supply (clean out the supplier's remaining inventory)?
5. Is there something we should do on a larger scale regarding drug shortages, aside from just working with the hospital pharmacy?

J.S. Jacobs, MD
Department of Anesthesiology, Cleveland Clinic Florida, 2900 Cleveland Clinic Boulevard, Weston, FL 33331, USA
e-mail: jjgas@bellsouth.net

B.G. Jericho (ed.), *Ethical Issues in Anesthesiology and Surgery*,
DOI 10.1007/978-3-319-15949-2_9

Overview

Shortages of medications used in the perioperative period have become the new normal. Specifically, generic injectable drugs are the most common subset of this group. In a 2012 survey conducted by the American Society of Anesthesiologists (ASA), over 97% of respondents experienced at least one medication shortage in the past year [1] (Fig. 9.1). Despite being widespread, shortages are often unpredictable requiring physicians to make rapid pharmaceutical substitutions. While inconvenient for the physicians, it can be much worse for the patients. Complications of short-supplied drugs range from an increase in postoperative nausea and vomiting to death.

Prior to delving into the causes of and concerns with drug shortages, it is important to define the term. Surprisingly, the meaning changes depending upon who is defining the word "shortages". The Food and Drug Administration (FDA) states that a shortage is "a situation in which the total supply of all clinically interchangeable versions of an FDA-regulated drug is inadequate to meet the current or projected demand at the patient level" [2]. Alternatively, the American Society of Health-Systems Pharmacists (ASHP) defines a shortage as "a supply issue that affects how the pharmacy prepares or dispenses a drug product or influences patient care when prescribers must use an alternate agent" [3]. While these definitions are subtly different, shortages may be more widespread depending on who is asked. Also, crucial to this definition is legislation that allows compounding pharmacies to make medications that are on the shortage list. This could be a concern to public health due to less national oversight of these pharmacies with the potential for contamination and public health dangers [4].

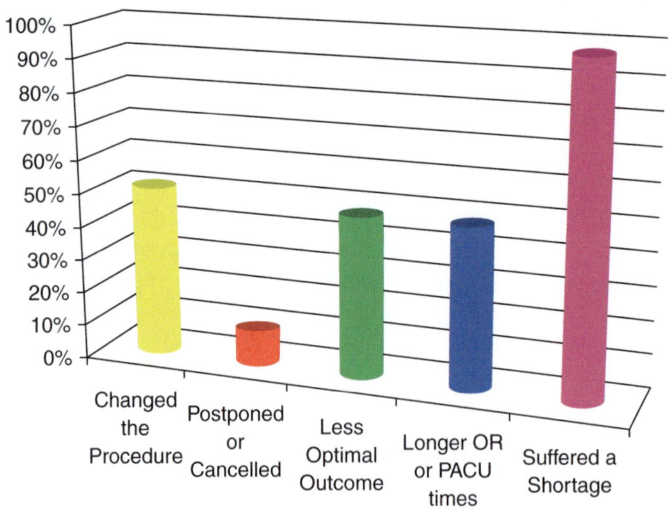

Fig. 9.1 Surveyed anesthesiologists affected by drug shortages

Manufacturing and Supplying Medications

To understand the causes of drug shortages, it is useful to explore the creation of a medication from the manufacturing and distribution points of view (Fig. 9.2). A pharmaceutical company needs to acquire raw products and then combine them to create the finished medication. Problems with the procurement of raw materials, such as civil unrest or a labor strike could be the initial hurdle. Despite the fact that 80% of the active ingredients used in pharmaceuticals come from outside of the United States, disruptions in delivery accounted for less than 10% of shortages from 2010 to 2011 [5]. Transportation of these materials to the factory could result in delays. Once all necessary materials are in the factory, reliable equipment is crucial. Machinery malfunction, loss of sterility, contamination with particulate matter, and other unacceptable outcomes can arise (Fig. 9.3). Once packaged, the medication is then transported to regional distribution centers across the United States. It is possible that due to inadequate planning or a sudden change in regional demand, one such center may be without the medication while other distribution centers have ample stock. These regional variances in supply could still result in national shortages. For example, when an anticipated shortage is announced, 89% of hospital purchasing agents buy excess inventory, which could increase the duration of a shortage [6]. From these regional distribution centers, the medications find their way into health care pharmacies for dispensation.

The story is also valuable from the procurement side. Clearly, a health care facility's pharmacy staff doesn't call multiple factories to obtain pricing and place orders for the thousands of products used. Rather, group purchasing organizations (GPOs) have been developed to handle this complex task. The GPOs then negotiate pricing and place orders with factories on behalf of their customers. What's important to understand is that health systems, since they are businesses, want to pay the lowest possible price for their products. While this sounds intuitive (nobody goes shopping and offers to pay higher prices), it has led to unintended consequences. Because there are few GPOs that handle the vast majority of health care systems, they have

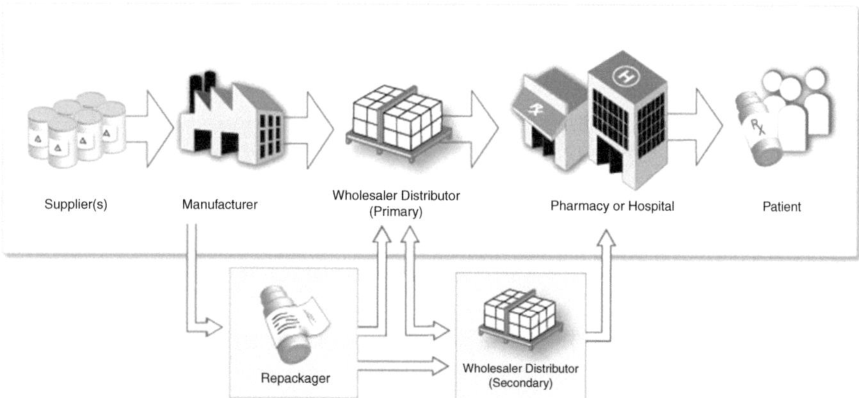

Fig. 9.2 Pharmaceutical supply chain. US Food and Drug Administration http://www.fda.gov/Drugs/DrugSafety/DrugShortages/ucm277626.htm

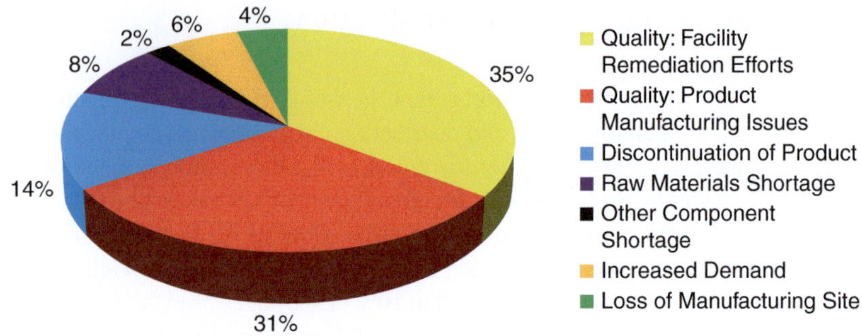

Fig. 9.3 Causes of drug of shortages

tremendous negotiating power with the manufacturers. In fact, they have so much power that the profit margins of most medications in short supply are razor thin. This has many effects: (1) with such small profit margins, there is no value for competing manufacturers to enter the market; (2) with GPOs controlling such large swaths of the market, it would be equally challenging and risky for a new manufacturer to enter the market without guaranteed contracts [7]; (3) when a machine breaks down for one of the low-profit generics, there is less incentive to repair the machinery; (4) because drug manufacturers make multiple products, if machinery breaks down for one of the more profitable medications, a manufacturer will often move this product to a generic line's equipment, when possible, to reap greater rewards; and (5) there is minimal incentive to provide more than the basic necessary maintenance of the equipment on the generic lines.

The other challenge is the practice of just-in-time inventory. Because the health care pharmacy and the regional distributors do not want cases of medications stored on site (lack of space and too much capital tied up), factories have followed suit. Therefore, medications are made and shipped rapidly. There is no "extra fat" built into the system. Thus, when a product manufacturing line goes down for whatever reason, existing stores of medications are used up at their normal rate, but there is no replacement forthcoming. All of the above issues lead to the major cause of drug shortages: lack of redundancy in the manufacturing supply chain [8]. Three manufacturers account for 70% of the sterile injectable market in the United States, and in some cases, one company is responsible for 90% or more of a drug [9]. For these critical medications, that's just not safe.

Ethical Discussion: Generalities

When evaluating the ethical implications of a situation or intervention, it is helpful to partition the discussion into the main silos of bioethics: autonomy, beneficence, nonmaleficence, and distributive justice. For the topic of drug shortages, this becomes quite useful before dissecting the more practical questions that should be addressed.

Autonomy, as it relates to drug shortages, arises with the situation of informed consent of the patient when using replacement medications. While the specific discussion of informed consent will be covered below, what is important to realize is that when scheduling procedures or operations, patients are forced to change their routines. Patients need to be granted a leave from their job, they need to arrange for child care, and they may need relatives or friends available to help them after the procedure. In many instances, this involves travel for both the patient and those friends and relatives. Therefore, the threshold for a patient to postpone a procedure is often much greater than it might be when simply weighing the science involved in the decision. As long as the patient understands the potentially increased side effects or recovery, the patient can choose a path that may seem unpleasant or unrealistic to the caregiver. This is why a complete discussion with the patient is ideal prior to making unilateral decisions.

Beneficence is the notion that the provider always wants to do the best thing for the patient. However, the "best" thing from the provider's perspective may not be the "best" thing from the patient's perspective, when other factors are taken into account, as described above. Furthermore, absolutism may not be the best path to follow, despite the inherent fact that "best" is an absolute. As an example, in appropriate patients, succinylcholine is the "best" muscle relaxant to perform a rapid sequence induction. Should the absence of this medication force the institution to close the emergency room doors and transfer all emergency operations to another facility? In this sense, beneficence needs to be balanced against competing interests. Beneficence from a single perspective may not be beneficent at all.

Nonmaleficence is the theory of non-harm, and this is the topic where different providers of care may have different perspectives as to what is fair, safe, and appropriate. What one caregiver considers dangerous, another may deem safe. This notion of not proceeding without the full armamentarium of medications needs to be balanced with the potential psychological or physiologic damage to the patient kept waiting for surgery. As a tangible example, if a patient scheduled for a surgery to resect contained colon cancer is postponed until "better" medications become available to the facility, the risk is taken that the cancer will progress to a worse stage. It cannot be argued that postoperative nausea and vomiting is "less bad" than newly metastatic colon cancer, and care must be taken to evaluate the entire scenario and all competing interests.

Distributive justice plays a clear role when the ideas of rationing or hoarding arise. Drug shortages necessarily mean that someone will be without medications, and great care must be ensured to minimize that this allocation is done as fairly as possible. This will be discussed more robustly below.

Ethical Challenges: Specifics

One of the key issues with drug shortages is to define exactly how front-line physicians are affected by shortages (Fig. 9.4). At least one professional society, the American Society of Anesthesiologists, has addressed this topic [10].

Knowledge	The use of less familiar medications
Economics	The pressure to continue with "business as usual"
Outcomes	Prolonged emergence from anesthesia, side-effects, or death
Ethics	Accounting for all of the above issues while balancing a patient-centric approach

Fig. 9.4 Challenges with drug shortages

Anesthesiologists are often faced with the challenge to use medications that are less familiar, have more side effects, may be less efficacious, and in some circumstances may result in less than optimal patient outcomes. One example is a case in which propofol was unavailable, so the hospital ordered multidose vials of methohexital. The operating room pharmacist dispensed an inappropriate dose to the anesthesiology department, and the anesthesiologist incorrectly diluted the medication giving the patient an eight-fold overdose leading to cardiac arrest and death [11]. In addition to these potential and real tragedies, these adaptations need to be done minimizing the production pressures involved with operating room throughput. To frame this from a different perspective, imagine if a vascular surgeon needed to perform a distal bypass, but successfully do so without bulldogs, without three of the most commonly used sutures, without the correct blades, and still complete the operation in the usual amount of time. You can bet that surgeon wouldn't remain silent about the deficiencies but complain to every person with ears. Because of the direct effect on the practice of anesthesia, anesthesiologists do have an ethical and professional responsibility to participate in the development of solutions to this societal problem.

Another quandary commonly faced is deciding when and if to postpone or cancel a case due to the lack of a crucial medication. No rational person would argue that an elective operation should be postponed if the facility was unable to provide supplemental oxygen. With the exception of oxygen, it's less clear what medications are "must haves." Part of a physician's duty is to protect patients by using sound medical judgment to decide appropriateness of care. There are reasonable substitutes for some medications that are in short supply, but some medications do not have a suitable alternative. It is up to each individual provider, working with the surgeon and accounting for the patient's planned procedure and health status to decide what is safe. Anesthesiologists and surgeons should consider postponing an elective procedure when the risks of proceeding outweigh the risks of using alternative medications to those in short supply or unavailable. There is no "magic list" of must-have drugs, and many factors must be taken into account.

The next important ethical issue regarding drug shortages is how much needs to be disclosed to the patient? Some medication shortages may have a definite and profound impact on the patient's experience. For example, the use of certain intravenous induction agents is associated with an increased risk of postoperative nausea and vomiting when compared with other agents. Some medications have a longer half-life, which might lead to longer than normal effects. On the other hand, some medications may be seamless substitutes for the usual drug. A specific example of a negative experience may include caring for a 30-year-old woman with a history of postoperative nausea and vomiting without any serotonin antagonists available. This can be compared with the situation when caring for a patient and metoprolol is available but labetalol is not available. These are clearly different circumstances for the patient. In general, if the anesthesiologist judges the risk of increased morbidity or mortality by using alternative medications to be negligible, then there is no need to discuss this issue when obtaining informed consent. However, if the anesthesiologist judges the added risk to be significant, then the discussion of alternative plans should be part of the informed consent process.

If a patient suffers a less than ideal outcome due to a drug shortage, there is a responsibility to report the event. Part of the solution to drug shortages comes from the ability to track bad outcomes and complications due to the lack of a medication or from the use of a substitute. If bad outcomes go unreported, there is a misperception that the shortages have no impact on patient safety. Examples include defective automobile parts or dangerous toys; if users kept silent, there would never be recalls. Where should these complications be reported? One place is to the Anesthesia Quality Institute (AQI), which is a Federally Designated Patient Safety Organization. This means anything reported to them is anonymous, confidential, and not discoverable based on Federal law (https://www.aqihq.org/airs/airsIntro.aspx). A second place is the FDA via drugshortages@fda.hhs.gov. In general, the collection of adverse events occurring as a result of drug shortages provides important information useful in the pursuit of a solution. Health care providers should report these events to the appropriate entities for this purpose. Furthermore, the patient has a right to know the cause of adverse events in order to mitigate further suffering, whenever possible.

Waste at the provider level plays an important role with drug shortages. The first thing every physician should evaluate is his or her normal pattern for medication usage. In the face of shortages, it may be reasonable to question whether all possible emergency drugs need to be drawn into syringes (as opposed to having them available in their original packages). It may be reasonable to use smaller vials of medications, when available, to minimize wastage. It is *never* reasonable, however, to create your own rules when it comes to dividing ampules or bottles of medications in order to share the drugs among multiple patients. There are strict guidelines for how this should be accomplished, and if the rules do not make sense, anesthesiologists should advocate for amending them. Of note, the ASA supports the CDC's position on single-dose vials and has adopted their position for safe injection practices, which can be found at www.asahq.org/For-Members/Advocacy/Washington-Alerts/CDC-Releases-Report-on-Infection-Transmission-from-Single-Dose-Vial-Use-for-Multiple-Patients.aspx. On-site pharmacies should be involved in the discussion and solution to maximize the medications that are in short supply. Pharmacists have the ability to safely divide single dose vials into multiple patients in accordance with the US Pharmacopeia General Chapter 797 Guidelines [12], and this can easily double the number of uses. Planning and creative thinking can prolong the limited supply an institution has. In summary, in the face of specific drug shortages, anesthesiologists should reassess customary practice patterns of drug usage to minimize drug wastage and safely maximize any limited supply. Physicians should also utilize available hospital resources including other health care professionals to help navigate specific shortages.

An unusual topic that should be addressed is the irony that physicians may have indirectly but inadvertently contributed to the current situation. This may be due to physicians' training and breadth of knowledge. For example, suppose drug A is the preferred medication to treat a specific problem, but drug A is no longer available. A provider with less experience or knowledge may not be able to prescribe a suitable alternative, and that inability could potentially bring patient care to a slowdown or standstill. Conversely, a better-trained physician may be comfortable using drug B or drug C to treat that same problem, and the loss of drug A would therefore go nearly unnoticed. The problem with this situation is twofold: (1) the loss of drug A may go unreported, and (2) eventually alternate drugs B and C may also become short-supplied leading to no alternatives. Therefore, by being so adaptable, further problems may occur, and when they do, it could be far worse. Therefore, flexibility and adaptability in patient care may obscure the reality of potential harm created by drug shortages and should not be a substitute for pursuing a permanent solution. Using alternative medications for those in short supply is a function of excellent skill, judgment, and training, but this should complement, as opposed to substitute for, reporting shortages and seeking solutions.

Fortuitously, in addition to front-line physicians, there are others within health care who are also concerned with solving medication shortages. Specifically, medical and medically-related societies have been leaders in identifying and ameliorating these issues. Of note, the American Society of Anesthesiologists, the American Society of Health-System Pharmacists, and the American Society of Clinical Oncologists have all played leadership roles in uniting the key stakeholders, asking questions, and providing solutions. Some of the ideas identified by these groups have made their way into practice. One example is the Food and Drug Administration now has a department dedicated to medication shortages with the goal of early identification, manufacturing remediation, and rapid approval of overseas supplies when appropriate. Another success of the FDA is the requirement that manufacturers must provide maximum notice when they plan to discontinue the creation of a drug that has been identified as critical. This gives the FDA time to identify other potential sources and maintain supply. The FDA has been proactive in the past few years since requiring early notification by manufacturers of impending disruptions. They have (1) contacted other manufacturers to assess willingness and ability to pick up the slack, (2) expedited inspections of review of submissions, (3) exercised temporary enforcement discretion for new sources, (4) worked with manufacturers to find root causes, and (5) reviewed risk mitigation strategies for remaining inventory. These actions have helped prevent new drug shortages at a rate of over 200/year from 2012 to 2014 [13].

Hospitals can be an additional source of help, since they do not simply have a patient-centered interest in remedying the situation; they have financial concerns as well. In fact, hospitals have shouldered an estimated $229.7 million annually from 2011 to 2013, and these are just direct costs. The purchase of therapeutic alternatives, purchases from off-contract distributors, and the cost of added labor dramatically increase this number [14]. In one study, labor costs were estimated to be $216 million annually, nearly doubling the initial estimate [15].

A topic that commonly arises when speaking of drug shortages is hoarding. Is it appropriate to order extra medications that are in short supply so a given facility has enough for the foreseeable future? While having plenty of medication x is important for one institution, if that medication is in short supply, then it follows that other facilities will have less, which could potentially inconvenience or harm their patients. Unfortunately, there is no clear demarcation between preparedness and hoarding. As a generalization, if one facility has a significant amount of extra medication stored away while a nearby facility has none, it is very likely unethical. Some might call it good business, but because this particular business involves people's health, it crosses a line. Confounding this statement, however, is that those two example facilities may use different GPOs for their supplies, which may result in differing availabilities. In summary, while stockpiling medications may be beneficial for a given institution, excessive accumulation and storage of drugs can result in shortages to other institutions and may be unethical. What is quite obvious is that if one facility is purchasing and storing short-supplied medications with the intent to resell at a profit, it is clearly unethical. Unfortunately, an online 2011 survey found that 56% of hospital purchasing agents had received "daily" solicitations from resellers of medications that were not part of the normal supply chain [5]. This is often referred to as the "gray market." In addition to the unethical nature of "scalping" or "price gauging" medications, there is the inability to ensure that proper handling of the drugs was maintained (pedigree). Additionally, the gray market can worsen the impact of drug shortages. There is one recommendation to have a 6-month supply on hand of the medications deemed critical [16]. For the office setting, this recommendation may be practical, but if all offices planned like this, it would likely precipitate a widespread crisis of many medications.

One final ethical topic is rationing. While rationing often arises when discussing limited resources, this is more commonly identified with ventilator use during mass casualties and organ transplantation. However, rationing has occurred with oncology medications and flu vaccinations. Whether perioperative medication rationing will ultimately fall to the department level remains to be seen, but in the off-chance that it does, it will be crucial to identify a policy that encompasses fairness (similar patients will be treated the same, regardless of special status), transparency, enforcement, relevancy, and the provision for an appeals process [17].

What should be crystal clear is that medication shortages are not solely a practice management challenge. There are wide-reaching ethical issues that need to be discussed when this topic arises.

Other Potential Concerns

While the current discussion centers around medications, based on the current business model and market supply chain, it would not be far-fetched to see shortages in other medical supplies in the coming years. Thinking about one's local facility, it is not unusual to have an important device or piece of disposable equipment on backorder. These may become more frequent as well without a reexamination of the system that currently serves health care institutions. The demand for low prices with buying representation by few corporations ultimately leads to less redundancy in supply. This lack of redundancy is the common thread behind medication shortages, and this may spill over into other venues of health care supply.

Solution

Regrettably, there is no quick fix or simple remedy for the problem with medication shortages due to the complex nature of the cause. Stepping back into basic economics, there has to be a motive for businesses to make a product, and that motive is typically profit. Because profit margins are so slim, there is no interest to entering the market. Therefore, solutions should probably be directed toward this imbalance. One idea posed by the FDA is the recognition that there is no incentive for quality production. If there were economic incentives for quality, it may encourage manufacturers to provide better maintenance and controls at the production level. Publicizing manufacturing quality data may also provide non-financial incentives for factories [13]. This may entail multiple fixes such as examining the relationship between GPOs, health care facilities, and manufacturers; delving into the manufacturing plants themselves; and perhaps broaching the idea that subsidies should be made to support the minimally profitable generics. These repairs are all financial in nature and assume that there will continue to be a steady supply of raw materials, which is not always the case.

There are many ethical issues that surround medication shortages. Some of them are at the patient level, but many are societal. Addressing these issues preemptively will allow more streamlined care and decision-making when urgent situations arise. These discussions need to take place, because based on the current way medications are supplied along with lobbying efforts of these entities and their (rightful) pursuit of profit, complete rectification of the problem is unlikely any time in the near future. The search for a solution must be attempted for the sake of the patients; not just for the current ones but also for future patients as well. However, until that occurs, ethical preparation is an imperative.

References

1. American Society of Anesthesiologists. Drug Shortage Survey. 2012. http://www.asahq.org/advocacy/fda-and-washington-alerts/washington-alerts/2012/04/2012-asa-drug-shortage-survey-results. Accessed on 13 Mar 2014.

2. US Department of Health and Human Services, Food and Drug Administration, A Review of FDA's Approach to Medical Product Shortages. Silver Spring: US Dept of Health and Human Services, Food and Drug Administration; 2011. p. 8. http://www.fda.gov/downloads/aboutFDA/reportsmanualsforms/reports/ucm277755.pdf. Accessed 18 Feb 2015.
3. Fox ER, Birt A, James KB, Kokko H, Salverson S, Soflin DL. ASHP guidelines on managing drug product shortages in hospitals and health systems. Am J Health-Syst Pharm. 2009;66(15):1399–406.
4. Barlas S. Manufacturers and hospitals spar over drug shortage reporting. PT. 2014;39(3):152, 215.
5. Wilson D. Deepening drug shortages. Health Aff. 2012;31(2):263–6.
6. American Hospital Association. Survey on drug shortages. Washington, DC: American Hospital Association; 2011. http://www.aha.org/content/11/drugshortagesurvey.pdf. Accessed on 13 Mar 2015.
7. Bedard M. Drug shortages: can we resolve the problem? Can J Anesth. 2013;60:523–7.
8. Woodcock J, Wosinska M. Economic and technical drivers of generic sterile injectable drug shortages. Clin Pharmacol Ther. 2013;93(170–6):174–5.
9. Golembiewski J. Drug shortages in the perioperative setting: causes, impact, and strategies. J Perianesth Nurs. 2012;27(4):286–92.
10. American Society of Anesthesiologists. Statement on the ethical consideration with drug shortages. ASA Committee on Ethics. 2013. http://www.asahq.org/~/media/sites/asahq/files/public/resources/standards-guidelines/statement-on-the-ethical-considerations-with-drug-shortages.pdf#search=%22drug%22
11. O'Donnell JT, Vogenberg FR. Drug shortages pose problems for P&T committees in accountable care organizations. PT. 2013;38(7):404–6.
12. Center for Disease Control. Protect patients against preventable harm from improper use of single-dose/single-use vials. 2012. http://www.cdc.gov/injectionsafety/cdcposition-singleusevial.html. Accessed 19 Feb 2015.
13. Food and Drug Administration. Strategic plan for preventing and mitigating drug shortages. Food and Drug Administration. 2013. http://www.fda.gov/downloads/drugs/drugsafety/drugshortages/ucm372566.pdf
14. Premier, Inc. Drug Shortages Continue to Pose Patient Safety Risks and Challenge Providers, According to Premier, Inc. Survey. 2014. https://www.premierinc.com/drug-shortages-continue-pose-patient-safety-risks-challenge-providers-according-premier-inc-survey/.
15. Kaakeh R, Sweet BV, Reilly C, Bush C, DeLoach S, Higgins B, Clark AM, Stevenson J. Impact of drug shortages on US health systems. Am J Health Sys Pharm. 2011;68(19):1811–9.
16. Weaver JM. Why are there so many drug shortages? Anesth Prog. 2010;57:89–90.
17. Rosoff PM, Patel KR, Scates A, et al. Coping with critical drug shortages: an ethical approach for allocating scarce resources in hospitals. Arch Intern Med. 2012;172(19):1494–9.

Chapter 10
Ethical Challenges in High-Risk Innovative Surgery

Shuddhadeb Ray, Michael O'Connor, and Peter Angelos

Abstract The fields of surgery and anesthesia have storied histories with advances in care fueled by innovation by creative individuals striving to improve the care of their patients. Ethical dilemmas arise when contemplating how to allow innovation to continue for the benefit of future patients while mitigating harm to current patients. In this chapter, we explore ethical issues in high-risk innovative surgery from the perspectives of the key stakeholders: the surgeon, the patient, the anesthesiologist, the medical device industry, and other members of the healthcare team.

Keywords Innovation • Informed Consent • Medical Devices • High-Risk Surgery • Surgical Ethics

Case Presentation

After taking courses and workshops to learn an innovative surgical technique, a surgeon spends some time working at an outside institution with the innovator of this new surgical technique that is claimed to improve clinical outcomes for patients. The surgeon believes it to be better than the conventional

S. Ray, MD, MPHS (✉)
Department of Surgery, Washington University School of Medicine, 660 South Euclid Avenue, Box 8109, Saint Louis, MO 63110, USA
e-mail: sray@wustl.edu

M. O'Connor, MD, FCCM
Department of Anesthesia and Critical Care, The University of Chicago, 5841 S. Maryland Avenue, MC 4028, Chicago, IL 60637, USA
e-mail: Moc5@dacc.uchicago.edu

P. Angelos, MD, PhD, FACS
Department of Surgery, MacLean Center for Clinical Medical Ethics, The University of Chicago Medicine, Chicago, IL, USA
e-mail: pangelos@surgery.bsd.uchicago.edu

B.G. Jericho (ed.), *Ethical Issues in Anesthesiology and Surgery*,
DOI 10.1007/978-3-319-15949-2_10

technique although the risks are possibly slightly higher. The new procedure requires the anesthesiologist to insert a central line and infuse a new medication that may have severe complications. In addition, potential complications for the procedure require both ICU management and emergency intervention by interventional radiology. When the surgeon returns to his institution, he sees that the institution has advertised that this new surgical technique is now available and will be performed by him. One week later, he sees a patient in his clinic. The patient is requesting that the surgeon perform the innovative surgical technique to address the patient's problem. The patient asks the following: What are the risks and benefits of the procedure compared to the traditional technique? What is your experience with this technique? How many patients have you operated on using this innovative technique? While the surgeon looks forward to performing the innovative technique he just learned, what should he tell the patient? Additionally, how important is it for the surgeon to involve the anesthesiologist and other healthcare team members in the early discussions with the patient of this potentially risky and innovative approach?

Introduction

The fields of surgery and anesthesia have storied histories with advances in care fueled by innovation by creative individuals striving to take better care of their patients. Advances in surgical technique have led to surgeries considered commonplace today that would have been deemed impossible in the past. For instance, in the nineteenth and early twentieth century, it was considered taboo to even consider operating on the heart, and those that dared to do so were often met with disapproval, and often justifiably so. Of 10 reported cases of surgery attempted for mitral stenosis between 1923 and 1928, eight patients died. Of the two surviving patients, only one benefitted from the surgery [1]. Over two decades later, in 1948, Charles Bailey, having experimented with mitral valve operations on dogs, attempted mitral valve surgery on patients at different hospitals in Philadelphia [2]. His first success came on his fifth patient, after four mortalities, for which he received the nickname the "butcher of Hahnemann Hospital." Bailey's first success came while operating on a patient in the afternoon following the death of his fourth patient in the morning at a different hospital. Recounting those events, Bailey noted, "We…promptly drove to Episcopal Hospital to commence the other operation before the morning's news could be effective in possibly having the Episcopal Hospital administration forbid us from doing the procedure" [3]. This is one of many stories of surgical innovation that provokes numerous ethical questions.

Thousands of patients annually now benefit from mitral valve surgery pioneered in part by surgeons like Dr. Bailey. Regardless, this achievement does not justify the loss of life of the patients Dr. Bailey treated before his surgical technique was successful. While informed consent, as we currently use the term, was not commonplace at that time, it would be interesting to know what information was shared with the patients and their families prior to their surgery. Were these procedures approved by the hospitals? Were the procedures and their implications discussed with the other physicians and healthcare providers involved in the care of these patients? Many of these issues have been addressed to different degrees since the time of Dr. Bailey's first operations for mitral valve stenosis.

In the United States, patients must now give informed consent before undergoing any procedure, for instance. Yet, other questions remain largely unanswered with ongoing ethical challenges. The care of patients undergoing innovative surgical procedures requires more than the skills of the surgeon alone. Anesthesiologists must provide safe anesthesia for the surgical procedure and care for the patient in the postoperative setting, including sometimes in an intensive care setting. Nurses and other healthcare providers also care for the patient throughout this process. There are no set rules or any guidance on how a surgeon might engage these other crucial members of the surgical (and medical) team in carrying out an innovative surgical procedure. Furthermore, unlike pharmaceutical drugs or medical devices, which are regulated by the Food and Drug Administration, the introduction of new surgical techniques requires no formal oversight. Surgeons must self-regulate the introduction of new surgical techniques. In some instances, surgeons may develop a new procedure as part of a protocol overseen by an Institutional Review Board, but not always [4]. The ethical dilemma lies in determining how to allow surgical innovation to continue for the benefit of future patients while mitigating harm to patients and engaging all parties involved in the process of surgical innovation. This complex undertaking may be approached by considering ethical issues from the perspectives of the key stakeholders in the process of surgical innovation: the surgeon, the patient and the public, the anesthesiologist, the medical device industry, and other members of the healthcare team.

The Surgeon

To a great extent, the history of surgery is a story of iterative improvement of established procedures punctuated by the introduction of radical departures from past techniques. A surgeon has significant creative leeway in the operating room in developing innovative procedures. In fact, although surgical techniques are described in textbooks and journal articles, there is no single mandatory method of completing any particular surgery. Moreover, unlike innovation in the development of new pharmaceuticals, there is no governing body that regulates the creation of new surgical techniques [5]. Surgeons have the right, and perhaps even a duty, to alter surgical techniques or develop new surgical techniques for the benefit of their patients. However, in developing innovations, surgeons face ethical challenges as new techniques will create new complications and alter the incidence of known complications. Hence, how can a surgeon disclose the risks of an operation when they are unknown? Without external oversight, the patient must depend on the surgeon's self-regulation to assess the effectiveness of the technique and to protect patients from harm. Other ethical concerns of innovative surgical procedures include the appropriateness of healthcare resource utilization to implement the new surgical technique, and also the identification and disclosure of potential conflicts of interest that may arise as surgeons are often the creators and promoters of new surgical techniques.

Any new technique in surgery has the potential to either help or harm a patient. One of the key ethical tenets of patient care is "nonmaleficence", which is based on the maxim Primum non nocere: "Above all [or first] do no harm" [6]. New techniques developed by surgeons have the potential to cause significant patient harm as illustrated by a number of historical cases. Consider, for example, the idea of ligation of the internal mammary artery for the treatment of angina. Angina was thought to be caused by decreased blood flow to the coronary arteries that perfuse the heart muscle itself. The new innovative approach to treating this problem was based on the idea that ligation of the internal mammary artery could potentially increase perfusion to the coronary artery. Surgeons, many at large academic centers, started offering this surgery to large numbers of patients. Thousands of patients underwent this invasive surgical procedure and developed complications from the surgery, including infection and postoperative arrhythmias. Unfortunately, these risks were not associated with any benefit. Cobb and colleagues ultimately showed that internal mammary artery ligation was not an effective way to treat angina [7].

Evaluating risk and disclosing it to the patient in reference to an innovative surgical procedure creates a complex informed consent process. The paradox of informed consent in innovative surgery lies in the fact that many risks of a new surgical technique cannot be known at the outset. Risks of new procedures can only be estimated. Such risks are much more difficult to disclose to the patient. Furthermore, even when a procedure is well documented in the literature, a surgeon may not know what the exact risks of the procedure will be in his or her hands. The period of time during which a surgeon adopts a new surgical technique is sometimes referred to as the "learning curve." During this variable time period, as multiple studies have shown, complication rates generally improve as surgeons gain more experience with the procedure [8, 9]. It is the surgeon's duty, then, to disclose his or her own experience to patients undergoing a new procedure and technique. It is equally important that the surgeon discloses to the patient the lack of long-term outcome data for an innovative procedure. This lack of outcome data makes the balancing of risks and benefits particularly challenging to the patient. Only by disclosing what is known along with the uncertainties of the new procedure can the surgeon respect the autonomy of the patient to the fullest extent possible in these challenging situations.

Another ethical implication of innovative surgical procedures includes the disclosure of potential conflicts of interest. There is a natural conflict of interest that arises when surgeons develop new innovative surgical techniques. As the innovator, the surgeon may have an emotional investment as well as a significant investment of time in the success of the procedure. The surgeon might also benefit from the procedure economically and by gaining prestige. For these reasons, the surgeon may also feel pressure from his or her institution to have the procedure succeed. This conflict of interest can potentially bias results tracked for the procedure by the surgeon or the hospital. These concerns suggest the importance of an objective third party oversight of innovative procedures, which can be obtained by an institutional review board (IRB). The IRB must approve the protocol and the consent form, and oversee any adverse events associated with a research protocol. Although IRB oversight can be helpful in protecting research subjects and in reducing bias in evaluating an innovative procedure, this type of oversight is only present when innovative techniques are evaluated in formal research protocols. Frequently, the assessment of the new innovation remains the responsibility of the surgeon.

Innovation takes many forms. Sometimes it involves coming up with a truly novel procedure, whereas other times it involves doing a procedure that is novel to a hospital or region. In the latter situation, it is particularly important that surgeons keep track of patient outcomes and compare them with outcomes in areas where there is an established history of completing the procedure to assure there are no significant increases in the rate of complications. It is important to note that obtaining and evaluating outcome data in routine clinical practice is far more difficult than generally appreciated. For example, at the Bristol Royal Infirmary, between 1988 and 1995, pediatric cardiac surgeons continued to perform heart surgery on children despite a mortality rate of 55%, which was much higher than the national average at that time [10]. Interestingly, these patients were not undergoing innovative procedures. Although ultimately this problem was recognized and managed, it serves as an example of how challenging outcome data evaluation for innovative surgery might be.

Although the costs of health care in the American healthcare system were previously largely ignored, in recent decades increasing attention has been directed towards the value of healthcare resource expenditures and utilization. Accordingly, surgeons must now consider the costs associated with innovative surgical procedures. Surgeons have the obligation to balance the costs associated with new techniques against the healthcare resources that could otherwise benefit patients in some other manner. However, the cost to the healthcare system should be considered in the context of the potential benefit of the procedure in the long-term and not just short-term increased health resource utilization, which tends to occur early in the adoption of innovative surgical techniques. For example, after laparoscopic cholecystectomy was introduced in the 1980s, it quickly became one of the most popular operations performed in the United States. Although laparoscopic cholecystectomy eventually led to improved postoperative recovery and reduced pain, early studies revealed increased complication rates including longer operative times and higher rates of common bile duct injuries. Had the assessment of the procedure been completed early in the experience of many surgeons, the increased healthcare expenditures and increased risks in the short term may have led to abandonment of the technique [5, 11]. Had such an early assessment been undertaken, we would likely not have developed the wide range of laparoscopic techniques now benefiting thousands of patients every year.

Surgeons must contemplate and navigate through a wide variety of ethical challenges in developing and implementing innovative surgical procedures. Whether the innovative procedure is novel or novel to the surgeon or region, surgeons have an obligation to address key ethical issues to adequately inform and protect their patient, minimize their own bias, and optimize utilization of limited healthcare resources.

The Patient

Prior to the Belmont report, physicians were free to perform experiments on patients without their explicit informed consent. Additionally, there was no consensus about what constituted an acceptable explanation of a proposed treatment for a patient. For many decades, paternalism ruled, and patients surrendered themselves to the care of their physicians with little knowledge of the risks of the treatments. In this context, iterative improvements in treatment were not considered innovation, and new procedures that, in principle, had significant therapeutic promise were not regarded as experimental but rather as straightforward improvements. The distinction between these is not a bright line, but a gray area. Exactly how much innovation constitutes experimentation remains undefined, with the opinions of practitioners and ethicists varying enormously. Regardless, optimism about the benefits of innovative procedures has shaped the consent conversations of patients since obtaining consent became an expectation.

Arguably the most important stakeholder in surgical innovation is the patient and the public on which the new innovation will be used. A number of external and internal forces must be considered in addressing the ethical issues of surgical innovation from a patient's perspective. Although patients look to physicians for counsel and guidance in making medical decisions, medical marketing also plays an important role in shaping patient desires. A phenomenon exists in American medicine in which what is 'new' is also considered 'improved' by patients, often regardless of the evidence that exists to support such a claim. Patients are also frequently enticed by hospitals with the latest technology. What may be potentially misleading to patients is that while progress in the field of medicine is often aggressively marketed, different aspects of medical innovation have different methods of regulation and approval that may not be clearly evident to the patient or public. For example, the Food and Drug Administration (FDA) has significant oversight over the development and approval of new drugs, a completely separate and different process than for the approval of new medical devices, and no formal regulation of new surgical procedures [12]. It is plausible that patients may think that the stringent criteria applied to the approval of new drugs also apply to medical devices or surgical techniques. Take for example the rapid adoption of robotic-assisted surgery throughout the United States. Despite a relative paucity in evidence in support of improved outcomes using robot-assisted surgery, it has been heavily marketed by a number of hospitals nationwide. A recent study by Dixon and colleagues showed that patients were more likely to choose a robot-assisted procedure when it was described as "state-of-the-art" or "innovative" instead of a procedure with uncertain evidence in the current literature [13]. In the modern era of "direct-to-consumer marketing", such treatment seeking by patients is evidence of the success of such marketing and of benefit to those who engage in it.

The process of informed consent requires the surgeon to explain the proposed procedure, including its risks, benefits, and alternatives to the patient or the patient's surrogate decision maker. This process is already difficult when surgeons are trying to explain complex but well-established procedures. However, when informed consent is sought for an innovative procedure, patients are forced to weigh the known risks of the established procedure (with more thorough evidence supporting its use) against the uncertain risks and benefits of the innovative procedure. A major challenge the patient faces in the informed consent process is attempting to understand the disease process they have and the procedure that is being done to address it. Studies about informed consent for surgical procedures often reveal that patients do not adequately understand the information provided about the procedure or the risks associated with their surgery [14]. The consent process for an innovative procedure adds an additional layer of complexity, as it requires the surgeon to explain both the proposed procedure and its alternative, and to elucidate the uncertain risks and benefits of each.

The main source of information about an innovative surgical procedure beyond medical marketing the patients are exposed to is the surgeon who will be operating on the patient. As previously discussed, surgeons have an inherent conflict of interest in this relationship with their patient. In fact, the surgeon will potentially benefit from the risk the patient may undertake. Therefore, there is an incentive for the surgeon to undersell the risk during the informed consent process. In describing the informed consent process for high-risk surgeries, Schwarze and colleagues described the concept of surgical 'buy-in', a process in which patients enter a contractual relationship when they consent for surgery and are expected by their surgeon to also commit to the necessary postoperative care, which can involve significant complications [15]. Similarly, when patients are involved in innovative surgical procedures, they may be expected by their surgeon to commit to postoperative care and potential complications, even when postoperative complications may not be well-known. Patients may additionally feel that they are an important part of the process of surgical innovation and, as such, patients may mistakenly feel a duty to help advance the field for surgery for the general public. Conversely, in choosing the conventional approach instead of the innovative procedure, patients might mistakenly believe that they are not doing their part to advance medicine and may feel that they are disappointing their surgeon. Ultimately, patients trust that their surgeons will do everything within their power to produce the best possible outcome.

In the process of surgical innovation, the patient and public have the burden of trying to understand and make decisions about complex procedures that they may not fully understand, and that may or may not benefit them. At the same time, patients may not appreciate that the incentive for surgeons may be to promote the innovative procedure rather than give priority to patient understanding and outcomes. Surgeons have a great deal of influence on medical decisions made by patients. It is the ethical duty of the surgeons to inform patients of the risks and benefits of an innovative procedure to the best of their ability while minimizing the surgeons' own bias towards the procedure, even when this practice might not be the most beneficial to the surgeons.

The Healthcare Team

A surgeon performing an innovative procedure may require the cooperation of other members of the healthcare team to change their practice in important ways that may not have been disclosed to the patient. Such perturbations may be minor, such as requiring an operating room technician to learn how to operate new equipment and change their workflow. Yet, both of these actions of the technician have their own learning curve and may impact patient outcomes and safety. In other instances, a surgeon might involve another practitioner, such as the anesthesiologist, to participate in procedures involving patient care and outcomes that the anesthesiologist might find troubling. Moreover, cases involving bad outcomes or demonstrating significant gaps between the procedure as explained to the patient and the procedure as performed by the surgeon can compel other healthcare providers to take extreme measures. These healthcare team members might call the attention of leadership or authorities, which can in turn provoke years of tension and strife. For example, many years ago, pediatric anesthesiologists in Winnipeg, Manitoba reported to their clinical and hospital leadership a series of bad outcomes from a new surgeon [16]. The result was an inquiry of findings, significant institutional conflict, and compromised careers [16].

With innovative surgery, these tensions exist in a context in which the risks are ill-defined, and some of the complications have not been anticipated. In general, surgeons who participate in innovation should preemptively engage everyone on their care team to understand the implications of the proposed innovation, and ensure that all team members are comfortable with the responsibilities and actions that may fall upon them.

The Medical Device Industry

Throughout surgical history, innovation has been closely linked with the use of novel surgical instruments and devices in addition to novel surgical techniques.

Medical devices such as cardiac defibrillators can be enormously beneficial and even lifesaving for patients. However, they can also cause harm. Unlike surgical techniques, medical devices must undergo an FDA approval process to be cleared for use in patients. However, the process by which medical devices are approved in the United States is very different from the standard set for pharmaceuticals. While clinical trials are required for drugs, medical devices have different approval paths based on the risk to the patient and this varies from a tongue depressor (FDA Class I) or surgical mesh (FDA Class II), to cardiac defibrillators (FDA Class III). A Class III device is "one that supports or sustains human life or is of substantial importance in preventing impairment of human health or presents a potential, unreasonable risk of illness or injury" [17]. It has recently been suggested that due to its purpose as addressing physician error resulting in significant morbidity and mortality, electronic medical records and health information technology should be considered a Class III device [18]. Class II devices must meet the less stringent criteria of being "significantly equivalent" to an already existing product that has been approved by the FDA through an application process called the 510(k) [17]. The process is purposely permissive to encourage innovation, although it can also leave patients vulnerable to potential harm. One cautionary tale comes from the use of surgical mesh, a FDA Class II device, in the treatment of pelvic organ prolapse. The FDA cleared the ProteGen Sling from Boston Scientific, as "substantially equivalent" to other similar devices on the market without human testing via the 510(k) process. Adopted by numerous gynecologists nationwide, the sling was used in thousands of patients. The ProteGen Sling was soon found to cause significant complications such as erosions, bleeding ulcers, and infections. However, the product was not removed from the market until reports of the complications surfaced in peer-reviewed medical journals that raised concerns about safety. The product was eventually removed from the market after 2 years of use with hundreds of complications surfacing after the product was recalled [19].

This episode illustrates the enormous challenge of recognizing problematic outcomes with established medical devices, especially when complications are rare or not anticipated. In most instances, medical devices provide significant benefits to patients. Regulation that hinders innovation through overly strict standards may ultimately do more harm than good. Medical devices have been and will be an important component of surgical innovation. Regulation of medical devices should ideally find that balance that promotes innovation and improved outcomes in a responsible manner while maintaining patient safety as its highest priority.

Discussion

The many stakeholders involved in the development and implementation of new innovations in surgery interact with each other in a complex network that may involve a variety of ethical challenges. At the center of this interaction are the patient and the public who can benefit from, or be harmed by, the new surgical innovation. The surgeon plays a critical role in both the process of developing the surgical innovation to advance the field of surgery and in that of self-regulation. At the same time, the surgeon must properly inform the patient of the risks, benefits, and alternatives of the procedure and prevent harm to the patient. Anesthesiologists and other members of the healthcare team play an important role in the process of surgical innovation. The details of any new innovation should be fully disclosed preemptively to team members so they are informed about and approve of their role in the process. Medical devices also play an important role in advancing surgical innovation and a balance must be struck between promotion and regulation of these devices to maximize patient benefit while minimizing potential harm. Policies and regulation in surgical innovation should incentivize the different stakeholders to focus foremost on the well-being of the patient.

References

1. Khan MN. The relief of mitral stenosis. An historic step in cardiac surgery. Tex Heart Inst J. 1996;23(4):258–65; discussion 265–6.
2. Harken DE, Ellis LB. The surgical treatment of mitral stenosis; valvuloplasty. N Engl J Med. 1948;239(22):801–9.
3. Acierno LJ. The history of cardiology. New York: Parthenon Publishing Group; 1994. p. 597–697.
4. Siegler M. Ethical issues in innovative surgery: should we attempt a cadaveric hand transplantation in a human subject? Transplant Proc. 1998;30(6):2779–82.
5. Angelos P. Surgical ethics and the challenge of surgical innovation. Am J Surg. 2014;208(6):881–5.
6. Beauchamp TL, Childress JF. Principles of biomedical ethics. 7th ed. Oxford: Oxford University Press; 2009.
7. Cobb LA, Thomas GI, Dillard DH, Merendino KA, Bruce RA. An evaluation of internal-mammary-artery ligation by a double-blind technic. N Engl J Med. 1959;260(22):1115–8.
8. Dinçler S, Koller MT, Steurer J, Bachmann LM, Christen D, Buchmann P. Multidimensional analysis of learning curves in laparoscopic sigmoid resection: eight-year results. Dis Colon Rectum. 2003;46(10):1371–8; discussion 1378–9.
9. Bridgewater B, Grayson AD, Au J, Hassan R, Dihmis WC, Munsch C, et al. Improving mortality of coronary surgery over first four years of independent practice: retrospective examination of prospectively collected data from 15 surgeons. BMJ. 2004;329(7463):421.
10. Kavarana MN, Sade RM. Ethical issues in cardiac surgery. Future Cardiol. 2012;8(3):451–65.
11. Bernard HR, Hartman TW. Complications after laparoscopic cholecystectomy. Am J Surg. 1993;165(4):533–5.
12. U S Food and Drug Administration Home Page [Internet]. [cited 2015 June 5]. Available from: http://www.fda.gov/.
13. Dixon PR, Grant RC, Urbach DR. The impact of marketing language on patient preference for robot-assisted surgery. Surg Innov. 2015;22(1):15–9.
14. Falagas ME, Korbila IP, Giannopoulou KP, Kondilis BK, Peppas G. Informed consent: how much and what do patients understand? Am J Surg. 2009;198(3):420–35.
15. Schwarze ML, Bradley CT, Brasel KJ. Surgical "buy-in": the contractual relationship between surgeons and patients that influences decisions regarding life-supporting therapy. Crit Care Med. 2010;38(3):843–8.
16. Province of Manitoba The Pediatric Cardiac Surgery Inquest Report [Internet]. [cited 2015 Jun 6]. Available from: http://www.pediatriccardiacinquest.mb.ca/. Accessed 13 June 2015.
17. United States Food and Drug Administration. Premarket approval application. General information. http://www.fda.gov/medicaldevices/productsandmedicalprocedures/deviceapprovalsandclearances/pmaapprovals/default.htm. Accessed 13 June 2015.
18. Richard IC. Health IT and patient safety: building safer systems for better care. Washington, DC: National Academies Press (US); 2011.
19. Wall LL, Brown D. The perils of commercially driven surgical innovation. Am J Obstet Gynecol. 2010;202:30.e1–4.

Chapter 11
Professionalism in the Operating Room

Alberto R. Ferreres

Abstract Acting on behalf of their patients, surgeons and anesthesiologists can be considered the moral and fiduciary agents of them. Surgeons and anesthesiologists optimize the care of their patients by exhibiting professionalism in their shared work environment. Professionalism in the operating room demands not only competence in a physician's discipline but also a strict work ethic, adherence to the ethical principles of the profession, diligence, and effective communications skills. The prevention of potential conflicts and the resolution of existing conflicts are necessary to optimize the care and safety of patients in the operating room.

Keywords Professionalism • Operating Room • Surgeon-Anesthesiologist Relationship • Ethics • Conflict Resolution

Case Presentation

A 76-year-old female with colon cancer was admitted for an elective laparoscopic colon resection the day prior to her scheduled surgery date. The patient has diabetes mellitus, a body mass index of 36, and a vague history of coronary artery disease. The surgeon's plan was to have the patient complete her bowel preparation as well as a preoperative evaluation/workup on the admission day. The day before her surgery, an attending anesthesiologist and a senior anesthesia resident evaluated the patient, assigned the patient's American Society of Anesthesiologists Physical Status as III, stated there was no need at that time to arrange a postoperative admission to the intensive care unit, and advised the surgeon that the patient was "cleared and ready for surgery." The patient then began her bowel preparation. The next morning, the patient was brought to the operating room in the preoperative ward and

A.R. Ferreres, MD, PhD, JD, MPH, FACS(Hon), ASA(Hon)
Department of Surgery, University of Buenos Aires, Vicente Lopez 1831 P.B. (1128), Buenos Aires, Argentina
e-mail: albertoferreres@gmail.com

B.G. Jericho (ed.), *Ethical Issues in Anesthesiology and Surgery*,
DOI 10.1007/978-3-319-15949-2_11

met the anesthesiologist assigned to care for her. The anesthesiologist evaluated the patient and determined that the patient was not medically optimized for the surgical procedure given the patient's medical history and vague cardiac history. The anesthesiologist requested a cardiac evaluation of the patient and discussed with the surgeon the need to reschedule the surgery. After acknowledging the situation, the surgeon became particularly annoyed and enraged since the surgeon believed that he had taken all the steps necessary in order to prevent the surgery being cancelled. The surgeon then started complaining and shouting, the situation escalated, and disruptive behavior was displayed towards the anesthesiologist. The surgeon's behavior was witnessed not only by the patient but also by the operating room staff.

The people's good is the highest law (Cicero, 106–43 BC, De Legibus)

Introduction

In 2001, the Institute of Medicine published a landmark report that redefined patient care as the "provision of care that is safe, effective, efficient, timely and patient centered for all those who are in need" [1]. This concept of healthcare delivery placed the patient's safety and welfare at center stage. For surgeons and anesthesiologists this concept of care expands care from one that simply consists of a "flawless technique during the performance of an operation" to care that also includes all of the needs of the patient and his or her family. The application of this concept of patient-centered care requires the further consideration of enhanced communication skills and the practice of ethical principles in the care of patients [2]. Patient-centered healthcare delivery emphasizes both the surgeon and the anesthesiologist as fiduciary agents who act on behalf of their patients. Thus, in addition to strong clinical and technical skills, an anesthesiologist and surgeon should have a thorough knowledge of bioethics and the practice of humanism to provide the best care for their patients. Ethics, therefore, lies at the center of professionalism.

Surgeons and anesthesiologists work together in the same environment, the operating room. The operating room is the hospital unit where surgical procedures are performed and each operating room is designed and equipped to provide surgical care to patients with specific conditions. In an efficient, optimal operating room, there should be the guarantee of the highest quality of surgical care and patient safety; the ease of scheduling patients for procedures; an atmosphere of trust and a respectful working environment; the maximization of operating room efficiency and efficacy with a decrease in delays and cancellations of surgical procedures; and satisfaction among patients, personnel and physicians. If these issues of the operating room are considered ahead of time, on the day of surgery, the teams delivering care can focus on the patient without distractions that could lead to conflicts and compromise patient safety. Therefore, the operating room environment requires teamwork to delivery high quality care.

In order to provide this high quality care, there is a team consisting of physicians of different specialties, nurses, technicians, and support personnel. This team approach is essential for patient care. Unusual to other areas of the hospital, though, the operating room involves two physicians (the surgeon and the anesthesiologist) sharing concurrently the management and responsibility of a single patient. This responsibility underscores important decisions, usually involving life and death. Other factors that can impact this provision of care include fatigue, sleep deprivation, and pressure on production and on outcomes [3].

Acting on behalf of their patients, surgeons and anesthesiologists can be considered the moral and fiduciary agents of their patients. Surgeons and anesthesiologists optimize the care of their patients by exhibiting professionalism in their shared work environment. Professionalism in the operating room demands not only competence in a physician's discipline but also a strict work ethic, adherence to the ethical principles of the profession, diligence, effective communications skills, and working as a member of a team. In the operating room, the prevention of potential conflicts and the resolution of existing conflicts are necessary to optimize the care and safety of patients.

In this chapter, we will review principles that promote professionalism in the operating room, provide elements that can identify the roots of potential conflicts, and introduce strategies for the prevention and resolution of such conflicts.

Professionalism and Ethical Principles

Teamwork is paramount for patient care in the operating room. Surgical and anesthesia teams work hand in hand in many procedures, be it elective or emergent, low complexity or high complexity. Mutual respect among all healthcare providers in the operating room should be the rule and excellent communication among all team members improves patient safety and promotes good patient outcomes.

Competence, diligence, legal issues and concerns, ethics, and concern for patient safety in the operating room are important considerations for all members of the perioperative team. These are concepts embodied in professionalism. In fact, professionalism comprises a "set of values reflected in the philosophy and behavior of individuals whose calling is first and foremost to serve individuals and populations whose care is entrusted to them, prioritizing the interests of those they serve above their own" [4].

John Gregory (1724–1774), a Scottish physician and moralist, must be credited as the one who allowed the transformation of medicine from a trade to a profession. A profession is a group of individuals who are bound by a common ethic or code of conduct. Gregory, in fact, introduced the foundation of medical ethics and defined medicine as "the art of preserving health, of prolonging life, of curing diseases and of making death easy" [5]. He also introduced the concept of the physician as a fiduciary agent to the patient by being "the person having duty, created by his or her understanding to act primarily for another's benefit in matters connected with such undertaking" [5].

The concept of the surgeon and anesthesiologist as the patient's moral fiduciary agent can be captured in several reflections. For instance, the surgeon/anesthesiologist should have the patient's interest as the primary consideration in the physician–patient relationship, as well as in surgical research and education. Similarly, this commitment divests self-interest and makes it a secondary consideration. Self-interest is thus blunted and makes the fiduciary's role morally demanding.

Ethics Remains at the Center of Professionalism in Both Surgery and Anesthesiology

Presidents of the American College of Surgeons have addressed widely the issue of professionalism in surgery. Dr. Copeland mentioned the importance of a surgical way of life and defined it as "the art and practice of surgery staying in your conscious thought continually" [6]. McGinnis quoted H. Debas stating that "Professional status is not an inherent right, but one granted by society and this obligates surgeons to put their patients' interests above their own. It must not be forgotten that ethical codes are the major characteristic that differentiate professions from occupations" [7].

Ralph M Waters (1883–1979) is considered a great contributor to the development of professionalism in anesthesiology. He considered it critical to establish a systematic body of scientific knowledge, scientific organizations, and a continuous improvement in clinical practice, represented by high quality anesthesia training programs [8]. In addition, Henry Beecher (1904–1976) was also a significant contributor to professionalism and medical ethics. His role was pivotal in medical research and innovation [9].

Professionalism is the basis of the contract between medicine and society and is guided by three fundamental principles [10]: (1) **The supremacy of patient welfare**, which is the dedication of physicians to serving patients' interests. Physicians are considered the moral and fiduciary agents of their patients; (2) **Patient autonomy**: surgeons and anesthesiologist should empower patients to make informed decisions about their treatment. Nonetheless, there are clinical situations which leave room for paternalism, such as trauma patients presenting for emergency surgery who do not have decision-making capacity and do not have a known surrogate decision maker; (3) **Social justice**: Aristotle first conceptualized justice as "the rendering to each individual of what is due to him or her" -justice is interpreted as the fair, equitable, and appropriate distribution of what is due or owed to persons. More recent works on social justice originate from John Rawls' "A Theory of Justice", in which he argues that a social arrangement forming a political state is a communal effort to advance the good of all individuals [11].

Other elements that define a profession include the possession of specialized knowledge and skills that are continually honed, ethics, and the evidence of competence (including licensing and certification). Professionalism describes certain attitudes, values, and behaviors that are expected from physicians. The essential characteristics of professionalism include: accountability (the physician is responsible and liable for his or her practice of medicine); competence and diligence; humanism integrated with integrity, compassion, sympathy; effective and proper communication; and respect of and practice of ethical principles. Furthermore, terms often significantly associated with professionalism include altruism, honor, compassion, integrity, dedication, empathy, responsiveness, prudence, and an ethos of self-regulation. The set of professional responsibilities include professional competence; scientific knowledge, honesty; respect for patient confidentiality; appropriate relationships with patients; the improvement of quality of care; easy and universal access to health care; maintaining trust by managing conflicts of interest; and fair distribution of limited resources.

The Four Principles of Bioethics

The principles of biomedical ethics as stated by Beauchamp and Childress are utilized when addressing bioethical issues and analyzing clinical ethical situations [12]. The four principles of biomedical ethics are autonomy, beneficence, nonmaleficence, and justice [12]. In addition to the four principles of bioethics, truthfulness, fairness, integrity, dignity, respect of an individual's rights, and honesty are all virtues of ethical behavior physicians should also uphold. The following are the four principles of bioethics as applied to professionalism in the operating room.

Autonomy

Autonomy derives from the Greek roots *autos* (self) and *nomos* (rule, governance, law) and makes reference to the original self-determination of city-states in Greece. A patient's autonomy is respected in regard to decisions related to medical care. The autonomy of the surgeon and anesthesiologist, in addition to the patient's autonomy, should be respected (for example, circumstances involving conscientious objection) as long as their professional responsibilities are fulfilled and patient care is not compromised.

Beneficence

Beneficence involves actions for the best interest of others.

Nonmaleficence

Nonmaleficence is derived from the *Primun non nocere* dictum and includes not only the duty not to inflict harm but also the duty not to impose a risk of harm. In cases where the patient has been put at risk, both law and morality set a standard that determines if the agent causally responsible for the risk is legally or morally liable. Conversely, negligence involves an act or omission of an act that is a departure from the professional standards of medical practice. The term negligence covers two situations: (1) an act intentionally imposing unreasonable risks of harm (advertent negligence or recklessness) and (2) the omission of an act imposing risks of harm (inadvertent negligence). Cases of negligence involve a behavior that falls below a standard of care established by the law to protect patients from the careless imposition of risks. Essential elements of negligence include the following: the physician (surgeon or anesthesiologist) must have a duty to the affected party; the physician must breach the duty; the affected party (the patient) must experience harm; and the harm must be caused by the breach of duty. "Professional malpractice" is negligence that involves departing from professional standards of care. The line between due care and inadequate care (which falls below what is due) may sometimes be difficult to draw.

Justice

Justice refers to the fair allocation of resources.

Sir David Ross (1877–1971) was the first to develop the *prima facie* ethical duties. Originally in the number of 5, these duties were fidelity, reparation, gratitude, promotion of a maximum of aggregate good, and nonmaleficence [13]. Not all of these duties bear the same importance. In his argumentation, Ross stated that the duty of nonmaleficence is the initial step prior to the duty to promote a maximum of aggregate good. Also, Ross stated that the duties of fidelity, reparation, and gratitude were more preeminent than the duty to promote good. Furthermore, Ross considered that four elements are basically good: virtue, knowledge, pleasure (all considered states of mind), and justice, which represents the relationship between the first three. Following the Kantian "*moral imperative*", Ross illustrates how moral decision-making sometimes requires us to think about the past and act according to a sense of duty rather than focus on the projected outcome. Ross' duties-based (deontological) ethics served as a foundation for the work of Beauchamp and Childress.

Therefore, the principles of Ross and Beauchamp and Childress are a foundation for the ethical duties of the surgeon and the anesthesiologist. Furthermore, the ethical duties of physicians include an implicit social and moral contract within the members of the medical profession, which includes the physician's responsibility to society and their specialty; self-regulation of their profession; the professional obligation to utilize scientific knowledge for the service of others; earning public trust in the practice of medicine; and optimizing the healthcare delivery system to uphold these moral and ethical responsibilities.

The Surgeon-Anesthesiologist Relationship

Traditionally, the degree of a surgeon's responsibility in the operating room has been compared to that of the captain of a ship and this was the ruling doctrine to judge a surgeon's behavior and liability in the operating room, considering him or her responsible for those assistants under his or her supervision. The legal doctrine, a variation of the "borrowed servant doctrine" considered that during any surgical procedure the surgeon was liable for all actions performed in the course of the operation and by anyone in that operating room. In fact, in early times, the anesthesiologist was considered one of the surgeon's dependents and the surgeon was considered the owner of the patient [14].

The doctrine of "*the captain of a ship*" was coined in McConnel v. Williams, 361 Pa. 355, 65 A.2d 243, 246 (1949), in which the Supreme Court of Pennsylvania ruled that "It can readily be understood that in the course of an operation in the operating room of a hospital, and until the surgeon leaves that room at the conclusion of the operation… he is in the same complete charge of those who are present and assisting him as in the captain of a ship over all on board, and that such supreme control is indeed essential in view of the high degree of protection to which an anesthetized, unconscious patient is entitled…" [15]. This doctrine was popular for a long time and assimilated in other judicial systems, yet its sustainability has diminished. In "Truhitte v. French Hospital," (1982 128 Cal. App. 3d 332, 348) the court explained "the captain of the ship doctrine arose from the need to assure plaintiffs a source of recovery for malpractice at a time when many hospitals enjoyed charitable immunity, which is no longer the case" [16]. But most important, the court also stated that "the theory that the surgeon controls all activities of whatever nature in the operating room is unrealistic in present-day medical care where today's hospitals hire, fire, train and supervise their nurse employees, implement surgery protocols and can absorb the risks of noncompliance" [16].

To perform his or her duties the surgeon requires the collaboration from other hospital employees and staff who do not report to or are not employed by the surgeon. Among this staff is the anesthesiologist who also has his or her own professional and scientific autonomy. Not only do anesthesiologists provide the benefits of unconsciousness, sedation, analgesia, and relaxation, but also resuscitate patients and provide life-sustaining measures to facilitate the surgeon's ability to care for the patient. The surgeon and anesthesiologist must work as a team, working jointly during the perioperative phases of care to achieve the best quality of care, the highest patient safety level, and the best outcome for the patient. This shared responsibility demands a clear definition of roles and a mutual respect of competencies.

Anesthesia is a unique medical specialty as it has a limited direct patient relationship. The anesthesiologist provides care to a patient who is referred primarily by a surgeon. Furthermore, the time-limited care provided by the anesthesiologist occurs during the perioperative period. After the immediate postoperative recovery of the patient, this relationship ceases and the surgeon most often resumes the sole care of the patient. Therefore, the patient's outcome in the immediate postoperative period depends, in addition to other factors, on how well the surgeon, anesthesiologist, and healthcare team work together as a team and communicate with each other. Sound ethical practices in the operating room are imperative and must be recognized by all providers involved in the patient's care.

Conflicts in the Operating Room

The healthcare environment is particularly prone to conflicts. It has been estimated that conflicts occur during the management of 50–78% of patients, and that 38–48% involve interpersonal conflicts among health care staff [17, 18].

The potential for interpersonal conflicts is heightened in the operating room where a broad range of healthcare professionals perform their tasks with overlapping and sometimes poorly defined areas of responsibility. Furthermore, the operating room is the only area of the hospital where two physicians of different specialties – each with its own professional autonomy – concurrently share direct responsibility for the same patient. Moreover, the roles of these physicians are such that one cannot perform his or her task without the other. In these situations, a conflict may arise. A conflict may be considered as "a state of disagreement or disharmony between persons or ideas" [19]. The conflict usually causes an emotional stir among those individuals involved. The conflict may arise between the anesthesiologist and surgeon, but also between these specialists and other operating room personnel such as nurses and technicians. Conflicts may also progress to harassment and disruptive behavior. Operating room and hospital leadership should establish and communicate the appropriate code of conduct in the operating room and be uncompromising in its corrective decisions and actions. The implementation and enforcement of operating room policies and regulations require the cooperation of all those involved in patient care. As conflicts in the operating room can compromise surgical and anesthetic care, successful conflict resolution will promote better patient care and safety, improved quality of care, and better patient outcomes.

The leading causes of conflict between surgeon and anesthesiologist include personal and cultural factors. Among the personal factors are poor communication skills; different personality traits; different personal values and beliefs; lack of appreciation by the other profession; and different models of salary and/or reimbursement for procedures. Furthermore, caring for sicker patients undergoing more complex surgical procedures may bring potential conflicts involving futility, appropriate versus inappropriate indications for procedures, do not resuscitate orders in the perioperative period, advance directives [20], as well as the care of Jehovah's Witness patients.

Operating room delays and cancellations are the most frequently felt source of conflict. The incidence of cancellations is around 2–14% of cases, but it can reach 21.8% in a tertiary care center [21]. Some of the common causes for delays and cancellations are the need for additional tests and consultations, shortage of blood supply, food intake by the patient prior to surgery, lack of availability of beds in adequately monitored postoperative care units, absence of essential equipment, and poorly controlled systemic diseases.

There are various measures to improve the relationship between surgeons and anesthesiologists and to prevent potential conflicts in the operating room. For instance, there should be agreement regarding the risk stratification and optimization of patients for surgery. When there is a disagreement regarding whether a patient is optimized for surgery, physicians should focus on the care of a patient and not on personal issues. Furthermore, a second opinion from a peer can be sought. In addition, an effort should be made to start the cases on time, with both surgeons and anesthesiologists being monitored and disciplined when late. Furthermore, there should be truthfulness regarding the scheduling of cases and honesty with respect to the duration of a procedure. However, at times and appropriately so, the duration of a procedure may be increased by an intraoperative complication and by the nature of practicing in an academic setting involving the education of resident physicians. Frequent communication of the surgeon with the anesthesiologist and the operating room staff with updates during a procedure may provide the team with a more objective estimate of the duration of the operation. Another measure to improve the relationship between surgeons and anesthesiologists is to include anesthesiologists on important decisions, such as introducing a new technology or a surgical innovation [22].

The performance of surgical procedures in an accredited setting mandates an environment in which all participants (patients, staff, nurses, colleagues, residents, students, and other personnel) are treated with respect. Discrimination on any level (race, age, gender, sexual preference, disability, or religion), bullying behavior, and harassment must be banned in every day activities and reported to ensure the employment of corrective measures.

Conclusion

In summary, conflicts in the operating room can arise because of the complexity of the environment and the interactions of a diverse set of individuals involved in patient care. Acting on behalf of their patients, surgeons and anesthesiologists can be considered the moral and fiduciary agents of their patients. Surgeons and anesthesiologists optimize the care of their patients by exhibiting professionalism in their shared work environment. Professionalism in the operating room demands not only competence in a physician's discipline but also a strict work ethic, adherence to the ethical principles of the profession, diligence, and effective communications skills. The prevention of potential conflicts and the resolution of existing conflicts are necessary to optimize the care and safety of patients in the operating room. The following elements can improve professionalism in the operating room and be utilized for conflict prevention and resolution:

- Awareness of the organizational culture of the institution. Once this is understood, change and improvement can be implemented.
- Respectful attitude. For example, be helpful, nice, courteous, and polite. Be cordial and easy to work with. Do more than what is expected from you.
- Culture of safety. Try to prevent errors and be gentle with those of others.
- Communication. Keep clear and precise communication, verbal and written. Be prompt in replying to others.
- Reliability.
- Flexibility. Do not complain for every detail.
- Promotion of education at all levels.
- Being able to receive constructive criticism.
- Fulfilling responsibilities.
- Promoting ethical behavior.

References

1. Institute of Medicine. Committee on Quality of Health Care in America. Crossing the quality chasm: a new health system for the 21st century. Washington, DC: National Academy Press; 2001.
2. Nurok M, Sundt III TM, Frankel A. Teamwork and communication in the operating room: relationship to discrete outcomes and research challenges. Anesthesiol Clin. 2011;29:1–11.
3. Rogers DA, Lingard L, Boehler ML, Espin S, Mellinger JD, Schindler N, Klingensmith M. Surgeons managing conflict in the operating room: defining the educational need and identifying effective behaviors. Am J Surg. 2013;205:125–30.
4. ABIMFoundation. American Board of Internal Medicine. ACP-ASIM Foundation. American College of Physicians-American Society of Internal Medicine; European Federation of Internal Medicine. Medical professionalism in the new millennium: a physician charter. Ann Intern Med. 2002;136:243–6.
5. McCullough LB. John Gregory and the invention of professional medical ethics and the profession of medicine. Dordrecht: Kluwer Academic Publishers; 1998.
6. Copeland EM. Presidential address: the role of a mentor in creating a surgical way of life. Bull Am Coll Surg. 2006;91:9–13.
7. McGinnis L. Presidential address: professionalism in the XXI century. Bull Am Coll Surg. 2009;12:8–18.
8. McGoldrick KE. The history of professionalism in anesthesiology. AMA J Ethics. 2015;17:258–64.
9. Beecher HK. Ethics and clinical research. N Engl J Med. 1966;274:1354–60.
10. Medical professionalism in the new millennium: a physician charter. Ann Intern Med. 2002; 136(3):243–6.
11. Rawls J. A theory of justice, revised edition. Cambridge: Harvard University Press; 1999.
12. Beauchamp TL, Childress JF. Principles of biomedical ethics. 4th ed. New York: Oxford University Press; 1994.
13. Ross WD. The right and the good. Oxford: Oxford University Press; 1930.

14. Henderson VE. Relationship between anesthetist, surgeon and patient. Anesth Anal. 1932;11:5–10.
15. McConnel v. Williams, 361 Pa. 355;65 A.2d 243, 246. 1949.
16. Truhitte v. French Hospital, 1982;128 Cal. App. 3d 332, 348.
17. Burns JP, Mello MM, Studdert DM, et al. Results of a clinical trial on care improvement for the critically ill. Crit Care Med. 2003;31:2107–17.
18. Cm B, Abernethy AP, Abbott KH, Tulsky JA. Conflict associated with decisions to limit life-sustaining treatment in intensive care units. J Gen Intern Med. 2001;16:283–9.
19. The Free Dictionary. http://www.thefreedictionary.com/conflict. Accessed 5 July 2015.
20. Cahana A, Weibel H, Hurst SA. Ethical decision-making: do anesthesiologists, surgeons, nurse anesthetists and surgical nurses reason similarly? Pain Med. 2008;9:728–36.
21. Van Klei WA, Moons KGM, Rutten CLG, et al. The effect of outpatient preoperative evaluation of hospital inpatients on cancellation of surgery and length of hospital stay. Anesth Analg. 2002;94:644–9.
22. Katz JD. Conflict and its resolution in the operating room. J Clin Anesth. 2007;19:152–8.

Chapter 12
Honesty in the Perioperative Setting: Error and Communication

Puneet Singh, Baddr A. Shakhsheer, and Ross Milner

Abstract Since the Institute of Medicine report, "To Err is Human," there has been a great focus on medical errors and the creation of systems to prevent the occurrence of these errors. Error disclosure is critical to managing medical errors in order to uphold the ethical principles of autonomy and truth-telling, both integral to the physician-patient relationship. Surgeons feel responsible for their patients' outcomes and report that errors should be disclosed though the surgeon may not have the proper training in disclosure. Institutional support, both for the emotional disruption that physicians face and for disclosure training programs, is important to advance patient-centered communication and high-quality health care.

Keywords Medical Error • Disclosure • Communication • Physician-Patient Relationship • Ethics

Case Presentations

Case Presentation 1

Prior to a gynecological tumor resection, a 54-year-old woman underwent an inferior vena cava (IVC) filter placement due to a recent deep venous thrombosis (DVT) and pulmonary embolism (PE). She recovered well from both the IVC placement and the resection of her tumor. Now, she presents to the operating room for the removal of the IVC filter. The IVC filter is unable to be

P. Singh, MD (✉) • B.A. Shakhsheer, MD
Department of Surgery, The University of Chicago Pritzker School of Medicine, 5841 S. Maryland Avenue, MC 5030, Chicago, IL 60637, USA
e-mail: puneet.singh@uchospitals.edu; Baddr.shakhsheer@uchospitals.edu

R. Milner, MD
Department of Surgery, MacLean Center for Clinical Medical Ethics, The University of Chicago Medicine, Chicago, IL, USA
e-mail: rmilner@surgery.bsd.uchicago.edu

B.G. Jericho (ed.), *Ethical Issues in Anesthesiology and Surgery*,
DOI 10.1007/978-3-319-15949-2_12

removed due to a technical difficulty in the operating room. The unsuccessful procedure is described in detail to the patient and her family. A CT scan is obtained and there is no evidence of recurrent cancer, but the tip of the IVC filter is nearly embedded in the wall of the vena cava. The patient returns to the surgeon's office for a reevaluation and a mutual decision between the patient and surgeon is made to reattempt the removal of the IVC filter. In the operating room, the surgeon utilizes a new technique and the IVC filter is easily removed from the IVC wall, but the IVC filter is nearly released from the snaring mechanism. If lost, the IVC filter could have traveled to the patient's heart. After a few minutes, the IVC filter was successfully removed and there was no harm to the patient.

Case Presentation 2

A 64-year-old man presents to a surgeon for a second opinion regarding the management of an aneurysmal degeneration in the right iliac artery above a prior endovascular repair. The patient has a past medical history of cardiac disease and severe pulmonary disease for which he uses oxygen at home. The surgeon has a lengthy discussion with the patient and family regarding the repair of the aneurysmal degeneration and the possibility of a complex endovascular repair that will require multiple devices. The surgeon explains to the patient and the family that some of the devices will be used in an off-label fashion. The patient and his family understand the risks and benefits of this complicated approach and agree to proceed. The patient undergoes a surgical repair of the aneurysmal degeneration with the last step of the surgery being the removal of one sheath from a renal artery. However, the sheath in the renal artery is trapped on a new device that was placed in the aorta. Finally, after multiple careful attempts, the surgeon is able to dislodge the sheath, but the sheath pulls the newly placed aortic stent into the proximal descending thoracic aorta and a portion of the sheath remains attached to the stent in the thoracic aorta. Fortunately, the stent does not cover any of the great vessels, which would have likely caused the patient to have a stroke. The sheath is eventually separated from the stent and the surgical procedure is then completed with a different endovascular approach. The patient remained in the hospital for a short time and was discharged from the hospital with no neurologic sequelae.

Introduction

Medical error and its impact on the healthcare system were thrust into the spotlight by the 1999 Institute of Medicine (IOM) report, "To Err is Human." This report detailed the types of preventable medical errors, the number of resulting deaths, the costs of these errors, and strategies to improve patient safety and the healthcare system. Furthermore, the authors described the effects of errors on the patient and family, the physician, and the physician-patient relationship [1]. This report remains fundamental in the patient safety movement and critical to discussions about error and the disclosure of error.

The IOM defines medical error as "failure of a planned action to be completed as intended or use of a wrong plan to achieve an aim" [1]. Medical errors include serious errors, minor errors and near misses that can potentially cause an adverse event, "an injury resulting from a medical intervention" [2]. Serious errors, often resulting from ineffective team communication [3] (e.g. the operating room team), are most likely to occur in the operating room, emergency department, and intensive care unit [1]. It is part of human nature to err and, thus, it is essential to work toward solutions to minimize medical errors. A critical aspect of the management of medical errors, in order to uphold the ethical principles of autonomy and truth-telling, is error disclosure.

This chapter discusses the history of disclosure; the patient and physician perspective on medical error; the surgeon-patient relationship; the ethical dilemmas that might arise from medical errors, in particular perioperative errors; and how physicians might navigate these situations in the disclosure of medical error.

The History of Disclosure

In the 1930s, doctors were advised to "keep a cautious tongue" with regard to errors [4]. This attitude toward error disclosure persisted throughout much of the twentieth century until specific disclosure programs such as the Lexington Model emerged [5]. In 1987, the Lexington Veterans Administration Medical Center (VAMC) lost two medical malpractice cases and discovered that a patient death was due to medical negligence. Subsequently, the facility, including the chief of staff and staff attorney, decided that the "right thing to do" was to disclose the medical error to the family [5, 6]. Kraman and Hamm, who led this innovative disclosure program, described this approach to ethical dilemmas involving medical error as "humanistic risk management," in which the physician and facility continued the caregiver role in communicating the error to the patient and/or family [6]. While their policy did not significantly impact litigation, the litigation costs were lower. The Lexington VAMC continued to report a high number of tort claims compared to other VAMCs, but interestingly the Lexington VAMC placed in the lowest quartile for litigation costs [7]. More importantly, the physicians and the VAMC believed disclosure to be their ethical and professional responsibility. The success of the Lexington Model led the Veterans Administration National Center for Ethics in 2008 (updated in 2012) to write a disclosure policy based on their model, although there has been significant variation in the uptake of these disclosure policies [5, 6]. This development of a disclosure policy in the Veterans Administration also prompted the creation of a simulation-based disclosure training programming for the VAMCs [5].

The IOM report and the success of the Lexington Model motivated other institutions and organizations to create policies on error communication. The Joint Commission released the first national standard in 2001 that required physicians to disclose outcomes of any treatment when they "differ significantly from the anticipated outcomes" [8]. Though the Joint Commission provided little detail about what should be disclosed and how this information should be disclosed, the Joint Commission release of the first national standard on disclosure was an important step because of the Joint Commission's role in accrediting hospitals [9]. Furthermore, the National Quality Forum created a safe-practice guideline on the disclosure of serious unanticipated outcomes with the goal of promoting high-quality health care [10]. Other organizations such as the American Medical Association (AMA) developed their own standards in their Code of Medical Ethics to advise physicians to "deal honestly and openly with patients," provide full disclosure to patients to support patients' autonomy in medical decision-making, and not be influenced by legal liability [11]. Another prominent policy addressing error communication is the Charter on Medical Professionalism, which is endorsed by over 100 organizations and calls for open and honest communication with patients including discussions of medical errors [12].

Similar to the Lexington VAMC, other institutions and organizations have demonstrated a link between transparency in error communication and decreased litigation costs [13]. The University of Michigan Health Systems showed that their open disclosure program reduced the number of litigation cases and the cost of litigation over 5 years. At the University of Michigan, the open disclosure program accomplished these reductions in cases and costs by acknowledging medical errors, fairly compensating patients and families, defending cases that did not have merit, and studying prior events to determine prevention strategies [14]. In addition, the American College of Surgeons Closed Claims Study, which examined 460 claims against general surgeons, demonstrated that transparency and communication in the surgeon-patient relationship decreased litigation and prevented errors and bad outcomes [15]. These nationally recognized organizations demonstrate that disclosure policies can be beneficial for all parties involved.

The Patient Perspective on Medical Error

As an autonomous stakeholder in the physician-patient relationship, patients desire full disclosure of medical errors. Delbanco and Bell conducted focus groups with patients and families and three themes emerged [16]: (1) Family members have strong feelings of guilt after an error occurs. (2) Patients and their families may fear further harm and/or retribution if they ask questions about the error or voice their feelings. (3) The patient and family may also feel abandoned, perhaps in response to how the physician feels and behaves toward them [16]. The patients and family members that were interviewed expressed their desire for an apology and direct, honest communication [16]. Furthermore, Gallagher et al. and Marcus et al., after interviewing patients and families about what they wanted after an error had occurred, found that patients and families wanted full disclosure of the error including the implications on their health, a genuine apology and a commitment to prevention of the error in the future [17, 18]. Further supporting the fact that patients want full disclosure, Mazor et al. conducted a study of nearly 1000 patients who responded to a mail survey with vignettes describing medical errors and reported that 98.8% of patients wanted full disclosure and 88% wanted a sincere apology [19]. Of interest, Mazor et al. found that *nondisclosure* was associated with respondents obtaining legal advice, yet *disclosure* was associated with increased patient satisfaction and trust – both of which are critical to the physician-patient relationship [19]. Not surprisingly, they also found that the type of error and the severity of the outcome might influence patients to seek legal advice despite physician disclosure [19]. Nevertheless, these studies reinforce the idea that open and honest communication can address the patient's need for information after a medical error occurs.

The Physician Perspective on Medical Error

The disclosure gap persists despite the existence of many organizational and national policies and the patient's desire for information. Patients and their families continue to have unmet needs following a medical error. In contrast to institutional disclosure, which is conducted by the organization after an adverse event rises above a certain threshold of harm, clinical disclosure is conducted by the physician and should occur routinely in the physician-patient relationship [5]. Thus, physicians have the greatest potential impact on error disclosure. Several studies have examined physician attitudes on the communication of errors and the barriers that exist which may explain the disclosure gap.

Physicians continue to follow the historical adages of "keep a cautious tongue" and "choose words carefully" when it comes to disclosure. A large, national survey of physicians from diverse specialties demonstrated that approximately one-third did not completely agree with the need to disclose serious errors [12]. Physicians interviewed in focus groups stated that they felt the need to put a positive "spin" on the discussion of the adverse event [17] even though patients and families do not desire a "spin doctor" [16]. In certain situations, physicians may be advised by hospital administration, risk managers or insurers to avoid words such as "error," "harm," "negligence," "fault," "mistake," or "sorry" as these may trigger litigation [16]. Furthermore, Gallagher et al. found that physicians agree that errors causing harm should be disclosed, however they may limit the discussion, choosing not to reveal how or why the error occurred [17]. Also, despite patients' desire for information on error prevention, Gallagher et al. found that error prevention was another area that is not often communicated to patients [17].

If physicians want to disclose errors, then what prevents them from doing so in practice? One of the perceived barriers is the fear of legal liability. Clinicians fear that patients may interpret an apology as an admission of fault [17]. Gawande writes in *Complications* that the tort system creates an adversarial physician-patient relationship [20]. Approximately thirty states have enacted "I'm sorry" laws in response to this sentiment, which protect the physician by making an apology inadmissible in court as evidence of legal responsibility. However, these laws do not exist throughout the country and thus, physicians may be advised by hospital administration, lawyers, risk managers and insurers to avoid apologizing and using trigger words [16]. This atmosphere of "silence and evasion" [16] is fueled in part by the historically hostile relationship between the medical and legal systems and can lead to further mistrust in the physician-patient relationship. Whether real or perceived, potential litigation is a large concern for physicians and those advising them. Medical liability reform is necessary to foster an environment of open communication and remains an active area of advocacy for many organizations, including the AMA [21].

Similar to patients, physicians also fear medical errors [16, 17]. Physicians fear the harm or potential harm they have caused the patient, the loss of patient trust, and the impact of medical errors on their reputation and career including being reported to the National Practitioners' Databank. The physician's feeling of guilt can lead to individual suffering and isolation [5, 16, 22]. Moreover, medical errors can be damaging to a physician's self-confidence. As one physician described, medicine requires one to "hit a home run every time" [17] and other studies report that the fear and worry surrounding errors may lead to burnout [23]. Furthermore, surgeons, in particular, report decreased job satisfaction after an error [23].

Ethicist John Banja describes the concept of medical narcissism, which gives the physician control, creates emotional distance from the patient and puts the focus on objective clinical data [24]. Banja goes on to further explain that avoidance and rationalization of errors may be defense mechanisms to preserve self-esteem [24]. Compounding this, physicians report few outlets for them to discuss the feelings and emotions associated with medical errors. Morbidity and mortality conferences may be a venue for discussing emotions associated with making medical errors; however, these conferences may be limited to the presentation of a patient's case and a discussion of the prevention of errors rather than a dialogue of the emotional upheaval a physician may face. Physicians may seek out informal outlets such as significant others or trusted colleagues, but few professional sources of support exist. Although forgiveness from the patient or support from colleagues can help, it is often the physician's own high standards which make it difficult for them to forgive themselves [17]. Institutional recognition of these issues may facilitate better support systems and strengthen humanistic disclosure programs. Patients often feel that physicians are cold and lack empathy when disclosing adverse events and for some patients, a physician who can communicate and express his or her feelings implies a caring nature [17].

The Surgeon-Patient Relationship

> The only surgeon without complications
> is the surgeon who does not operate. –Unknown

The surgeon-patient relationship is a unique one that lies at the center of the field of surgical ethics. Throughout the history of the surgical profession, there has been increasing recognition that surgery is different from other specialties of medicine and that the specialty of surgery has a distinct ethical code. The ethics of the profession stem from the fiduciary relationship between the surgeon and the patient. In this unique physician-patient relationship, the surgeon must first cause harm to the patient by using a scalpel to make an incision before the surgeon can heal the patient. Furthermore, through the informed consent process and in a relatively short time, the surgeon must establish a physician-patient relationship which will continue into the operating room while the patient is asleep and continue throughout the perioperative period. This therapeutic relationship between a surgeon and a patient requires the physical presence of the surgeon unlike another physician who can remotely prescribe a medication to treat a patient's illness [25]. Thus, the patient places a significant amount of trust in the surgeon and surgeons often feel a great sense of responsibility for ensuring a good outcome for the patient. In other words, the surgeon takes on the "captain of the ship" role to direct the pre-, intra- and post-operative care. Sociologist Charles Bosk's *Forgive and Remember* highlights this intimate link between the surgeon's action and the patient's outcome: The internist whose patient dies is asked by colleagues "What happened?" versus the surgeon who is asked "What did you do?" [26].

Inherent to surgery are risks, which are presented to the patient in the informed consent process. These risks may become a surgical *complication* defined as "…any undesirable, unintended, and direct result of surgery affecting the patient which would not have occurred had the surgery gone as well as could reasonably be hoped" [27]. However, *error* as defined previously has a distinct undertone of culpability that *complication* does not. As such, *complications*, which are adverse events, can result from an error or be independent of error. Conversely, *errors* can occur without a resulting complication [28]. In spite of this distinction, Bosk's observation demonstrates the perceived responsibility of the surgeon for all outcomes whether good or bad [26].

Communication about errors is part of surgical culture from the beginning of a young surgeon's training in the form of morbidity and mortality conferences and role modeling by senior surgeons. When asked about disclosure of errors to patients, surgeons feel an obligation to disclose based on ethics and professionalism and report the need to disclose all errors [2, 12, 29]. Gallagher et al. conducted a mail survey of 2637 medical (nonsurgical) and surgical physicians with case scenarios of serious errors depending on the specialty of the physician [2]. The questions asked how physicians would handle the disclosure. Compared to nonsurgical physicians, surgeons were more likely to disclose the error (81% versus 54%, $P<0.001$) [2]. Interestingly, surgeons also thought a lawsuit was more likely after the surgical error compared to the medical physicians who were surveyed about a medical (i.e. nonsurgical) error (57% versus 40%, $P<0.001$) [2]. Furthermore, there were significant differences in how the disclosure was conducted as only 19% of surgeons used the word "error" (versus 58% of medical clinicians, $P<0.001$) [2]. Surgeons were also significantly less likely to communicate the details of the case, an explicit apology, and the details of error prevention [2]. This study demonstrates that despite intentions to provide full disclosure of errors, surgeons often provide less information than medical colleagues [2], which may be due to surgical culture in which the focus is on the resulting adverse event rather than the error itself [30]. Another study of 30 surgeons who were observed disclosing errors to standardized patients found that the surgeons performed best when describing the medical facts of the case [30]. However, only 57% of the surgeons used the word "error" and only 65% clearly took responsibility for the error in their discussion [30]. The two poorest areas of performance of the surgeons were empathetic communication with the standardized patient (47% offered an apology) and having a discussion with the standardized patient about the prevention of future errors [30]. These studies suggest that surgeons may not always communicate openly with patients about errors potentially leading patients to believe that adverse events are unpreventable complications of their surgical care.

The disclosure gap that exists in surgical care is due in part to the lack of training of physicians in the disclosure of medical errors as few physicians and surgeons receive formal training [30, 31]. Yet, medical trainees are even less prepared to discuss medical errors [32] despite interpersonal and communication skills being a core competency of resident education mandated by the Accreditation Council for Graduate Medical Education [33]. Morbidity and mortality conferences are one opportunity for surgical trainees to observe and participate in error discussion as a survey of academic surgical residency program directors found that during mortality and morbidity conferences 74% of programs discuss all deaths and 50% of programs discuss all complications [34]. To teach interpersonal and communication skills in the setting of disclosure of medical errors, a study described a single institution's approach to training surgical residents with a web-based didactic course followed by a filmed review of the resident disclosing an error to a standardized patient [35]. We also believe that surgical training programs should provide didactic education on how errors should be disclosed and simulations to provide live feedback on communication techniques with the goal of patient-centered communication. Furthermore, there should be an emphasis on how to provide an explicit, sincere apology to a patient. Though some surgeons believe an apology is an admission of medical negligence and is inappropriate in error disclosure [35], patients desire apologies that "…acknowledge an error and its consequences, take responsibility, and communicate regret for having caused harm…" [36]. Facing one's own mistakes and apologizing may require training [36] but doing so fosters an environment of honest and direct communication that can preserve the physician-patient relationship.

Conclusion

Since the IOM report "To Err is Human," there has been a great focus on medical errors and the creation of systems to prevent the occurrence of these errors. Once an error happens, physician disclosure of the error and the consequences to the patient is ethically and professionally mandated. Nevertheless, there is a wide range of what information to disclose and how physicians perform the disclosure. Surgeons feel a sense of responsibility for their patients' outcomes and report that errors should be disclosed though they may not be direct in their communication or provide an apology. Institutional support, both for the emotional disruption that surgeons and physicians face and for disclosure training programs, is critical in advancing patient-centered communication and high-quality health care.

Case Resolutions

Case Presentation 1

In case presentation 1, the patient suffered a near miss when the IVC filter was nearly released from the snaring mechanism during filter removal. Despite the technical challenge, there was no harm to the patient and no disclosure of the intraoperative challenges was felt to be necessary. This case highlights the dilemma of disclosing near misses without complications.

Case Presentation 2

In case presentation 2, the patient suffers a serious error intraoperatively that also does not result in harm. This case demonstrates the internal dilemma surgeons may face when having to disclose a medical error. The patient did well but he suffered a significant intraoperative error, which could have led to significant harm. Although a stroke was described to the patient as a potential *complication* of the procedure during the consent process, a stroke was not described as a complication of the *error* that had occurred. In this case, the technical error was completely disclosed to the patient's family immediately after the surgery was completed. The following day when the patient's trachea was extubated and the patient was alert, the surgeon informed the patient of the technical error during surgery. The patient had done well since surgery and the patient and his family were very comfortable with the explanation of the problems that occurred in the operating room. The surgeon's open communication and disclosure of the technical error to the patient and family helped to maintain an honest relationship between the surgeon, the patient, and his family. Thus, full disclosures of medical error should be provided to every patient and their family to preserve the physician-patient relationship and uphold ethical principles.

Acknowledgment Edward Dunn, MD for providing expertise on error disclosure and the development of the disclosure training program at the Lexington VAMC.

References

1. Kohn L, Corrigan J, Donaldson M. To err is human: building a safer healthcare system. 1st ed. Washington, DC: Institute of Medicine, National Academy Press; 2000.
2. Gallagher TH, Garbutt JM, Waterman AD, Flum DR, Larson EB, Watern BM, et al. Choosing your words carefully. Arch Intern Med. 2006;166:1585–93.

3. Lingard L, Espin S, Whyte S, Regehr G, Baker GR, Reznick R, et al. Communication failures in the operating room: an observational classification of recurrent types and effects. Qual Saf Health Care. 2004;13:330–4.
4. Pinkus R. Learning to keep a cautious tongue: the reporting of mistakes in neurosurgery, 1890 to 1930. In: Rubin SB, Zoloth L, editors. Margin error: the ethics of mistakes in the practice of medicine. 1st ed. Hagerstown: University Publishing Group; 2000. p. 131–52.
5. Dunn EJ, McKinney KM, Martin ME. Empathic disclosure of adverse events to patients. Fed Pract. 2014;31(5):18–21.
6. Kraman SS, Hamm G. Risk management: extreme honesty may be the best policy. Ann Intern Med. 1999;131:963–7.
7. Hamm GM, Kraman SS. New standards, new dilemmas: reflections on managing medical mistakes. Bioethics Forum. 2001;17(2):19–25.
8. Joint Commission on Accreditation of Health Care Organizations. Revisions to Joint Commission standards in support of patient safety and medical health care error reduction: effective July 1, 2001. Oakbrook Terrace: JCAHO; 2001.
9. Gallagher TH, Studdert D, Levinson W. Disclosing harmful medical errors to patients. N Engl J Med. 2007;356:2713–9.
10. National Quality Forum (NQF). Safe practices for better healthcare-2010 update: a consensus report. Washington, DC: NQF; 2010.
11. Council on Ethical and Judicial Affairs. Code of Medical Ethics of the American Medical Association. 2014–2015th ed. Chicago: AMA; 2014.
12. Iezzoni LI, Rao SR, DesRoches CM, Vogeli C, Campbell EG. Survey shows that at least some physicians are not always open or honest with patients. Health Aff. 2012;31(2):383–91.
13. Griffen FD. The impact of transparency on patient safety and liability. Bull Am Coll Surg. 2008;93(3):19–23.
14. Clinton HR, Obama B. Making patient safety the centerpiece of medical liability reform. N Engl J Med. 2006;354(21):2205–8.
15. Griffen FD. ACS Closed Claims Study reveals critical failures to communicate. Bull Am Coll Surg. 2007;92(1):11–6.
16. Delbanco T, Bell SK. Guilty, afraid, and alone – struggling with medical error. N Engl J Med. 2007;357(17):1682–3.
17. Gallagher TH, Waterman AD, Ebers AG, Fraser VJ, Levinson W. Patients' and physicians' attitudes regarding the disclosure of medical errors. JAMA. 2003;289:1001–7.
18. Marcus L, Dorn B, McNulty E. Renegotiating health care: resolving conflict to build collaboration. 2nd ed. San Francisco: Jossey-Bass; 2011.
19. Mazor KM, Simon SR, Yood RA, Martinson BC, Gunter MJ, Reed GW, et al. Health plan members' views about disclosure of medical errors. Ann Intern Med. 2004;140:409–18.
20. Gawande A. Complications: a surgeon's notes on an imperfect science. 1st ed. New York: Picador; 2002.
21. American Medical Association (AMA). Medical liability reform. 2015. http://www.ama-assn.org/ama/pub/advocacy/topics/medical-liability-reform.page?. Accessed 10 May 2015.
22. Harrison R, Lawton R, Perlo J, Gardner P, Armitage G, Shapiro J. Emotion and coping in the aftermath of medical error: a cross-country exploration. J Patient Saf. 2015;11:28–35.
23. Waterman AD, Garbutt J, Hazel E, Dunagan WC, Levinson W, Fraser VJ, et al. The emotional impact of medical errors on practicing physicians in the United States and Canada. Jt Comm J Qual Patient Saf. 2007;33(8):467–76.
24. Banja J. Medical errors and medical narcissism. 1st ed. Sudbury: Jones and Bartlett Publishers; 2005.
25. Namm JP, Siegler M, Brander C, Kim TY, Lowe C, Angelos P. History and evolution of surgical ethics: John Gregory to the twenty-first century. World J Surg. 2014;38:1568–73.
26. Bosk CL. Forgive and remember: managing medical failure. 2nd ed. Chicago: The University of Chicago Press; 1979.
27. Sokol DK, Wilson J. What is a surgical complication? World J Surg. 2008;32(6):942–4.

28. Angelos P. Complications, errors, and surgical ethics. World J Surg. 2009;33:609–11.
29. Bell SK, White AA, Yi JC, Yi-Frazier JP, Gallagher TH. Transparency when things go wrong: physician attitudes about reporting medical errors to patients, peers, and institutions. J Patient Saf. 2015. doi:10.1097/PTS.0000000000000153.
30. Chan DK, Gallagher TH, Reznick R, Levinson W. How surgeons disclose medical errors to patients: a study using standardized patients. Surgery. 2005;138:851–8.
31. Pichert J, Hickson G, Trotter T. Malpractice and communication skills for difficult situations. Amb Child Health. 1998;4:213–21.
32. White AA, Bell SK, Krauss MJ, Garbutt J, Dunagan WC, Fraser VJ, et al. How trainees would disclose medical errors: educational implications for training programmes. Med Educ. 2011;45:372–80.
33. Accreditation Council for Graduate Medical Education. ACGME common program requirements. 2013. http://www.acgme.org/acgmeweb/Portals/0/PFAssets/ProgramRequirements/CPRs2013.pdf. Accessed 11 May 2015.
34. Gore DC. National survey of surgical morbidity and mortality conferences. Am J Surg. 2006;191(5):708–14.
35. Raper SE, Resnick AS, Morris JB. Simulated disclosure of a medical error by residents: development of a course in specific communication skills. J Surg Educ. 2014;71(6):e116–26.
36. Robbennolt JK. Apologies and medical error. Clin Orthop Relat Res. 2009;467:376–82.

Chapter 13
Futility and the Care of the Perioperative Patient

Scott B. Grant, Parth K. Modi, and Eric A. Singer

Abstract Futility in healthcare is an area of significant debate. Generally, a futile treatment is one that is incapable of producing a beneficial result. The degree of benefit required has been contentious in the ethics literature. Different definitions of futility have been proposed to arrive at a consensus regarding which treatments would be provided and to agree on futile interventions that could be withheld. However, each of these definitions has flaws. Some hospitals, healthcare organizations, and states have implemented policies to create a procedural approach to futility disputes. Several authors have advocated discarding the language of futility as it often is an expression of physician frustration and impedes communication between care providers, patients and their surrogates. Many resources are available to assist in difficult cases involving futility including preoperative risk calculators and institutional ethics committees, but, ultimately, the best tool in approaching these challenging situations is open and honest communication between the patient, or surrogate, and the physician.

Keywords Futility • End-of-Life Care • Inappropriate Treatment • Surgery • Anesthesiology • Perioperative

---

Scott B. Grant and Parth K. Modi have contributed equally to this chapter.

S.B. Grant, MD, MBE
Department of Surgery, Rutgers Robert Wood Johnson Medical School,
1 RWJ Place, MEB 596, New Brunswick, NJ 08901, USA
e-mail: Scott.B.Grant@gmail.com

P.K. Modi, MD
Department of Surgery, Division of Urology, Rutgers Robert Wood Johnson Medical School,
1 RWJ Place, MEB 584A, New Brunswick, NJ 08901, USA
e-mail: modi.parth@gmail.com

E.A. Singer, MD, MA, FACS (✉)
Department of Surgery, Section of Urologic Oncology, Rutgers Cancer Institute of New Jersey, Rutgers Robert Wood Johnson Medical School, 195 Little Albany Street, Room 4563, New Brunswick, NJ 08903, USA
e-mail: eric.singer@rutgers.edu

B.G. Jericho (ed.), *Ethical Issues in Anesthesiology and Surgery*,
DOI 10.1007/978-3-319-15949-2_13

Case Presentations

In order to frame the issues covered in this chapter, we have compiled several seminal cases involving futility conflicts and their resolution. While numerous technological advances have been made in the four decades since the Quinlan case, the challenges faced by health care providers and families remain stubbornly constant.

1975 – Karen Quinlan – Karen Ann Quinlan was a 21-year-old female who was celebrating a friend's birthday at a bar, when she began to fall asleep [1]. Her friends brought her home. When they realized that she was not breathing, they gave her mouth-to-mouth resuscitation and called an ambulance [1]. She arrived at Newton Memorial Hospital on April 15, 1975, was placed on a ventilator, and subsequently developed pneumonia [1]. After five months and a fifty-pound weight loss, Karen was still on the ventilator. Her adoptive parents sought legal help to withdraw the ventilator [1, 2]. Karen had irreversible brain damage and would never recover. Her parents agreed with the religious advice of Pope Pius XII, from his 1957 pronouncement, that there is no moral obligation to maintain life via "extraordinary means" [1]. Karen's parents signed a form authorizing the attending physician to withdraw the ventilator [1]. The medical team decided not to withdraw the ventilator. The Quinlans then asked the court to declare Karen incompetent and appoint her father, Joseph, as her guardian so that he could order the withdrawal of the ventilator [1]. The court took the petition on October 20, 1975 and a Morris County New Jersey (NJ) Superior Court Judge appointed a public defender to watch out for Karen's interests [1, 2]. The NJ Superior Court rendered a decision on November 10, 1975 denying Karen's father to be appointed her guardian so he could authorize the withdrawal of the ventilator [2, 3]. The NJ Supreme Court rendered a unanimous decision written by Chief Justice Richard J. Hughes (announced March 31, 1976), which overturned the NJ Superior Court ruling and ruled in the Quinlan's favor [3]. The NJ Supreme Court ruled in favor of the constitutional right of privacy with a patient's right to decline medical treatment in certain circumstances, and permitted this right of privacy to be exercised by proxy using substituted judgment (in this case by Karen's father) [3]. The court added two qualifications to the exercise of the right of privacy by proxy including: (1) a prognosis by the attending physicians and (2) concurrence in the prognosis by an "ethics committee" [3]. The NJ Supreme Court also applied an "ordinary-extraordinary" distinction as mentioned above by Pope Pius XII [3], and found no difference between terminating artificial nutrition and hydration and discontinuing a mechanical ventilator [4]. After withdrawal of the ventilator, Karen Quinlan continued to breath on her own for 9 years and died June 11, 1985 of pneumonia.

In re Quinlan, 70 NJ 10, 355 A. 2d 647, cert denied, 429 US 922 (1976)

1983 – Claire Conroy was an 83-year-old female who lived in a nursing home in New Jersey for three years with "organic brain syndrome". She later developed diabetic necrotic decubitus ulcers on her left foot and was transferred to the hospital on July 21, 1982 where doctors recommended an above the knee amputation of her left leg [4–6]. Her guardian (her nephew) refused to give consent for the amputation and later demanded that Claire Conroy's nasogastric feeding tube be removed. However, her physicians refused to remove the feeding tube, so the guardian petitioned the court for the authority to remove it [5, 6]. At that time, Claire Conroy weighed 50 pounds and was unable to speak. After the court proceedings, Judge Stanton (who had visited the patient) ordered removal of the feeding tube on February 2, 1983 (In re Conroy, 188 N.J. Super. 523 [Ch. Div. 1983]); however, his decision was held, pending appeal [5, 6]. On February 15, 1983, the patient died with the nasogastric tube still in place [5]. On July 8, 1983, the New Jersey appellate court reversed the lower court's decision [5]. The appellate court opinion read: "The trial judge authorized euthanasia … If the trial judge's order had been enforced, Conroy would not have died as the result of an existing medical condition, but rather she would have died, and painfully so, as the result of a new and independent condition: dehydration and starvation. Thus she would have been actively killed by independent means" [5]. The guardian ad litem then brought the case to the NJ Supreme Court, who in January 1985 declared that terminating any medical treatment, including artificial nutrition and hydration, on incompetent patients is lawful if certain criteria are met [4]. As a result, it is now widely accepted legally and in medical ethics, that artificial nutrition and hydration are medical interventions that can be withheld or withdrawn in the same manner as any other medical intervention (see also Cruzan below).

In the matter of Claire Conroy, Sup Ct. N.J. App. Div., A-2483-82, July 8, 1983; 486 A.2d 1209 (1985)

1990 – Nancy Cruzan – Nancy Beth Cruzan was in a motor vehicle collision in January 1983 [7]. She was in a persistent vegetative state after the accident and was maintained on artificial nutrition and hydration via a gastrostomy tube inserted with the consent of her husband [7]. Nancy's parents sought to end her tube feedings, being convinced that she would not want to continue living in a persistent vegetative state [7]. A Missouri trial court authorized the withdrawal of Nancy Cruzan's artificial nutrition and hydration, but this decision was overturned in November 1988 by the Missouri Supreme Court [7]. The Missouri Supreme Court argued that the state had an "unqualified" interesting in preserving life which should supersede the right of guardians to refuse treatment in the absence of "clear and convincing evidence" that this would be the patient's wish [7, 8]. Cruzan became the first "right to die" case heard by the United States (US) Supreme Court, which rendered its decision in June 1990 [7, 8]. The US Supreme Court affirmed the Missouri Supreme Court's decision, but established at least three important holdings [8]. First, there is a constitutional right to refuse treatment based on a protected "liberty interest" [8, 9]. Second, the right to refuse treatment persists despite a patient becoming incompetent [8]. Third, states may create different procedural safeguards and standards of evidence to ensure that withdrawal of treatment reflects the patient's wishes when the patient lacks the capacity to make medical decisions [8]. Finally, Justice Sandra Day O'Connor wrote a concurring opinion in Cruzan with four other members of the Supreme Court stating, "artificial feeding cannot readily be distinguished from other forms of medical treatment" [9]. After testimony by witnesses that withdrawing artificial nutrition reflected Nancy Cruzan's wishes, artificial nutrition and hydration were withdrawn in December 1990. Nancy Cruzan died two weeks later.

Cruzan v. Harmon, 760 S. W. 2d 408 (1988)

Cruzan v. Director, Missouri Dept of Health, 110 S. Ct. 2841, 497 US 261 (1990)

US Supreme Court decision 1990

1991 – Helga Wanglie was an 85-year-old female patient residing in a nursing home. On January 1, 1990, she was transferred to Hennepin County Medical Center with complaints of dyspnea. At the medical center, Helga Wanglie was intubated, she was placed on a ventilator, and she remained in a persistent vegetative state for over a year [10, 11]. Physicians recommended stopping mechanical ventilation suggesting that it was "nonbeneficial" [11]. The hospital went to court after Steven H. Miles, MD, the ethics committee consultant at the Hennepin County Medical Center who evaluated the patient, and the medical director and hospital administrator petitioned to get permission to withdraw treatment [10, 11]. The patient's husband, daughter, and son successfully asserted that substituted judgment about the patient's view of what constitutes appropriate medical intervention should take precedence over the medical team's view that mechanical ventilation was not beneficial [10, 11]. Helga Wanglie subsequently died of sepsis on July 4, 1991 [10, 11]. The court decision occurred 3 days prior to her death [10]. This case created the legal hierarchy of authority regarding medical decision making so that the patient and his or her next of kin or a designated health proxy take precedence over the physician's recommendation [10].

In re Helga Wanglie, Fourth Judicial District (Dist. Ct., Probate Ct. Div.) PX-91-283. Minnesota Hennepin County.

1993–1994 – Baby K– Baby K was diagnosed prenatally with anencephaly and pregnancy termination was recommended by both the obstetrician and neonatologist [12]. Nonetheless, Baby K was born by cesarean section on October 13, 1992 [12]. Baby K had difficulty breathing at birth, was intubated, and mechanical ventilation was begun [12]. Within days of the birth, the physicians urged the mother (since the father was only remotely involved) to discontinue mechanical ventilation because it was medically inappropriate and to place a Do Not Resuscitate order, but the mother refused [12]. The hospital ethics committee and a subcommittee became involved, and the subcommittee decided on October 22 that if the difference of opinion continued, the hospital should seek legal resolution [12]. Baby K was transferred to a nursing home on November 30 not on mechanical ventilation. On January 15, 1993, Baby K returned to the hospital for mechanical ventilation and stayed until February 12 [12]. Fairfax Hospital went to federal court to seek a ruling that they were not obligated to provide "inappropriate" treatment if Baby K were to return to the emergency department in respiratory distress [12]. The mother argued that "all human life has value," whereas the hospital, the guardian ad litem appointed by the court, and Baby K's father all thought that further mechanical ventilation was medically and ethically inappropriate [12]. District Court Judge Claude Hilton used the Emergency Medical Treatment and Active Labor Act (EMTALA), section 504 of the Rehabilitation Act, and the Americans with Disabilities Act to argue that hospitals cannot discriminate against anencephalic infants who present with an emergency medical condition such as respiratory distress and must provide treatment [12].

Furthermore, when there is no "finding of neglect or abuse," parents have the right to make medical decisions for their children, and when parents disagree, courts should support the parent who decides "in favor of life" [12]. On February 10, 1994, the US Court of Appeals, in a two-to-one opinion, affirmed Judge Hilton's ruling, arguing the EMTALA did not provide an exception for anencephalic infants and required continued mechanical ventilation for Baby K [12]. Baby K died April 5, 1995 at the hospital.

In re Baby K, 832 F. Supp. 1022 (E.D. Va. 1993), 16 F. 3d 590 (4th Cir. 1994

1995 – Gilgunn v. Massachusetts General Hospital – Catherine Gilgunn was a 71-year-old female who fell in her home in mid-May 1989, but only presented to Massachusetts General Hospital (MGH) on June 7, 1989 with a diagnosis of a recurrent left hip fracture [13, 14]. Nine days into her hospitalization, Catherine experienced multiple seizures that left her comatose [13, 14]. Dr. Cassem, who directed MGH's optimal care committee (MGH's ethics committee), issued a do not resuscitate (DNR) order, which was withdrawn after the patient's daughter Joan Gilgunn objected. Catherine had a tracheostomy and a gastrostomy tube placed with the family's consent [15]. After obtaining approval from MGH's optimal care committee and assuming care of Catherine, a month later Dr. Dec reinstated the DNR order for Catherine [13, 15]. Dr. Dec had begun weaning the ventilator support provided to Catherine starting on August 7, Catherine was extubated, and she was placed on CPAP for more than ten hours [13, 14, 16]. Catherine Gilgunn died three days after Dr. Dec placed the DNR order on August 10 1989. Joan Gilgunn claims she was never told of the second DNR order, although two of her four siblings agreed with the hospital's decision [13]. Joan Gilgunn then sued Dr. Cassem and Dr. Dec, seeking damages for the mental anguish that she suffered because her mother's wishes were not followed [13]. Judge David Roseman presided over the Suffolk Superior Court that vindicated Dr. Cassem and Dr. Dec, where the jury found that although Catherine Gilgunn would have wanted treatment continued, such care was ultimately "futile" [13]. This case ruled that cardiopulmonary resuscitation need not be provided to a patient dying with multiple organ system failure, even if requested by the patient's family, since CPR is ineffective in these circumstances and would cause harm [15]. However, this ruling did not create a legal precedent since it was only a jury verdict, was not heard at an appellate level, and the plaintiff withdrew her appeal on January 21, 1998 [15].

Gilgunn v. Massachusetts General Hospital, Super. Ct. Civ. Action No. 92–4820, Suffolk Co., Mass., verdict, 21 April 1995

Joan Gilgunn v. Massachusetts General Hospital, et al. Massachusetts Appeals Court case no. 97-P-2150

1995 – Baby Sun Hudson – Baby Sun Hudson was a full-term baby born with thanatrophic dysplasia, which is a lethal genetic condition [17]. The condition is characterized by underdeveloped lungs, small ribs, and a narrow small chest [17]. The mother had not received prenatal care, the physicians were unaware of the fetus' medical status at birth, and thus the physician's resuscitated the newborn at delivery [17]. Once the diagnosis was made, the physicians recommended withdrawal of treatment but the mother refused [17]. The mother had a psychiatric history and claimed that the "Sun" fathered her child [17]. The doctors felt that continued treatment was inhumane because the infant was "slowly suffocating because his lungs lack the capacity to support his body" [17]. The hospital invoked the Texas Advance Directives Act of 1999 (see chapter for more details), and some 40 hospitals declined to accept the child in transfer [17]. Texas Children's Hospital was reluctant to unilaterally withdraw treatment given the mother's questionable mental status, and so sought legal resolution [17]. A Harris County Probate judge ruled that Texas Children's Hospital had no obligation to continue medical treatment. However, the ruling was appealed and the First Texas Court of Appeals in Houston sent the case back to the probate judge on a procedural question [17]. That issue was resolved and the probate judge again ruled that the hospital could withdraw treatment, which occurred nearly 6 months after Sun Hudson's birth [17]. Sun Hudson died moments later [17].

Hudson v. Texas Children's Hospital. Court of Appeals of Texas, Houston (1st Dist.). No. 01-05-00143-CV. March 1, 2005.

Introduction

Even Hippocrates, in *The Art*, recognized the limits of medicine and discussed the concept of medical futility: "Whenever a man suffers from an illness, which is too strong for the means at the disposal of medicine, he surely must not expect that it can be overcome by medicine" [18]. However, while trying to treat a certain disease in one generation may be futile, scientific and medical progress permit the same disease to be effectively treated in subsequent generations. For instance, in the last century, antibiotics, antivirals, and antifungals were developed to treat infections; insulin and other classes of medications were developed to treat diabetes; dialysis and kidney transplantation were developed to counteract end-stage renal disease; and intubation, mechanical ventilation and tracheostomy can permit survival despite pulmonary failure.

While medical and technological advances have made the treatment of many diseases and the prolongation of life more successful, every person will eventually die. At some point in the course of a person's life, aggressive, invasive, or toxic medical treatments are no longer appropriate, and providing them are no longer in his or her best interest. In our current medical system, disagreements often arise as to when that point has been reached, for which interventions, and who should make that determination. These disagreements commonly revolve around a powerful, but vague, term: Futility.

What Is "Futility"?

The Oxford English Dictionary defines futile as something that is "Incapable of producing any result; failing utterly of the desired end through intrinsic defect; useless, ineffectual, vain" [19]. While this strict dictionary definition is what comes to mind when most people think of futility, many authors have attempted to define medical futility by various criteria.

The strictest such conception is *physiologic futility*. Clark and Minkus define physiologic futility as "treatments that fail to achieve their intended physiological effect" [20]. Alternatively, *quantitatively futile* treatments are those that have an exceedingly low probability of success [21]. Examples of physiologically futile treatments include performing CPR on a patient who has exsanguinated and treating a patient suffering from the common cold with antibiotics (not antivirals). This definition of futility seems, on its face, to be easy to accept. Who would want a treatment that is certain not to achieve its intended effect? Why should society pay for such an intervention? However, the determination that a treatment will have no effect is sometimes a probabilistic calculation [22] and rational people may disagree as to what probability of effect is worth pursuing. On the other hand, while proponents of quantitative futility decision-making models cite its objective and scientific basis, empiric data does not exist for every clinical situation and specific probabilities cannot always be calculated.

The counterpart to quantitative futility is *qualitative futility*, which can be defined as treatment that fails to lead to an acceptable quality of life for the patient [20].

While mechanical ventilation of a patient in a persistent vegetative state would not be quantitatively futile (as it has the intended physiological effect of oxygenation), it would be considered qualitatively futile by those who do not find the resulting quality of life acceptable. This is one of the most contentious areas of futility, as an "acceptable quality of life" varies greatly across patients and societies. In a medical culture that places great value in patient autonomy, establishing a universal standard for acceptable quality of life has so many pitfalls as to be virtually impossible.

Imminent demise futility refers to treatments for patients who are expected to die in the near future regardless of the success of that intervention [23]. While such an intervention may improve the functioning of one or more organ systems, it is considered futile if it will not prevent the impending death of the patient. A similar category is *lethal condition futility* that includes interventions for patients who have a terminal illness but for whom treatment may prolong life without improving the patient's chance for survival from his or her disease [24, 25].

Opponents of these futility definitions argue that they may often be used to distance the provider from difficult cases and patients at the end of life rather than promoting valuable, though challenging, conversations between the medical team and the patient's family and surrogates [24]. Furthermore, these conceptions of futility place a strong emphasis on the ability of the physician to predict survival. With new and emerging treatment modalities, limited empirical data and an ever-complex variety of patients and clinical situations, the accuracy of survival prognostication is far from certain [26, 27].

Principle-Based Approach to Futility

Autonomy has become arguably the most important ethical principle in our current health care system, often taking priority over others. Schneiderman and colleagues argue that the moral and legal importance of patient self-determination came about as a response to the previous model of paternalistic medicine [21]. The right of a patient to choose for himself or herself whether to receive or refuse treatments is a well-accepted result of this focus on patient autonomy. This autonomy can become problematic, however, when patients (or surrogates) insist on care that is considered futile by health care providers. While patients have the ethical and legal right to accept or reject treatment, autonomy does not give patients the right to demand any medical treatment they choose [20]. Patient autonomy must be balanced with physician conscience – the right of a physician to practice medicine in a responsible and rational way, consistent with professional norms. As moral agents, both physicians and patients have the right to self-determination, but not the right to impose their will on the other [28].

The complementary ethical principles of beneficence (an obligation to do good for another) and nonmaleficence (an obligation to prevent harm or injury) are also central to this discussion of futility. Absolute nonmaleficence is impossible, with many possible side effects and harms associated with any treatment or intervention. Often, balancing these benefits and harms is necessary. Clark and Minkus argue that physicians, with their medical and scientific expertise, are best suited at evaluating the quantitative benefits and harms of a proposed therapy, while patients and surrogates, with their insight into the patient's wishes, are best suited to determine the qualitative benefits and harms [20]. This analysis provides support for a shared decision making model of futility determination and emphasizes the need for open and honest communication among physicians and patients/surrogates.

Finally, the ethical principle of justice states that all people should be treated fairly and equally. In the area of medical futility, distributive justice is central. Medical resources are finite and providing futile care consumes those resources without benefit, potentially depriving others of their use. This principle highlights the importance of the concept of futility in general and in avoiding futile interventions and care. In addition, it establishes society as a stakeholder in the conversation about medical futility.

Virtue-Based Approach to Futility

Aristotle described the virtue of "phronesis", meaning practical knowledge or wisdom [29]. Phronesis is not scientific knowledge or technical ability, but the knowledge of how to act in complex situations by both understanding the facts of the situation and correctly judging the appropriate goals [30]. Pellegrino, informed by the writings of Saint Thomas Aquinas who integrated the Aristotelian virtue of phronesis with the Catholic virtue of prudence, applied the virtue of prudence to the problem of futility. Pellegrino argued that futility should be used as a "prudential guide" – the weighing of a treatment's effectiveness, benefits, and burdens in the context of a patient's clinical situation [24, 28].

In this context, Pellegrino avers that a treatment's benefits are not quantifiable by the physician, but are instead based on the values and subjective view of the patient or his surrogate [24, 28]. Treatment burdens, on the other hand, have both objective and subjective aspects and therefore must be considered by both patient and physician. Finally, treatment effectiveness is objective in nature, relies on empirical evidence, and is within the realm of the physician's expertise. The assessment of these three criteria, combining the subjective and objective inputs from appropriate participants, ultimately leads to a joint decision on futility questions [28]. This approach, argues Pellegrino, avoids the automatic labeling of certain clinical conditions or categories of a patient as "futile" and instead recognizes that multiple aspects of a situation must be carefully considered by both the patient/surrogate and the treatment team [28].

Patient Autonomy Versus Surgeon Conscience

The Society of Critical Care Medicine, in its 1997 consensus statement regarding futile treatment, described three contexts in which the language of futility is used [31]: First, when the patient or surrogate and the physician agree that the benefits of treatment are outweighed by its burdens; second, when the patient or surrogate desire an intervention which the caregiver regards as having no benefit and believes should be withheld; finally, when a community or insurer wishes to allocate limited and costly resources and labels certain controversial and/or expensive treatments as futile to justify denying coverage for them. Of these three categories, the first rarely results in conflict and the third is now considered a problem of rationing, and not truly a question of futility. The second scenario, one of conflict between patient and physician, is most commonly thought of when discussing medical futility.

Helft and colleagues have asserted that physicians have historically used futility as a justification for unilaterally withholding certain treatments from patients against their (or their surrogates') will [32]. Several authors have argued that while physicians may understand the scientific basis of disease and therapy, futility is at its root a subjective question of value and is best answered by the patient [32–35]. Champions of physician conscience, however, argue that the physician, like the patient, is a moral agent [36]. Allowing the patient's autonomy to override the physician's conscience is to reduce the physician to simply an extension of the patient's wishes [36]. Consensus has not been reached on this debate, as it is not simply a question of which side is right or wrong, but, as Helft et al. put it, "a complex network of relational obligations" [32].

How Do We Resolve Futility Disputes?

Virtually every hospital ethics committee has heard end-of-life cases in which a surrogate decision maker insisted that "everything" be done. In the early 1990s, representatives of ethics committees in the greater Houston area met during monthly meetings of the Houston Bioethics Network and had discussions about medical futility policy, and in August 1993 convened an ad hoc group to create a multi-institution futility policy [25]. The group relied on a procedural approach rather than a definition of futility, focusing on an open and fair process grounded on professional and institutional integrity balanced by patient autonomy [25]. The Houston multi-institution collaborative policy on medical futility (HMICPMF) sought to minimize four problems: "nonparticipation by the patient or surrogate, unilateral physician action, ignoring patient transfer options, and the potential for patient abandonment" [25]. The policy was designed to supplement existing policies permitting autonomous refusal or limitation of unwanted interventions, seeking to provide a conflict resolution mechanism for when a patient or surrogate decision maker requested an intervention a responsible physician assessed as medically inappropriate [25].

The HMICPMF permits a medically inappropriate intervention to be withheld or withdrawn without the consent of the patient or surrogate decision maker if the procedural approach is followed [25]. This approach starts with the physician discussing options, including palliative and hospice care, explaining the reasons the intervention is medically inappropriate, and assuring the patient and surrogate(s) that not providing the intervention does not mean they are being abandoned [25]. The physician also needs to discuss the possibility of patient transfer to another physician or another institution, and provide the patient or surrogate(s) with a copy of the HMICPMF guidelines [25]. If, after reasonable effort, agreement is not reached, the physician must obtain a second opinion from another physician and must then present the case for review by an institutional interdisciplinary body [25]. The physician must then notify the patient or surrogate(s) that the process has been started, and describe what it involves, possible outcomes, the possibility of transfer before the interdisciplinary review, and that the meeting will not take place for at least 72 hours unless the patient or surrogate(s) consents to an earlier time [25]. The patient or surrogate(s) are encouraged to attend the review process [25]. If the review process finds that the intervention is medically inappropriate, the intervention may be stopped, but only the intervention deemed inappropriate may be stopped (all other medically appropriate interventions are continued) [25]. Furthermore, transfer within the same institution to another physician to provide the intervention deemed medically inappropriate by the review committee will not be allowed [25].

The Texas Advance Directives Act of 1999 (TADA) went into effect on September 1, 1999, and supplanted the HMICPMF. TADA provides a legal safe harbor for the treatment team and institution if they follow the provisions below [37]:

1. The patient/surrogate(s) must be given written information on hospital policy on the ethics consultation process.
2. The patient/surrogate(s) must be given 48 hours advanced notice and invited to participate in the ethics consultation process.
3. The ethics or medical committee or consultation team must provide a written report of their findings to the patient/surrogate(s).
4. If the ethics consultation process fails to resolve the futility dispute, the hospital must work with the patient/surrogate(s) to attempt to arrange transfer to another physician and institution who are willing to provide the requested care refused by the current treatment team.
5. If no accepting physician or institution can be found after 10 days, then the treatment team can unilaterally withhold or withdraw the interventions determined to be futile by the ethics consultation process.
6. The patient/surrogate(s) may appeal to the Texas state court and request an extension from the judge before treatment is withdrawn. This extension will be granted by the judge only if the judge determines that there is a reasonable likelihood of finding an accepting physician or institution for transfer if more time is granted (not on the merits of whether the treatment is futile).
7. If an extension is not sought or not granted by the judge then futile treatment may be unilaterally withdrawn or withheld with immunity from civil or criminal prosecution.

Provision seven provides the "legal safe harbor" for physicians, institutions, and ethics committees, and is the first in the country regarding futility [37]. The Texas Hospital Association distributed written information to its member hospitals in March 2000 on the essential provisions of TADA, and notified its members in June 2003 when the law was amended [38].

Smith et al. performed a study to determine awareness and experience with TADA among Texas Hospital Association hospitals during the first 5 years of implementation (9/1999–7/2004) [38]. They sent a 20-item written survey to 409 hospital members of the Texas Hospital Association in 2004, and 200 surveys were returned with 197 usable for analysis (48.2% response rate) [38]. Smith et al. found that 81% of respondents (n=159) were aware of the TADA review process, and only 30% (n=58) had reviewed actual cases [38]. Forty hospitals reported reviewing 256 cases – 213 adult cases (83%) and 42 pediatric cases (16%) [38]. Hospitals reviewed anywhere from only 1 to 77 cases, although Smith et al. acknowledged that it is possible that the hospital reporting 77 cases conflated ethics consultations regarding inappropriate treatment with the formal TADA process [38]. Review committees agreed with physicians that treatment was inappropriate in 70% of the 256 cases reviewed [38]. In cases where the treatment was determined to be inappropriate, before the end of the 10-day waiting period, 78 patients died, 71 patients or surrogates agreed to withdraw the inappropriate treatment, 30 patients were transferred to another institution, and eight patients from three hospitals (six from one hospital) improved and appropriateness of treatment was reassessed [38]. After the 10-day waiting period, 33 patients had treatment discontinued and 45 patients had treatment continued [38]. The reality that in eight cases patients improved suggests that the determination of inappropriate treatment was inaccurate, and these cases should serve as a caution for future reviews to assess the clinical facts with empirical data and evidenced-based medical judgments [38]; quality assurance in these judgments is critical because if the committee is wrong the patient will likely die.

The "vast majority of states' advance directives statutes include language affirming healthcare providers' ethical right to decline to comply with patients' advance directives" [38]. Eight states have statutes that affirm a physician's ability to forgo providing requested treatment [38]: California [39], Maine [40], Maryland [41], Massachusetts [42], New York [43], Tennessee [44], Virginia [45], and Washington [46].

The American Medical Association (AMA) Council on Ethical and Judicial Affairs (CEJA) also created a report on medical futility in end-of-life care, with guidelines recommending a process-based approach [47]. They describe the range of ways in which "futile" has been used in a medical context, as described above, including quantitative futility, the intent of prolonging dying, and community or institutional standards of futility [47]. They reference other CEJA reports, including establishing the ethical permissibility of withdrawing and withholding interventions, the benefits of advance care planning in preventing contentious situations, and orders not to intervene such as do not resuscitate (DNR) or do not attempt resuscitation (DNAR) orders [47]. They correctly identify that the root of many futility disputes is a "discrepancy between the values or goals of the involved parties," with patients or surrogates wanting to pursue treatment whereas physicians see death as inevitable and prefer comfort care only, or vice-versa [47]. The report carefully distinguishes futility and resource allocation from rationing, acknowledging that while both futility judgments and allocation decisions need to be made, futility arguments should not resort to resource-saving criteria as their basis, and that "rationing needs should not motivate declarations of futility" [47]. CEJA cautions not to use futility as an excuse to avoid difficult discussions [47].

The fair process approach with due process standards proposed by AMA CEJA focuses on the process between parties rather than defining futility and imposing that definition on the parties [47]. The process would be adjudicated by a regulatory body of the institution or community with membership composition legitimizing its authority, likely including both patient/public representation and healthcare professionals [47]. The regulatory body would need transparency in its development and in its fair process policies [47]. The first recommended step is deliberation and negotiating a shared understanding between patient or proxy and physician about what constitutes futile care and what are acceptable limits for the physician and institution; ideally this should occur before critical illness [47]. If a shared understanding is not reached, transfer of care can be arranged to preempt conflict later [47]. Second, joint decision making using outcomes data whenever possible in an informed consent process should occur between patient or proxy and physician [47]. Third, an individual consultant and/or patient representative can be brought in to facilitate discussions that will help resolve the conflict [47]. Fourth, an institutional committee such as an ethics committee can be involved if disagreements have not been resolved. The format of this committee (ad hoc, preidentified subgroup, or whole committee) must be structured so that the patient or proxy's side is represented, either by community representation on the committee, permitting the patient or proxy to call for ethics committee involvement, and/or permitting the patient or proxy to attend the meeting [47]. Fifth, if the committee decides with the patient/proxy but the physician is unpersuaded, transfer to another physician within the institution may be arranged; conversely, if the committee decides with the physician but the patient/proxy is unpersuaded, transfer to another institution may be sought. Finally, transfer to another physician or institution may not be possible because none can be found willing to follow the patient/proxy's wishes. Perhaps this transfer is not possible because the request violates medical ethical normative values. In this case, ethically, the intervention need not be provided, "although the legal ramifications of this course of action are uncertain" [47]. Many times the healthcare team feels that certain treatments are futile and should be stopped, but is reluctant to do so if the family does not consent to withholding or withdrawing treatment because of the potential legal ramifications that will ensue.

In 2015, a group of professional societies (American Thoracic Society, American Association for Critical Care Nurses, American College of Chest Physicians, European Society for Intensive Care Medicine, and Society of Critical Care), developed recommendations to "prevent and manage intractable disagreements" about potentially inappropriate treatments in an intensive care unit setting [48]. This consensus statement included four recommendations:

1. "Institutions should implement strategies to prevent intractable treatment conflicts, including proactive communication and early involvement of expert consultants.
2. The term "potentially inappropriate" should be used, rather than futile, to describe treatments that have at least some chance of accomplishing the effect sought by the patient, but clinicians believe that competing ethical considerations justify not providing them. Clinicians should explain and advocate for the

treatment plan they believe is appropriate. Conflicts regarding potentially inappropriate treatments that remain intractable despite intensive communication and negotiation should be managed by a fair process of conflict resolution; this process should include hospital review, attempts to find a willing provider at another institution, and opportunity for external review of decisions. When time pressures make it infeasible to complete all steps of the conflict-resolution process and clinicians have a high degree of certainty that the requested treatment is outside accepted practice, they should seek procedural oversight to the extent allowed by the clinical situation and need not provide the requested treatment.

3. Use of the term "futile" should be restricted to the rare situations in which surrogates request interventions that simply cannot accomplish their intended physiologic goal. Clinicians should not provide futile interventions.
4. The medical profession should lead public engagement efforts and advocate for policies and legislation about when life-prolonging technologies should not be used" [48].

The Futility Conflict

Rowland et al. published a hypothetical case analysis regarding aggressive surgery on a severely demented patient who lacks decision-making capacity and has a thigh sarcoma with pulmonary metastasis [49]. They discuss several important points regarding surgical futility distinguishing between the following: what can be done, including aggressive surgery; what should be done including less aggressive palliative surgery; or declining to perform surgery and offering nonoperative palliative care [49]. Rowland et al. highlight the surgical futility concept that sometimes the patient or surrogate(s)' goals of therapy are not possible outcomes of surgical intervention. Therefore, surgeons play a vital role in educating patients and surrogate decision makers on prognosis, burdens of treatment, and realistic expectations for recovery and functionality and how this could impact postoperative quality of life [49]. Furthermore, in patients with dementia, operative interventions may exacerbate diminished cognitive capacity and worsen mental status. Demented patients also have greater difficulty recovering from surgery because of their inability to participate in postoperative care [49]. Additionally, patients with advanced dementia may lack decision-making capacity, necessitating surrogate decision makers [49]. The surrogate decision makers must be reminded that they must choose the treatment the patient would choose for himself or herself. Furthermore, even if the family wants everything done because it is difficult to potentially lose a close family member, the family must consider whether the patient would feel the same way [49]. Rowland et al. also discuss the hierarchy by which decisions should be made, starting first by examining advance directives, next using substituted judgment to act in accordance with the patient's unstated wishes, and finally following a best interest standard, based on achieving the best outcome for a patient given the range of anticipated treatment outcomes [49]. Best interest does not necessarily mean pursuing the most aggressive treatment, since a poor quality of life and little ability to engage in surroundings postoperatively may be worse than palliative options [49].

Although it is not often invoked in the US, the ethical concept of distributive justice and allocation of scarce resources or health care rationing, based on the expected quality of life achievable, is one other consideration [49]. It is also important to acknowledge that whereas surgeons may know the achievable and likely outcomes of operative intervention better than the patient or surrogate(s), the patient or surrogate(s) may not have the same perspective on the value of a certain postoperative quality of life and thus may disagree about whether the proposed intervention is futile [49]. Rowland et al. discuss an "ethics bottom line," including that the first question to ask in discussions of surgical futility should be: "Is this appropriate care for the patient?" [49]. The answer to this question hinges on whether surgery can realistically meet the desired treatment goals. Furthermore, in cases where the utility of surgical intervention is questioned, it is important to distinguish between inappropriate surgical therapy (e.g. attempting cure with unresectable disease), and "effective surgical therapy with controversial beneficial outcome" (e.g. aggressive surgery with low likelihood of cure and significant detriment to postoperative quality of life) [49]. It is also important to distinguish withdrawing on a futility basis with physician-assisted suicide. The difference is the cause of death: underlying end-stage disease in withdrawing for futility versus the drug(s) prescribed in physician-assisted suicide [50].

Disagreements in these situations are simply about a failure to communicate or a lack of trust in the prognosis described by the healthcare team. Zier et al. found that 88% of surrogate decision makers of critically ill patients doubted the physician's poor prognosis [51]. Grossman and Angelos titled their paper "Futility: What Cool Hand Luke Can Teach the Surgical Community," because of the iconic line from the movie with Paul Newman "What we've got here is a failure to communicate" [52]. Angelos relates a case in which he told a patient's family that additional treatment of the patient would prolong suffering and be futile. Angelos recommended that aggressive treatment cease and comfort care measures be initiated. The family became suspicious and distrustful, questioning how a stranger could know when the burdens outweighed the benefits of the treatment [52]. Using the term "futile" created a disconnect, isolating the family from the healthcare team [52]. Grossman and Angelos believe the concept of medical futility is a by-product of the deteriorating physician-patient relationship as a result of the once paternalistic relationship now being based primarily on patient autonomy. Futility is a power-grab by physicians to retake decision-making power and thus marginalize and limit patient or proxy participation in future decision making [52].

Invoking "futility" risks creating feelings of patient abandonment. Most importantly, declaring a situation "futile" does not achieve the intended goal, and instead often leads to patient and proxy confusion and stress and physician frustration [52]. Grossman and Angelos ultimately conclude that futility be struck from the professional lexicon since the term "worsens communication, and lessens patient care" [52]. Instead, they recommend "that increased efforts be made to educate patients and their families regarding realistic expectations of the patient's disease and its prognosis" and, if necessary, invoke the term "medically and surgically inappropriate" [52]. Grossman and Angelos recommend that we communicate, honestly disclose status and prognosis, "offer our best medical advice, and never hide behind the term *futility*" [52].

Another issue in the conflict surrounding futility is healthcare providers' moral distress when they are compelled to provide treatments that cause suffering without the ability to cure, or to provide treatments that prolong the dying process without achieving palliation, thus violating the principles of beneficence and nonmaleficence. This view led to a discussion of physician autonomy and conscientious objection to providing interventions that would cause suffering at the request of family or surrogate decision makers. It must be acknowledged, however, that when healthcare providers refuse to provide care, the families and the patients are those who live with the long-term consequences of those decisions. Thus, if a physician cannot in good conscience provide a treatment, it is the physician's obligation to arrange for a transfer of care to another provider.

The role of anesthesiologists in providing or participating in futile perioperative interventions has received little attention in the medical literature. However, Nurok and Sadovnikoff discuss the different roles that the anesthesiologist can play while observing the fiduciary duty to the patient, including: service provider, consultant, or gatekeeper [53]. They reject the anesthesiologist as service provider, since viewing an anesthesiologist as a mere technician diminishes the moral responsibility of the anesthesiologist [53]. Anesthesiologists can be seen as consultants, and Nurok and Sadoynikoff credit the National Health Service of Great Britain where patients with significant comorbidities facing high-risk surgery are first seen by anesthesia to determine their fitness to tolerate major surgery [53]. Finally, anesthesiologists can serve not only as gatekeepers with the right to cancel surgeries when patients are too vulnerable, but also can be ombudsman who postpone a case, permitting a thoughtful review, possibly with the input of others such as the patient's primary care doctor, the hospital ethics committee, and/or the chaplaincy [53].

One additional strategy that can both help reframe the conflict and help resolve it is to bring additional human resources to the situation. Requesting a second medical or surgical opinion can help assuage concern from the patient or family that the prognosis provided is inaccurate, or could result in a transfer of care if the second opinion disagrees that the situation is futile. Palliative care consultation can be helpful, as the palliative care specialists excel at facilitating goals of care discussions, and, obviously, at palliating symptoms. It is important, however, to inform the patient and family and surrogate(s) about this consultation prior to their arrival, and to clearly state that palliative care involvement is not necessarily equivalent to transition to comfort care only and hospice or to patient abandonment by the primary team. Ethics committee or consult service involvement can help clarify the ethical conflict and tension of the case, and delineate the ethically permissible options in the present circumstance. Involving social work and/or the chaplain can be helpful in answering questions regarding making arrangements for home hospice, and also providing psychosocial and spiritual support during truly difficult emotional times. Finally, one strategy that may be utilized but is not ethically appropriate is avoiding confrontation and simply acquiescing to patient or surrogate demands.

Costs Associated with "Futile" Care

It is widely known that care at the end of life is expensive. Barnato et al. sampled inpatient claims for 20% of all Medicare elderly decedents and 5% of all survivors between 1985 and 1999 and found that 30% of Medicare resources are expended on the 5% of beneficiaries who die each year [54]. Emanuel et al. examined Medicare data for beneficiaries in California and Massachusetts who died in 1996 and found that one-third of costs during the last year of life occurred during the last month of life [55].

Given how poorly coordinated end-of-life care can be, and also how inattentive this care can be to patient preferences, it is vitally important to assess a patient's end-of-life preferences and deliver value-congruent care. Zhang et al. conducted a longitudinal multi-institutional study of 627 patients with advanced cancer, and found that of the 188 participants of 603 in the final analysis (31.2%) who had end-of-life discussions, aggregate costs of care were $1876 compared with $2917 for patients who did not have end-of-life discussions. Thus, the cost of care was 35.7% lower among patients who had end-of-life discussions, and furthermore, patients with higher costs had worse "quality of death" [56].

Preoperative Risk Stratification Systems: Facilitating Informed Decisions

Given that before every surgical procedure an informed consent discussion of risks, benefits, and alternatives must occur, patients or their surrogates are always asked to weigh the potential benefits against the known risks. With ever increasing data sets on surgical outcomes, including even surgeon-specific and procedure-specific outcomes, patients or their surrogates are in a better position than ever before to make informed decisions. It is well known that certain operations are high-risk in general, and that certain patient factors make an operation high-risk for that specific patient.

Schwarze et al. performed a retrospective cohort study in which they used the Pennsylvania Health Care Cost Containment Council (PHC4) data set of all non-Veterans Affairs hospital admissions in Pennsylvania from April 1, 2001 to December 31, 2007 to identify all procedures by the International Classification of Diseases, Ninth Revision, Clinical Modification (ICD-9-CM) codes associated with a mean crude in-hospital mortality of at least 1% among patients 65 years and older [57]. They then eliminated procedures that were markers of severe illness, such as tracheostomy, rather than procedures that intrinsically carry a high-risk of mortality. Schwarze et al. found that 227 procedures were associated with a 1% or more mortality and these 227 operations are performed on more than half a million patients 65 years or older annually [57]. Additionally, they found that the pooled inpatient mortality for these 227 high-risk procedures was double in the 65 years and older group compared to the same procedures in younger patients (6% versus 3% mortality) [57]. The list of procedures is available as supplemental content to their article, and could be used by surgeons to understand which operations they perform that are high-risk in the elderly, and thus facilitate better decision making and patient counseling [57]. Recognizing that some operations are high-risk may lead to more careful deliberation and consideration of nonoperative treatment [57]. This might also help elderly patients to pause before a high- risk operation and more carefully consider the value of the surgery. If the patient chooses to proceed, the patient can be better prepared for potentially adverse outcomes [57].

There are additional preoperative risk stratification systems that have been validated as predictors of postoperative outcomes and mortality, including cardiac risk predictors [58–60], the American Society of Anesthesiologists classification system [61, 62], or more recently, measures of clinical frailty [63, 64]. Additionally, a multiple organ dysfunction score is another tool used to predict survival in a critical care setting [65]. Furthermore, a recently developed and readily available tool is the surgical risk calculator of the American College of Surgeons National Surgical Quality Improvement Program (ACS NSQIP) [66]. This calculator utilizes the NSQIP database to estimate patient morbidity or mortality after surgery [67]. This surgical risk calculator considers, in addition to other factors, the patient's age, sex, functional capacity, American Society of Anesthesiologists Physical Status, and past medical history as well as the surgical procedure and the emergent nature of the procedure to project the surgical risk for a patient [66, 67]. The surgical risk calculator is yet another preoperative risk stratification tool that can provide patients and surrogate decision makers specific outcome data regarding their surgery and a tool that can facilitate preoperative discussions between physicians and their patients [67].

Conclusion

As the tools and techniques of modern medicine improve, so too must our ability to communicate with patients. As Schuster summarizes, we must be able to distinguish between "everything that *can* be done" and "everything that *should* be done" [68]. No less importantly, we must also be able to make that distinction clear to our patients without abandoning compassion. The language of futility has been too vague and its use too adversarial for the profession of medicine and society to come to an understanding for effectively resolving the disputes that frequently arise when considering the appropriateness of a medical treatment or surgical intervention. For this reason, some authors have proposed that the term futility be removed from our professional lexicon [52]. Instead of shortening conversations to one word that summarizes how the physician may feel, we need to expand our discussions with patients and surrogates and, in so doing, strengthen the physician-patient relationship and ultimately provide better care to our patients.

References

1. Powledge TM, Steinfels P. Following the news on Karen Quinlan. Hastings Cent Rep. 1975;5(6):5–6. 28.
2. Branson R, Casebeer K. Obscuring the role of the physician. Hastings Cent Rep. 1976;6(1):8–11.
3. Annas GJ. In re Quinlan: legal comfort for doctors. Hastings Cent Rep. 1976;6(3):29–31.
4. Annas GJ. When procedures limit rights: from Quinlan to Conroy. Hastings Cent Rep. 1985;15(2):24–6.
5. Annas GJ. Nonfeeding: lawful killing in CA, homicide in NJ. Hastings Cent Rep. 1983;13(6):19–20.
6. Capron AM. Ironies and tensions in feeding the dying. Hastings Cent Rep. 1984;14(5):32–5.
7. Wolf SM. Nancy Beth Cruzan: in no voice at all. Hastings Cent Rep. 1990;20(1):38–41.
8. Orentlicher D. From the office of the general counsel. The right to die after Cruzan. JAMA. 1990;264(18):2444–6.
9. Gostin LO. From Quinlan to Cruzan, Glucksberg, and Vacco- a brief history and analysis of constitutional protection of the 'right to die'. JAMA. 1997;278(18):1523–8.
10. Angell M. The case of Helga Wanglie. A new kind of "right to die" case. N Engl J Med. 1991;325(7):511–2.
11. Miles SH. Informed demand for "non-beneficial" medical treatment. N Engl J Med. 1991;325(7):512–5.
12. Annas GJ. Asking the courts to set the standard of emergency care – the case of Baby K. N Engl J Med. 1994;330(21):1542–5.
13. Rutter TL. US doctors win life support lawsuit. BMJ. 1995;310(6989):1223–4.
14. Capron AM. Abandoning a waning life. Hastings Cent Rep. 1995;25(4):24–6.
15. Paris JJ, Cassem EH, Dec GW, Reardon FE. Use of a DNR order over family objections: the case of Gilgunn v. MGH. J Intensive Care Med. 1999;14(1):41–5.
16. Orr RD. The Gilgunn case: courage and questions. J Intensive Care Med. 1999;14(1):54–6.
17. Paris JJ. What standards apply to resuscitation at the borderline of gestational age? J Perinatol. 2005;25:683–4.
18. Hippocratic corpus. The art. In: Reiser S, Dyck A, Curran W, editors. Ethics in medicine: historical perspectives and contemporary concerns. Cambridge, MA: MIT Press; 1977.
19. Dictionary OE. "futile, adj.": Oxford University Press.
20. Clark PA, Mikus CM. Time for a formalized medical futility policy. Mercy Health System's procedures will help free its physicians from legal concerns. Health Prog. 2000;81(4):24–32.
21. Schneiderman LJ, Jecker NS, Jonsen AR. Medical futility: its meaning and ethical implications. Ann Intern Med. 1990;112(12):949–54.
22. Veatch RM, Spicer CM. Medically futile care: the role of the physician in setting limits. Am J Law Med. 1992;18(1–2):15–36.
23. Grant SB, Modi PK, Singer EA. Futility and the care of surgical patients: ethical dilemmas. World J Surg. 2014;38(7):1631–7.
24. Singer E. Medical futility: hippocratic fact or contemporary fiction? Washington, DC: Georgetown University; 2001.
25. Halevy A, Brody BA. A multi-institution collaborative policy on medical futility. JAMA. 1996;276(7):571–4.
26. Clarke MG, Ewings P, Hanna T, Dunn L, Girling T, Widdison AL. How accurate are doctors, nurses and medical students at predicting life expectancy? Eur J Intern Med. 2009;20(6):640–4.
27. Yourman LC, Lee SJ, Schonberg MA, Widera EW, Smith AK. Prognostic indices for older adults: a systematic review. JAMA. 2012;307(2):182–92.
28. Pellegrino E. Decision at the end of life: use and abuse of the concept of futility. Sgreccia JDDVCaE, editor. Citta del Vatticano: Libreria Editrice Vaticano; 2000.
29. Rowe CJ, Broadie S, editors. Nicomachean ethics. New York: Oxford University Press; 2002.
30. Svenaeus F. Empathy as a necessary condition of phronesis: a line of thought for medical ethics. Med Health Care Philos. 2014;17(2):293–9.

31. Consensus statement of the Society of Critical Care Medicine's Ethics Committee regarding futile and other possibly inadvisable treatments. Crit Care Med. 1997;25(5):887–91.
32. Helft PR, Siegler M, Lantos J. The rise and fall of the futility movement. N Engl J Med. 2000;343(4):293–6.
33. Brett AS, McCullough LB. When patients request specific interventions: defining the limits of the physician's obligation. N Engl J Med. 1986;315(21):1347–51.
34. Veatch RM. Why physicians cannot determine if care is futile. J Am Geriatr Soc. 1994;42(8):871–4.
35. Youngner SJ. Who defines futility? JAMA. 1988;260(14):2094–5.
36. Paris JJ, Reardon FE. Physician refusal of requests for futile or ineffective interventions. Camb Q Healthc Ethics. 1992;1(2):127–34.
37. Fine RL. Medical futility and the Texas Advance Directives Act of 1999. Proc (Bayl Univ Med Cent). 2000;13(2):144–7.
38. Smith ML, Gremillion G, Slomka J, Warneke CL. Texas hospitals' experience with the Texas advance directives Act. Crit Care Med. 2007;35(5):1271–6.
39. California Health Care Decisions Law. 2005.
40. Maine Uniform Health-Care Decisions Act. 2005.
41. Maryland Health Care Decisions Act. 2006.
42. Massachusetts Health Care Proxies – Physicians; refusal to honor proxy. 2006.
43. New York Health Care Agents and Proxies. 2006.
44. Tennessee Health Care Decisions Act, Determination of capacity – Compliance by health care provider or institution. 2006.
45. Virginia Health Care Decisions Act. 2006.
46. Washington Natural Death Act. 2006.
47. American Medical Association Council on Ethical and Judicial Affairs. Medical futility in end-of-life care. JAMA. 1999;281(10):937–41.
48. Bosslet GT, Pope TM, Rubenfeld GD, Lo B, Truog RD, Rushton CH, et al. An official ATS/AACN/ACCP/ESICM/SCCM policy statement: responding to requests for potentially inappropriate treatments in intensive care units. Am J Respir Crit Care Med. 2015;191(11):1318–30.
49. Rowland KJ, Kodner IJ, Cashen M, Schwarze ML. Surgical futility: "Aggressive" surgery on the severely demented. Surgery. 2009;145(4):351–4.
50. Jones JW, McCullough LB. I know about Jack and you're no Jack Kevorkian. J Vasc Surg. 2010;52(2):489–90.
51. Zier LS, Burack JH, Micco G, Chipman AK, Frank JA, Luce JM, et al. Doubt and belief in physicians' ability to prognosticate during critical illness: the perspective of surrogate decision makers. Crit Care Med. 2008;36(8):2341–7.
52. Grossman E, Angelos P. Futility: what Cool Hand Luke can teach the surgical community. World J Surg. 2009;33(7):1338–40.
53. Nurok M, Sadovnikoff N. Why are we doing this case? can perioperative futile care be defined? Curr Opin Anaesthesiol. 2013;26(2):176–81.
54. Barnato AE, McClellan MB, Kagay CR, Garber AM. Trends in inpatient treatment intensity among Medicare beneficiaries at the end of life. Health Serv Res. 2004;39(2):363–75.
55. Emanuel EJ, Ash A, Yu W, Gazelle G, Levinsky NG, Saynina O, et al. Managed care, hospice use, site of death, and medical expenditures in the last year of life. Arch Intern Med. 2002;162(15):1722–8.
56. Zhang B, Wright AA, Huskamp HA, Nilsson ME, Maciejewski ML, Earle CC, et al. Health care costs in the last week of life: associations with end-of-life conversations. Arch Intern Med. 2009;169(5):480–8.
57. Schwarze ML, Barnato AE, Rathouz PJ, Zhao Q, Neuman HB, Winslow ER, et al. Development of a list of high-risk operations for patients 65 years and older. JAMA Surg. 2015;150(4):325–31.
58. Lee TH, Marcantonio ER, Mangione CM, Thomas EJ, Polanczyk CA, Cook EF, et al. Derivation and prospective validation of a simple index for prediction of cardiac risk of major noncardiac surgery. Circulation. 1999;100(10):1043–9.

59. Goldman L, Caldera DL, Nussbaum SR, Southwick FS, Krogstad D, Murray B, et al. Multifactorial index of cardiac risk in noncardiac surgical procedures. N Engl J Med. 1977;297(16):845–50.
60. L'Italien GJ, Paul SD, Hendel RC, Leppo JA, Cohen MC, Fleisher LA, et al. Development and validation of a Bayesian model for perioperative cardiac risk assessment in a cohort of 1,081 vascular surgical candidates. J Am Coll Cardiol. 1996;27(4):779–86.
61. Menke H, Klein A, John KD, Junginger T. Predictive value of ASA classification for the assessment of the perioperative risk. Int Surg. 1993;78(3):266–70.
62. Wolters U, Wolf T, Stützer H, Schröder T. ASA classification and perioperative variables as predictors of postoperative outcome. Br J Anaesth. 1996;77(2):217–22.
63. Robinson TN, Wu DS, Sauaia A, Dunn CL, Stevens-Lapsley JE, Moss M, et al. Slower walking speed forecasts increased postoperative morbidity and 1-year mortality across surgical specialties. Ann Surg. 2013;258(4):582–8; discussion 8–90.
64. Makary MA, Segev DL, Pronovost PJ, Syin D, Bandeen-Roche K, Patel P, et al. Frailty as a predictor of surgical outcomes in older patients. J Am Coll Surg. 2010;210(6):901–8.
65. Marshall JC, Cook DJ, Christou NV, Bernard GR, Sprung CL, Sibbald WJ. Multiple organ dysfunction score: a reliable descriptor of a complex clinical outcome. Crit Care Med. 1995;23(10):1638–52.
66. American College of Surgeons National Surgical Quality Improvement Program (ACS NSQIP) surgical risk calculator. Available from: http://riskcalculator.facs.org/.
67. Bilimoria KY, Liu Y, Paruch JL, Zhou L, Kmiecik TE, Ko CY, et al. Development and evaluation of the universal ACS NSQIP surgical risk calculator: a decision aid and informed consent tool for patients and surgeons. J Am Coll Surg. 2013;217(5):833–42.e1–3.
68. Schuster DP. Everything that should be done – not everything that can be done. Am Rev Respir Dis. 1992;145:508–9.

Chapter 14
End-of-Life Issues: Management of Cardiac Implantable Electronic Devices

Cynthiane J. Morgenweck

Abstract It has become increasingly acceptable for clinicians to disable cardiac devices placed in a patient if the patient so requests. When deactivation was first proposed, there was significant resistance. However, with the rise of patient autonomy, the recognition that quality of life is a patient judgment and the increased burdens of multiple chronic illnesses patients face as they live longer, device deactivation is a reasonable approach in end-of-life care. The three intracardiac devices (pacemaker, automatic implantable cardioverter defibrillator and ventricular assist device) have different benefits, burdens and deactivation trajectories. This chapter will review the commonalities and differences and suggest some talking points when there is a request for deactivation.

Keywords End-of-Life • Ethics • Deactivation • Pacemakers • Automatic Implantable Cardioverter Defibrillators • Ventricular Assist Devices

Case Presentation

A 65-year-old man has been admitted to the hospital for an exacerbation of his congestive heart failure for the sixth time in 18 months. Careful management by your intensive care unit (ICU) team has once again improved his condition and the plan is to discharge him from your ICU. He has an automatic implantable cardioverter defibrillator (AICD), which has shocked him on occasion, and he is grateful for the 'extra' opportunities for life the shocks have given. However he has also told you that he is more interested in palliative care, that he is tired of the 'revolving door' of his disease process. He notes that time out of the hospital is becoming shorter and although he is not fully aware of the passage of time while

C.J. Morgenweck, MD, MA
Center for Bioethics and Medical Humanities, Medical College of Wisconsin, 8701 Watertown Plank Road, Milwaukee, WI 53226, USA
e-mail: cmorg@mcw.edu

B.G. Jericho (ed.), *Ethical Issues in Anesthesiology and Surgery*,
DOI 10.1007/978-3-319-15949-2_14

in the ICU, his family tells him that the time it takes for him to improve is becoming longer. You offer to have a discussion with him about treatment limitations and suggest a palliative care consult in conjunction with the rest of his family. When the consultation occurs, he agrees to a do not resuscitate (DNR) bracelet but he and his family ask that his AICD remain active through one or two shocks, after which, if the shocks are not beneficial, it would be reasonable to deactivate the defibrillator. Is this an acceptable request? What else would you like to know? What would you like to tell the patient and family?

Introduction

Cardiac devices are becoming more ubiquitous. Current devices are the small, fairly benign pacemakers (PM), the small (and uncomfortable for some) automatic implantable cardioverter defibrillators, and the larger, obvious and life-changing ventricular assist devices (VAD). These devices were all introduced with the intent of helping patients live better lives by assisting the functioning of a failing heart, through the maintenance of appropriate rhythms (PMs and AICDs), rapid defibrillation (AICDs) or assisting circulation (VADs). Each of these devices has helped patients. However, as the end of life approaches, some patients and families view the device as a barrier to high quality end-of-life care. Patients and families will then ask for these devices to be deactivated as death nears.

Initially these requests were considered to be ill-advised, that placement of the device was a permanent, non-negotiable aspect of care. However, with increasing emphasis on patient participation in decision making and with increased understanding of the negative aspects of the devices, there has been a greater acceptance of the potential reasonableness of such requests. Each of these three devices has different functions and a different profile of interference in the patient's life, so requests for deactivation create different responses in physicians who are being asked about deactivation.

It is important that the physician understand his or her own responses to such requests and the reasons for and against deactivation. With a clear foundation of personal views, a general response to such requests can be crafted that is then fine-tuned according to the individual request. In this chapter, the generic reasons for not honoring a deactivation request will be followed by a brief review of each device with a discussion of the concerns with specific device deactivation. Some suggestions for the deactivation process will be provided.

Reasons to Refuse Device Deactivation

There are arguments supporting the position that these devices should not be deactivated. Deactivation is done via electronic reprograming, thus there is no need to excise the device. Physicians may construe deactivation as worsening the patient's health, which is not a goal of medicine. Patients and physicians may believe that a device deactivation request is really a disguised suicide attempt. Physicians assert that the written order for deactivation would be assisting in the suicide. If the order writing is not considered suicide assistance, then it is euthanasia. The written order will allow for the killing of the device-dependent patient. The Heart Rhythm Society (HRS) considered these concerns and in 2010 issued a consensus statement that explains why deactivation should not be construed as assisting suicide or euthanasia [1]. HRS acknowledged conscientious objection by physicians with the caveat that care of the patient should be transferred to a provider who is willing to honor the request.

Currently, emphasis is placed on patient-centered or shared decision making, which focuses on understanding the goals of the patient and designing a plan of care that is as respectful of those goals as is possible [2]. When patients are asked about how they would like to die, they most frequently describe a 'low tech' death – at home, surrounded by loved ones and being kept comfortable. Patients and families may believe the devices unnecessarily prolong cardiac function as the rest of the body is shutting down, thus extending the dying process beyond that which might otherwise be expected.

The HRS statement declares that decisional patients have the power to assess ongoing therapies particularly in light of their changing health status to determine the continued usefulness of the particular therapy. If the patient is not decisional, then information about the appropriateness of deactivation should be shared with the legally authorized representative (LAR) of the patient. If there is no LAR, then family members engaged in the care of the patient should be involved in end-of-life conversations. In this chapter, "surrogate" will be used to indicate LAR or engaged family members. When receiving a terminal diagnosis, the patient may decide that cardiac devices are no longer as beneficial as they once were. HRS analysis supporting deactivation focuses on the patient's perception of device benefits and burdens in the context of the patient's goals and values for end-of-life care.

Although the HRS consensus statement does not explicitly mention VADs, the overarching term used to describe PMs and AICDs is 'cardiovascular implantable device,' which easily includes VADs. Ethical analysis by Mueller et al. supporting VAD deactivation proceeds similarly to the HRS analysis [3]. Both focus on patient driven assessments of benefits and burdens and a legally supported distinction between killing and allowing to die.

Pacemakers

Although PMs are the oldest of the three cardiac devices, familiarity with the device has not created the most robust consensus about deactivation. PMs continue to create unease when physicians are asked about deactivation. Usually, the longer a medical intervention is used, the easier it becomes to consider its removal. For example, initial requests for ventilatory support removal were met with strong opposition. Now most clinicians are reasonably comfortable with such requests. This is also true of dialysis discontinuation as well as artificial nutrition and hydration, to a large extent. The fundamental issue that creates a negative response to PM deactivation requests is that there is no apparent burden to its continued functioning. The PM is small, with no external wires and it paces in an unobtrusive manner. There is the potential for infection at the time of placement and lead fracture may occur, but rarely. Faulty pacing can be detected and the PM is easily reprogramed for better pacing. Battery lifetime is now about 10 years and battery replacement is usually an outpatient procedure.

Huddle et al. suggest that since there is no active role played by a physician once the PM is implanted, there can be no deactivation as this would be either assisting suicide or euthanasia [4]. This denies the ongoing care a patient receives after PM placement. If Huddle's analysis is accepted, devices might return to short-term batteries, wherein a discussion could be had before each battery replacement. This would be similar to the placement of a timer on a ventilator as described by Kinzbrunner, thus requiring the active intervention Huddle deems necessary for deactivation [5]. Miller et al. have suggested that withdrawal of care is indeed killing, that we have created moral fictions to ease our discomfort with such actions, and that it is acceptable in some circumstances to do so [6].

Some surrogates are not aware that a PM can be deactivated; other surrogates may view the PM as an impediment to a natural death by prolonging the patient's life in an inappropriate manner – the forced beating of a heart in a dying patient. This certainly is the contention put forth by Butler [7]. Physicians find it difficult to deactivate a device that seemingly has no downside – PMs do not limit the patient's day-to-day activities, unlike an AICD or a VAD. The physician may believe that the PM only enhances cardiac function so that the patient can enjoy life. However, at the end of life, the PM may not be furthering opportunities for the enjoyment of life [8, 9]. To deny deactivation is to insist that neither the physician nor the patient can come to a different definition of health care as the patient's health status changes.

Deactivation might not create any change in a dying patient's health, which might be disappointing to the patient and surrogate if that is what was anticipated. An intrinsic rhythm of 40 may be sufficient for a bed bound patient. Or, there may be increasing symptoms once the PM is deactivated, such as fluid retention. The slow intrinsic rate may prevent sitting or standing easily. Of course if the patient had undergone ablation prior to the PM implantation, there might not be any rhythm and the non-paced heart will stop.

These varied outcomes should be discussed with the patient and surrogate before the PM is deactivated. Whitlock et al. reported that death subsequent to deactivation occurred within "a few hours" [10]. Mueller et al. also reported that the time to death was less than a day [11]. Contingent plans for supporting the patient after deactivation should be created since there are so few reports of what actually occurs. Palliative care consultation can provide assistance in symptom management once the PM is deactivated as well as support of the family. It is also important that all of the staff providing care for the patient understand the rationale for the deactivation. When considering PM deactivation, the conversation ought to include a discussion of a do not resuscitate order (DNR), which should be in place before the deactivation process occurs. Clear documentation of the reasons for the deactivation must be available for the person who will deactivate the PM, as well as the actual order for deactivation. This will mitigate concerns about the deactivation decision particularly if the request is made during one shift with one set of physicians and the actual deactivation does not transpire until another shift with another set of physicians.

Automatic Implantable Cardioverter Defibrillators

These devices became available in the 1980s and were approved by Medicare shortly thereafter. As indications for the AICD have expanded, an increasing number have been implanted every year. These devices are about the same size as a PM. In actuality, many devices are currently manufactured with the ability to function as both PM and AICD. The potential short-term complications are the same as for PM – infection and lead fracture. However, what became well known within cardiology circles shortly after AICDs were implanted is that some patients are completely aware of the shocks they receive [12]. At their most intense, the shocks are described as mule kicks or baseball bats to the chest. Cardiologists do alter medication regimes as well as reprogram the device so that the shocks are fewer and less uncomfortable, but these maneuvers do not always help the patient. Some patients will alter their lifestyle in the hope of fewer shocks. They may give up once pleasurable activities to avoid the traumatic shocks. Various counseling modalities have been useful in diminishing patient anxiety, however the counseling does not decrease the number of shocks [13]. It is important to remember that not all patients who have an AICD implanted are shocked and that not all patients who are shocked are bothered by the shocks.

As patients age and other chronic illnesses become more prominent, patients may decide that the AICD is no longer a welcome treatment modality. If there is a new life limiting diagnosis, patients may find the potential swift trajectory of death from a sudden cardiac arrhythmia more appealing than the long, slow downward trajectory of the newly diagnosed terminal illness. A device that initially was welcome as preventing sudden cardiac death is now unwelcome as preventing sudden cardiac death. On this basis and perhaps especially if the patients have experienced significant unpleasantness with the shocks, the patients may request deactivation of the AICD.

Paola et al. have suggested that the AICD is a biofixture, thus it has become part of the patient and ought not be deactivated [14]. However, Sulmasy counters that the location of the device is not in and of itself reason to eschew deactivation [15]. HRS also does not accept location of a device as a reason for deactivation refusal.

When patients are asked to describe a good death, many will talk about dying in one's sleep, presumably of an arrhythmia. Thus, deactivating an AICD would now make this 'good death' more possible. Some clinicians believe that it is assisting suicide to deactivate the AICD. In the case of a terminal diagnosis and a decisional patient's request for deactivation, this is not assisting suicide but demonstrating respect for patients. If the clinician has concerns about a patient's abilities to make such a decision, it would be reasonable to ask for a psychiatric evaluation.

The conversation with a patient who is requesting AICD deactivation ought to include the information that deactivation does not guarantee a quick death from a fatal arrhythmia. There might be an arrhythmia that is not fatal - making the patient worse off but not dead. There may be no arrhythmia after the device is deactivated, especially if it fired infrequently or not at all. So, in spite of deactivation, the patient may experience the downhill decline he or she hoped to avoid. Thorough conversations with the patient and surrogate describing these possibilities before deactivation enable better decision making. Concerns can also be addressed with input from the palliative care team [16, 17]. DNR orders should also be clarified during the conversation about deactivation.

Ventricular Assist Devices

VADs were initially introduced as a bridge to heart transplantation but have become destination therapy for some patients. The implantation of a VAD is high-risk surgery, with significant complications – strokes, multisystem organ failure, bleeding and infections [18]. The need for post placement anticoagulation keeps the patient at risk for bleeding - gastrointestinal bleeding can be chronic in nature and a cerebral bleed can, of course, be devastating. External wires create an ongoing increased risk for infection. Management of the device requires support from a caregiver, family or friends as well as the advanced heart failure team.

Physicians may be reluctant to deactivate these devices for the same reasons as PMs and AICDs – deactivation is assisting suicide and perhaps even more so than AICDs, deactivation really will (within a short period of time) directly cause the death of the patient. This latter objection, the legal concept of proximate cause, may be a powerful influence in the consideration of VAD deactivation but it is balanced by the unwanted, unacceptable devastation some patients experience with placement.

Unlike the surgery for PM or AICD placement, VAD placement is major surgery with the above-mentioned complications that can permanently impair the patient. Deactivation has more rapidly become acceptable perhaps because physicians have learned from their experiences with PMs and AICDs. Physician concerns with assisting suicide and euthanasia are the same as with PMs and AICDs so the ethical and legal support framework provided by the HRS is applicable and valid. There are articles describing VAD deactivation [5, 19]. Although it is a small sample, Mueller et al. deactivated 20% of VADs placed in a nearly 6-year time frame [5]. None of the requests for deactivation were denied. Mueller et al. suggested that familiarity with deactivation of PMs and AICDs allayed concerns about the "permissibility of meeting these requests" [5]. A significant addition to their approach to VAD placement is that all the potential recipients now "receive consultation with a palliative medicine specialist who engages the patient in the process of advance care planning" [5]. The potential recipients are encouraged to voice their wishes should there be "device failure, catastrophic complications, development of a secondary comorbid condition, or ongoing poor quality of life" [5].

As palliative care has become an increasingly valuable part of patient care, particularly in ICUs, the tough conversations needed to explore VAD deactivation requests can be collaborative in nature with input from both the palliative care team as well as the ICU team in conjunction with the patient or surrogate [20, 21]. Furthermore, the palliative care team can assure the patient that management of all symptoms, not just cardiac symptoms will be in the plan of care. Integration of palliative care into heart failure care has been well described in the literature [17, 22, 23]. If there are wishes to transfer to home or residential hospice care, again the palliative care team has the expertise to coordinate such a request including a discussion of holding off on the VAD deactivation until the transfer has occurred.

Although not inherently needed in each deactivation conversation, an ethics consultation may provide value particularly when deactivation is new to the team or institution. VAD placement is performed after a multidisciplinary advanced heart failure team has thoroughly evaluated the patient and the team continues to monitor the patient after placement, thus there is continuity of care with ongoing assessments of the VAD's value.

VAD deactivation is either turning off the device or letting the batteries run down. Although VAD patients are dependent on the VAD, there still is some functioning heart muscle, so it is inappropriate to assume that VAD deactivation will cause immediate death. Palliative care can help support the patient and the family during this time. Again, DNR status should be discussed and documentation of the reasons for the deactivation is necessary to avoid misunderstandings.

Device Deactivation Process

Personal Values

The very first concern in considering device deactivation is the physician's response to such a request. Awareness of the potential for deactivation is increasing. A physician should anticipate such requests and reflect upon personal values. HRS acknowledges conscientious objection, however HRS supports an obligation to transfer care to a colleague willing to deactivate, should the patient or surrogate ask for deactivation. The physician also has an obligation to inform the patient of his or her non-deactivation stance from the start of the patient-physician relationship so the patient has the opportunity to seek another physician with an approach to deactivation that is in more alignment with the patient's goals and values.

Timing of General Information: From Physician to Patient

As HRS advocates, during the pre-implantation conferences, there ought to be a brief statement to the effect that as the patient's health status changes deactivation is a possibility. It is difficult for some physicians to inform patients that a device can be deactivated before it has even been placed, but a short sentence is all that is needed during the initial informed consent conversation. If appropriate, this is also the time for the physician to inform the patient that deactivation will not be performed because of conscientious objection. This information provides the patient the opportunity to find another provider.

PM and AICD placement surgeries are considered minor surgeries and ongoing care is transitioned from the implantation specialist to the primary cardiologist to the primary care physician. If these physicians are uncomfortable communicating deactivation possibilities, each may assume another has discussed the information such that a patient remains uninformed. Butler and Puri advocate for "an ethical *responsibility* to inform patients that devices can be painlessly deactivated, when in the patient's view, burdens outweigh benefits" [24]. It is important to remember that informing a patient is not inherently an agreement to do so.

The heart failure team, who regularly communicate with each other and the patient, manages the patient who undergoes VAD placement surgery. This continuity of care increases the likelihood that patient and surrogate are informed of the deactivation possibility. In some institutions, palliative care specialists are part of the team and they can help with deactivation information [21].

As the device parameters are adjusted, as batteries are changed and as the patient's health status changes, simple reminders are appropriate. If a patient or surrogate asks more questions about deactivation, then a fuller description of what would likely happen is appropriate. If the physician will not deactivate a device, the patient should be so reminded, along with a referral to another physician who would be willing to honor the request.

Timing of General Information: From Patient to Surrogate and Physician

During the informed consent conversation for implantation, the patient should be encouraged to fill out an Advance Directive (AD), if he or she has not already done so. If the AD names a surrogate, the patient should have discussions with the surrogate about when, if ever, deactivation should be considered. Pasalic et al. conducted a 2-year retrospective review of patients who underwent PM implantation to determine whether or not the patients had an AD and if so, comments if any about the PM [25]. Over half of the 205 patients had ADs, but only one AD mentioned the PM [25]. While this might be a reflection of lack of knowledge about the potential for PM deactivation, Tajouri reviewed the content of ADs in patients with AICDs and found similar results [26]. Thirty percent of the patients who had AICDs implanted during the yearlong study had ADs and only two ADs specifically mentioned the AICD [26].

Deactivation requests may become a consideration when the patient is given a second life limiting diagnosis, the first being the heart disease. This is another opportunity to urge the patient to update an existing AD or create one. Information in the AD should include when, if ever the patient would deem it appropriate, to deactivate the device. Written guidance is beneficial when patients cannot communicate and there is general unease about deactivation. Placing the information in the patient's chart can enhance a patient-physician alliance should the time come for a specific discussion about deactivation.

Education of Patient and Family

Although it is increasingly common for a patient to be aware of deactivation possibilities, there are still many patients who have not been so informed. Some patients may be surprised and grateful for the option, other patients may be uninterested in which case no further conversation is needed. When the medical team, the patient and surrogate all agree that device deactivation is the most appropriate care for the particular patient, there ought to be an educational conference about the process of deactivation. The patient and surrogate may assume that when the device is deactivated, the patient dies immediately. This may or may not happen. It is most likely to happen, based on the few reports available, for a PM or a VAD. An AICD may or may not shock frequently so there may be a more variable time frame to patient death. This educational session is an excellent time to introduce the palliative care specialists, if it has not already happened. While the immediate topic is providing care for the patient during and after deactivation, it is important to remember that the patient may be experiencing noncardiac symptoms that the palliative care team can help manage. Reported PM and VAD deactivation have been followed by patient death within a day, so the patient might remain in the hospital.

A patient may wish to go home with hospice care or go to a residential hospice. If so, it is reasonable to maintain the device until the transfer occurs, but this must be discussed with the patient and the family. DNR status must also be explicitly addressed. With careful planning and thorough communication with the receiving parties, successful transfer may be possible. There are a few protocols for the deactivation process [27], so if a hospice is new to this kind of care sharing of information will enhance the likelihood of a successful deactivation. Conscientious objection from hospice nurses and the allied health care professionals who will be called upon to do the deactivation should be supported, but there also must be reassurance that there will be health care providers who will honor the request at the receiving institution before the transfer is made.

Deactivation at Home Hospice or Residential Hospice

If home or residential hospice is preferred and is feasible, the patient and family should meet the palliative care team who will assist in the transfer of care and help coordinate the deactivation in the new location. Allied health care professionals are more likely to deactivate in nonhospital settings, so it becomes important for these personnel to understand the reasoning for the deactivation [28]. Good documentation is key. The scheduling of the deactivation should be in accord with plans the family may have for saying their goodbyes as well as the work schedule of the deactivator. Clear communication about role responsibilities is vital. Palliative care teams may be new to the deactivation of cardiac devices, but they are not new to the transfer of care to hospice, to ensuring the most comfortable death possible and to encouraging the difficult end-of-life conversations. Having the palliative care team involved, whether an in-hospital or out-of-hospital deactivation is planned, will allow for the best possible conversations with the patient and family, including the possibility of the patient not dying immediately after deactivation. The palliative care team will also address the noncardiac symptoms of the patient.

Deactivation at End of Life: Pacemakers

As described earlier, this is the most controversial device to deactivate. The process of deactivation involves resetting the PM to parameters such that there is no device pacing. Patient and surrogates must be informed that the time of death cannot be completely predicted. There is no active registry of deactivation stories; of those that are described, death occurred within a day. Concerns have been raised that if a patient is bedbound, the deactivation may not accomplish much since little is known about what kind of cardiac output is necessary for such patients. The patient may develop a slow intrinsic rhythm that prevents the anticipated death, but does cause more heart failure. As Bevins explains, the pacemaker was placed for a cardiac disease so heart failure should not be a complete surprise [29]. If palliative care has been involved, they will of course be available to manage new symptoms that appear after the PM is deactivated. Before the PM is deactivated, there also needs to be a conversation about a DNR order, if one has not yet been written. Deactivating a PM and writing a DNR order are linked, but each requires formal acknowledgement so there is no miscommunication.

Deactivation at End of Life: Automatic Implantable Cardioverter Defibrillators

The potential for painful shocks is well known and much work is done to minimize them. A patient can have his or her medications adjusted, have the threshold for defibrillation adjusted and the patient is encouraged to undergo psychological support to diminish the trauma of the shocks. As the patient's heart disease continues to progress, if the patient receives another life limiting diagnosis or if the number of shocks increases in spite of excellent medical management, a patient may declare that the benefits of the device are no longer worth the burdens. A patient anticipates that if there are no defibrillatory shocks, there will be a lethal arrhythmia with death ensuing immediately. This may not occur and has to be explained and explored with the patient or surrogate who are requesting deactivation. The AICD can be deactivated, and the patient may not suffer a lethal arrhythmia, thus continuing to live as has been reported by Buchhalter et al. [30]. The AICD can be deactivated and the patient may suffer a non-lethal arrhythmia, which may leave the patient more debilitated, but not dead. If the patient is actively dying and the AICD is deactivated, there will be no further shocks and the more natural death being sought by the patient and surrogate is more likely to occur.

If the device implanted is being used as both a PM and an AICD, then all functions of the device must be reviewed with the patient or surrogate. Some physicians are willing to deactivate the defibrillator but not the PM. This plan must be presented to all participants for understanding and approval. If the patient or surrogate wishes to have all functions deactivated, the physician must have a further discussion with all participants or assist in the orderly transfer of care if there is conscientious objection by the physician. DNR status is part of the deactivation conversation.

As with PMs, all of this information must be documented so that all team members participating in the care of the patient can understand the decision-making process and the care plan.

Magnets for PMs and AICDs

If the plan is for the patient to remain in the hospital during and after the deactivation, then there will be access to a cardiology team that is familiar with the patient as well as the device and can aid in correcting unexpected deviations from the plan of care. If the patient is transferred to home hospice or residential hospice, especially if this is new territory for the hospice team, education about the use of magnets is imperative. Magnets create asynchronous pacing, however magnets are also able to stop the defibrillator function of an AICD [31]. If there is a single device that is both pacing and defibrillating, careful discussion about what is being deactivated (tachyarrhythmia pacing, bradyarrhythmia pacing, defibrillation – some or all) and the effect of a magnet on each function is needed to assure that the planned deactivation is achieved.

Deactivation at End of Life: Ventricular Assist Devices

At minimum, advanced heart failure teams are composed of cardiologists, surgeons, intensivists, social workers, psychologists and nurses. Most of these clinicians are involved in all aspects of patient care - evaluation, implantation and post-implantation management. Ethicists, chaplains and palliative care specialists may also participate in patient care. Although the team may experience some reluctance to immediately honor the patient's request for deactivation, the ongoing relationship with the patient creates a real-time understanding of the patient's concerns.

After deactivation there may be some heart function left, but it likely will not be sufficient to sustain the patient for many days. Mueller et al. reported on 14 deactivations, and all died within a day [3]. Brush et al. reported death occurred within 20 minutes [19]. If a patient or surrogate wishes to transfer to home or residential hospice, the physicians must plan for the orderly transfer of care in conjunction with the family. This planning should cover among other topics, refraining from deactivation until after the transfer, DNR status and exactly who is going to deactivate. Unfortunately, a patient may not be stable enough for transfer and the patient and family will have to be so informed.

Future Concerns

Kramer et al. elicited nursing concerns with deactivation [32]. Nurses are the providers who spend the most time at the bedside, so their observations ought to be examined closely. Nurses want better communication about deactivation at the implantation conference, at the time of life limiting events and when a device is deactivated. Nurses are physician allies who provide important information about patient and family concerns. They help defuse conflicts between physicians and families, so acting on these observations about cardiac devices will most likely result in an enhanced partnership. Brush et al. interviewed VAD patient caregivers who appreciated the comprehensive end-of-life care plans but also advocated for increased education for the hospice providers who were not always as savvy as the caregivers [19].

As these devices continue to be used, as the deactivation potential becomes more widely known and as hospice care becomes more sought after, sharing of successful deactivation protocols will enhance the dying experience for patients and families. It must be remembered that the protocol should be device specific – each device treats a different aspect of cardiac disease. Plans for transfer of care in cases of conscientious objection must be in place.

It would also be beneficial to continue reporting on patient deaths after device deactivation to further the understanding of how to approach deactivation. For example, concerns are raised about heart failure after deactivation of a PM, however the few reports available do not indicate that this occurs. A formal registry where data could be archived would inform the physicians of the more common scenarios after deactivation.

Conclusion

When Karen Ann Quinlan's parents requested the removal of her ventilator in 1975, there were significant objections to the request from the medical community as well as the lay community. The issue of removal of medical therapies has been reasonably settled with an understanding that patients have an ethically well-grounded ability to refuse medical therapies even if removal will likely result in their death. In the last 30 years, this controversy, although settled, appears to have reinvented itself as cardiac devices are increasingly used to enhance the lives of patients with heart disease. As the devices have become more common, specialty societies, ethicists and the lay have for the most part, again come to the understanding that patients can ask to have therapies removed, even after started. Physicians may object, but do have an obligation to assist in orderly transfer of care. In the future, when implantable hearts are available outside of research protocols, these concerns will again come to the fore. Analysis of the concerns raised by current devices as well as the concerns raised in the research trials of artificial hearts will enable the formulation of ethically and legally sound deactivation protocols [33, 34]. As always, there will be difficulties, but we can best move forward by examining our past, learning from the prior errors and anticipating some of the new concerns.

References

1. Lampert R, Hayes DL, Annas GJ, Farley MA, Goldstein NE, Hamilton RM, et al. HRS expert consensus statement on the management of cardiovascular implantable electronic devices (CIEDs) in patients nearing end of life or requesting withdrawal of therapy. Heart Rhythm. 2010;7(7):1008–26.
2. Allen LA, Stevenson LW, Grady KL, Goldstein NF, Matlock DD, Arnold RM, et al. Decision making in advanced heart failure: a scientific statement from the American Heart Association. Circulation. 2012;125(5):1928–52.
3. Mueller PS, Swetz KM, Freeman MR, Carter KA, Crowley ME, Severson CJ, Park SJ, Sulmasy DP. Ethical analysis of withdrawing ventricular assist device support. Mayo Clin Proc. 2010;85(9):791–7.
4. Huddle TS, Bailey FA. Pacemaker deactivation: withdrawal of support or active ending of life. Theor Med Bioeth. 2012;33(6):421–33.
5. Kinzbrunner BM. Jewish medical ethics and end-of-life. J Palliat Med. 2004;7(4):558–73.
6. Miller FG, Truog RD, Brock DW. Moral fictions and medical ethics. Bioethics. 2010;24(9):453–60.
7. Butler K. Knocking on heaven's door: the path to a better way of death. New York: Scribner; 2014. p. 1–3.
8. Rhymes JA, McCullough LB, Luchi RJ, Teasdale TA, Wilson N. Withdrawing very low-burden interventions in chronically ill patients. JAMA. 2000;283(8):1061–3.
9. Pelligrino ED. Decision to withdraw life-sustaining treatment. JAMA. 2000;283(8):1065–7.
10. Whitlock SN, Goldberg IP, Singh JP. Is pacemaker deactivation at the end of life unique?: a case study and ethical analysis. J Palliat Med. 2011;14(10):1184–8.
11. Mueller PS, Hook C, Hayes DL. Ethical analysis of withdrawal of pacemaker or implantable cardio-defibrillator support at the end of life. Mayo Clin Proc. 2003;78(8):959–63.
12. Jauhar S. Jolts of anxiety. New York Times. 5 May 2002.
13. Kohn CS, Petrucci RJ, Baessler C, Soto DM, Mosowitz C. The effects of psychological intervention on patient's long-term adjustments to the ICD: a prospective study. PACE. 2000;23(4):450–6.
14. Paola FA, Walker RM. Deactivating the implantable cardioverter-defibrillator: a biofixture analysis. South Med J. 2000;93(1):20–3.

15. Sulmasy DP. Within you/without you: biotechnology, ontology and ethics. J Gen Intern Med. 2008;23(S1):69–72.
16. Matlock DD, Stevenson LW. Life-saving devices reach the end of life with heart failure. Prog Cardiovasc Dis. 2012;55(3):274–81.
17. Hauptman PJ, Havranek EP. Integrating palliative care into heart failure care. Arch Int Med. 2005;165(4):374–8.
18. Yuan N, Arnaoutakis GJ, Georg TJ, Allen JG, Ju DG, Schaffer JM, et al. The spectrum of complications following left ventricular assist device placement. J Card Surg. 2012;27(5):630–8.
19. Brush S, Budge D, Alharethi R, McCormick AJ, MacPherson JE, Reid BB, et al. End-of-life decision making and implementation in recipients of a destination left ventricular assist device. J Heart Lung Transplant. 2010;29(12):1337–41.
20. Bruce C. A review of ethical considerations for ventricular assist device placement in older adults. Aging Dis. 2013;4(2):100–12.
21. Swetz KM, Freeman MR, AbouEzzeddine OF, Carter KA, Boilson BA, Ottenberg AL, et al. Palliative medicine consultation for preparedness planning in patients receiving left ventricular assist devices as destination therapy. Mayo Clin Proc. 2011;86(6):493–500.
22. Hupcey JE, Penrod J, Fenstermacher K. A model of palliative care for heart failure. Am J Hosp Palliat Med. 2009;26(5):399–404.
23. Quaglietti S, Pham M, Froelicher V. A palliative care approach to the advanced heart failure patient. Curr Card Rev. 2005;1(1):45–52.
24. Butler K, Puri S. Deathbed shock: causes and cures. JAMA Int Med. 2014;174(1):88–9.
25. Pasalic D, Tajouri TH, Ottenberg AL, Mueller PS. The prevalence and contents of advance directives in patients with pacemakers. PACE. 2014;37(4):473–80.
26. Tajouri TH, Ottenberg AL, Hayes DL, Mueller PS. The use of advance directives among patients with implantable cardiac defibrillators. PACE. 2012;35(5):567–73.
27. Fromme EK, Stewart TL, Jeppesen M, Tolle SW. Adverse experiences with implantable defibrillators in Oregon hospices. Am J Hosp Palliat Med. 2011;28(5):304–9.
28. Mueller PS, Ottenberg AL, Hayes DL, Koenig BA. "I felt like the angel of death": role conflicts and moral distress among allied professionals employed by the US cardiovascular implantable electronic device industry. J Interv Card Electrophysiol. 2011;32(3):253–61.
29. Bevins MB. The ethics of pacemaker deactivation in terminally ill patients. J Pain Symp Manage. 2011;41(6):1106–10.
30. Buchhalter LC, Al O, Webster TL, Swetz KM, Hayes DL, Mueller PS. Features and outcomes of patients who underwent cardiac device deactivation. JAMA Intern Med. 2014;174(1):80–5.
31. Jacob S, Panaich SS, Maheshwari R, Haddad JW, Padanilam BJ, John SK. Clinical applications of magnets on cardiac rhythm devices. Europace. 2011;13(9):1222–30.
32. Kramer DB, Ottenberg AL, Gerhardson S, Mueller KA, Kaufman SR, Koenig BA, Mueller PS. "Just because we can doesn't mean we should": views of nurses on deactivation of pacemakers and implantable cardio-defibrillators. J Inter Card Electrophysiol. 2011;32(3):243–52.
33. Stolberg SG. On medicine's frontier: the last journey of James Quinn. The New York Times. 8 Oct 2002.
34. Jolly D. Recipient of artificial heart goes home. The New York Times. 9 Jan 2015.

Chapter 15
End-of-Life Issues: Spirituality

Cynthiane J. Morgenweck

Abstract There is an increasing emphasis in medicine for healthcare providers to treat the whole patient. Whole patient care includes the physical, psychosocial and spiritual care of the patient. Contemporary medicine has focused on the physical illnesses of the patient, creating a large armamentarium of tools to combat disease processes. In addition, addressing the spiritual needs of critically ill patients is an important part of intensive care, particularly when the patients are dying in the hospital. This chapter will describe some differences between spirituality and religiosity, suggest some self-education tactics for physicians interested in expanding their understanding of spirituality and discuss approaches to some common requests of a spiritual nature in the intensive care unit (ICU).

Keywords End-of-Life • Spirituality • Religion • Ethics • Prayer

Case Presentation

A 71-year-old man is in your intensive care unit (ICU). He was admitted with altered mental status, hypotension and sepsis due to his widely metastatic cancer. His daughter, his power of attorney for healthcare asked that he receive all possible medical interventions. He was intubated, started on pressor support as well as antibiotics. He has not improved in the last 5 days. His oncologist told the daughter and you that there are no more curative or palliative options available for him. He remains septic and you believe he is going to die soon. You have kept his daughter informed of his condition and you had another conversation with her about his impending death. She expressed her appreciation for your care of her father. She understands he is terminal; she is

C.J. Morgenweck, MD, MA
Center for Bioethics and Medical Humanities, Medical College of Wisconsin, 8701 Watertown Plank Road, Milwaukee, WI 53226, USA
e-mail: cmorg@mcw.edu

B.G. Jericho (ed.), *Ethical Issues in Anesthesiology and Surgery*,
DOI 10.1007/978-3-319-15949-2_15

resigned to his death. She tells you that she and her father are of the same religion. She asks you to be present when she and the chaplain recite the customary prayers said for a dying person of their faith tradition. You have relayed this request to the chaplain assigned to the ICU. This chaplain states that it would be inappropriate to perform these prayers because the chaplain and the patient have had many pleasant conversations over the course of his chemotherapy during which the patient made it abundantly clear that he had forsaken his religious upbringing and does not want to receive any of the traditional rites of passage. What are your next steps? What are you going to tell the daughter?

Introduction

As has been said innumerable times, medicine is both an art and a science. If the direction of medicine in the last 100 years is examined, there has been a distinct scientific turn. This science has helped many live. With the discovery of anesthetics, vaccinations, antibiotics and the application of aseptic techniques, many lives have been saved. Since World War II there have been extraordinary advances in the scientific aspects of medical care. Many acute diseases are now reliably cured and there is always great interest in the next discovery that will enhance health. With this emphasis on the latest scientific discovery, there has been neglect of the art of medicine. The art of medicine includes creating and maintaining a healing relationship that sustains the patient throughout the course of the illness. In spite of scientific advances, patients still die and the last days of their lives can best be served by the art of medicine rather than the science of medicine.

There have been three trends in the last 15 years that are reshaping the approach to care of the critically ill patient. First, Rothman described a recent paradox [1]. More Americans are dying at home, as they would like, but if they die in a hospital, it is more likely to be in an ICU. Secondly, as Aslakson [2] and Cook and Rocker [3] have suggested, palliative care is an increasingly accepted part of the care of the ICU patient. The intensivist who may be more focused on helping those patients who still have a chance to survive the ICU frequently welcomes the communication skills as well as the symptom management expertise of the palliative care specialist. The third trend is the increasing emphasis on having healthcare teams treat the whole patient. The whole patient concept includes seeking to understand the medical, psychosocial, spiritual and religious concerns of the patient. This renewed interest in the spiritual and religious concerns of the patient is especially relevant as a patient nears death. Further, the Joint Commission expects a spiritual assessment of patients to be performed and has suggested some questions to ask [4]. Guidelines from the American College of Critical Care Medicine Task Force state that “all members of the interdisciplinary team need to recognize the impact of spirituality on the patient/family ICU experience, especially with regard to matters of faith at the end of life" [5]. The Task Force supports training "ICU clinicians to incorporate spiritual care of the patient and family into clinical practice" [5]. This is "an important step in addressing the goal of care for the whole person" [5].

When it is accepted that a patient is dying in the ICU, the patient and family may continue to seek the assistance of the intensivist. The intensivist's role changes from preventing death to enabling the best possible death. Knowledge of the patient's religious background is important since decisions about continuing aggressive care in the face of the medical likelihood of death are frequently based on an understanding of religious teachings [6]. These teaching may encourage the patient or family to insist on care that does not, according to the physician, appear to provide a benefit or prolongs the suffering and death of the patient. It is reasonable for the physician to become familiar with the most commonly encountered perspectives. There are many articles describing the different religious perspectives on end-of-life care [7–12]. Physicians should use the information in these and other articles as guides since many patients do not practice their faith in complete accordance with the tradition. Thus when discussing critical decisions, the physician should inquire about the particular patient's perception on end-of-life care.

Impending death causes many patients to wonder about their lives, what kind of impact they have had on others, as well as what happens during and after death. Some patients express interest in seeking reconciliation with those they believe to have harmed as well as helping their families cope with their death. Patients usually continue with the tradition that has given meaning to them during their lives. They may return to the religion of their youth, if they have moved away from formal religious practices. Physician knowledge of these traditions may ease the patient's transition from life to death and may enable better family acceptance of the death.

In the ICU, as the intensivist begins to accept the inevitability of a patient's death, the intensivist may wish to maintain his or her scientific role, devote his or her limited time to those patients he or she believes will live and increase the role of the palliative care team. This may be the result of the intensivist's own discomfort with failing to prevent the death of the patient. On the other hand, the intensivist can work with the patient and family to create a better death, which is in keeping with the whole patient model of care. In the ICU, the family is frequently the voice of the patient and, as the patient is dying, the family needs to receive care as well. This care will likely involve conversations about the spiritual and religious practices of the patient as understood by the family. Although this is not traditional medical therapeutics as conceived in the latter half of the twentieth century, this care reinforces the role of physician as healer.

Spirituality and Religion

When asked, most Americans consider themselves spiritual, if not religious. There is no universal definition of spirituality. In general, spirituality is "that which allows a person to experience transcendent meaning in life. This is often expressed as a relationship with God, but it can also be about nature, art, music, family or community – whatever beliefs and values give a person a sense of meaning and purpose in life" [13]. Patients who are facing their death may start to review their life, seeking meaning without reference to a religious tradition. This is a spiritual approach. A religious approach would be more oriented toward a life review in relation to the tenets of the patient's faith tradition. Religion may be defined as a shared understanding of the transcendent by a community of members. Religions attempt to organize and clarify the world, both seen and unseen. Religions give guidance on how to live one's life which includes how to relate to other human beings as well as how to relate to the transcendent. And of course, religions provide guidance on how to die.

Both religion and medicine are tools to enhance human flourishing. Spirituality is concerned with the thoughts and activities that enhance the person's flourishing. Like religions, medicine also tries to organize and explain the world, however medicine is oriented toward explaining the natural world, leaving out the transcendent. Medicine works to manipulate the natural world to enable better health. Medicine is not always able to prevent worsening health, and as a patient begins to die, spirituality may enhance the patient's sense of well-being and understanding of the events that are in progress more than further medical interventions. Medicine as a completely separate entity from spirituality is a relatively recent idea – it has come to prominence in the last 150 years or so. As Sulmasy [14], Groopman [15] and Richardson [16] have reminded us, there was a time when the priests were also the physicians, thus able to provide both physical and transcendent comfort during the dying process. Whole patient care suggests that (to paraphrase Hippocrates) when physician efforts to *cure* a patient are not possible via scientific medicine, then physicians continue to *care* for the patient in the form of spiritual support.

Pesut [17] describes three approaches to spirituality, making it clear that there is not a unifying definition but rather some common themes. Reading and evaluating multiple definitions of spirituality enables a physician to explore how he or she might best be able serve the whole patient meaningfully when encouraging the patient to talk about spirituality. Puchalski and Romer [13] support the taking of a spiritual history in order to know the patient more fully. As a patient nears the end of life, a spiritual assessment may be of benefit to both the patient and the physician. Taking the inventory signals that the physician understands the importance of spiritual issues. The patient's answers will help the patient review the lived life, more fully understand the impending death and perhaps uncover one or two more undertakings that the patient might accomplish before death.

With the increased emphasis on treating the whole patient, it is reasonable for the physician to start a dialogue about patient or family concerns. Asking about the spiritual concerns of the dying patient as well as concerns of family members with an offer of continued chaplain conversation as soon as the physician is out of his or her comfort zone reinforces the continued commitment to patient care.

If there are explicit questions about a particular faith tradition with which the physician is not familiar, a gentle statement that the physician is unable to supply a religiously specific answer is best. An offer of chaplaincy assistance or communication with the patient's personal religious leader should immediately follow the explanation. This explanation and offer can prevent an interpretation of discounting the faith concerns of the patient.

Preparation for Addressing Spiritual Concerns

Discussions with the patient and family about spirituality may be anxiety provoking for the physician who finds himself or herself to be the least knowledgeable person in the conversation. This lack of knowledge can be uncomfortable for the physician who is accustomed to leading conversations, demonstrating expertise about the medical aspects of disease processes. Being a team member (along with the patient, family, chaplains, nurses and social workers) as opposed to team leader may be a new experience for the physician. For conversation about spiritual issues to have value and meaning for the patient and family, it is necessary to learn about spiritual concerns at the end of life. Starting a discussion of spirituality will be appreciated by the patient; however, the physician must remain sensitive to the patient who does not wish to talk or prefers to talk with personal clergy.

Chaplains as Resources

When the physician decides to expand his or her support of the patient to include spiritual concerns, engaging the services of the chaplain is essential. Seeking support from the chaplain is necessary to prevent the perception of an attempt to take over the chaplaincy program. Discussions will help the physician discern what the chaplains believe would be the best use of the physician's time, the most effective communication route with the chaplains and common pitfalls encountered when helping the patient and family with their spiritual concerns. Chaplains can describe the most common religious traditions of the hospital patient population and direct the physician to local clergy who can expand the physician's knowledge base. The physician might shadow a chaplain initially and then ask the chaplain to observe the physician's interactions a few times, providing suggestions to improve the physician's skills. Chaplains must be informed of the physician's intentions so that when the physician reaches the limits of his or her abilities to help, the chaplain can reasonably seamlessly continue to provide support. Finally, the chaplains will also be able to recommend conferences, books, videos and other resources that the physician would find useful as the spiritual education process continues.

As the physician becomes increasingly comfortable engaging in spiritual conversations with the patient and family, the physician may wish to pursue further self-education. Todres, Catlin and Thiel describe a pastoral care program developed to train intensivists about spiritual distress [18]. While this program is rather unique, an interested intensivist could research local clinical pastoral educational opportunities. Undertaking a formal course of study may be more than the physician wishes to do; however, learning opportunities can be sought out, with perhaps weekend or weeklong conferences focusing on one or two aspects of spiritual care. Internet searches can elicit conferences to attend, online lectures as well as high quality readings to enhance the understanding of both spirituality and religion.

Self-Examination

As with so many other issues, an initial step would be an inventory of personal attitudes and beliefs about spirituality. The fundamental question is whether or not the physician believes it is appropriate to participate in the spiritual care of the patient. If the sincere answer is no, then the physician ought to craft a respectfully worded statement to that effect to be delivered to the patient and family should they ask for help. Along with the statement, the physician should offer to contact the hospital chaplains for assistance.

If the physician deems it reasonable to participate in the spiritual care of the patient, there are many questions to be considered. What level of participation is appropriate? What are the physician's personal definitions of spirituality and religion? If the physician has a faith tradition, how well does the physician understand it? How comfortable is the physician listening to the spiritual concerns of the dying patient? How comfortable is the physician listening to religious tenets that are either different from or in conflict with those of the physician? What is the appropriate response of the physician to this kind of conflict? Thorough evaluation of honest answers to these questions will direct next steps in the education process and also define limits of the physician's involvement in spiritual care.

Spiritual Assessment Tools

Before delving into the spiritual care of the patient, the physician should examine some current spiritual assessment tools. Saguil and Phelps identify three tools, FICA, HOPE and Open Invite [19]. Each of these contains a few questions that the physician can answer for himself or herself in order to determine which tool is most suited to his or her personal style of practice. Sulmasy suggests establishing an "empathic connection" before engaging in a spiritual assessment [20]. A patient may self-identify as both spiritual and religious and the physician can elect to focus on the spiritual, while simultaneously offering to contact appropriate chaplains or the patient's personal religious advisor for further religious interactions. Fitchett describes different levels of spiritual participation and suggests that it would be reasonable for a physician to do an initial spiritual screening and perhaps start the spiritual history taking, leaving the in depth spiritual assessment to the chaplain services [21]. In patient interviews, Yardley et al. noted that "[t]here was an expectation that any healthcare professional could deal with initial care to meet spiritual needs" and "no participant felt they would mind being asked questions about spirituality" [22]. If these questions are asked in an open and attentive manner, patients will most likely appreciate the asking. The patient should also be made to feel that it is completely acceptable to refuse such inquiries.

Competencies for Spiritual Support

The Marie Curie Cancer Care Organization [23] lists knowledge competencies as well as skill competencies for beginning to more advanced palliative care specialists [23]. Although this list was developed for palliative care, review of the competencies can assist the physician in assessing personal needs to deepen spiritual support skills. At every level of competency there is an emphasis on awareness of personal limits, recognition that this is a patient-centered, patient-focused activity with the patient directing the majority of the conversation and that active listening is key to a successful interaction. The physician must self evaluate in these key competencies.

Communication Skills

Communication skills are foundational to spiritual support and can be learned by attending conferences focused on communication, reading articles and observing those who already do it well. The communication skills for spiritual care are not the same communication skills needed for medical care. Medical communication is conceived of as conveying information in a patient appropriate manner and eliciting the patient's goals and values in order to craft a plan of care that is as respectful of the stated goals and values as is possible. A physician guides a medical conversation while the patient's hopes and fears guides the spiritual conversation. Spiritual care of the patient involves attentive listening as well as a willingness to ask for clarifying details as the patient expresses concerns.

When there has been careful preparation for the interaction with the patient, there is a greater likelihood of a successful interaction. There are helpful phrases to use that will encourage patients to express their thoughts. Sulmasy has provided several questions that might "engage the patient in significant spiritual sharing" [20]. Coulehan suggests, "Let me see if I have this right…" as a reflective response [24]. An alternative phrase might be "Help me to understand more about….". All phrases are respectful; demonstrating a real interest in what the patient or family is talking about. Careful listening to the responses of the patient will guide the conversation.

Other Considerations

Asking the patient about his or her spirituality implies that the patient can respond, and so a spiritual/religious assessment should take place as soon as is reasonable. If there isn't sufficient time for the assessment or the patient is unable to answer, then talking with family members and identified personal clergy are the next best options.

Physicians ought to learn about the beliefs of different religious groups relative to end-of-life care in order to have an appreciation of appropriate medical technology for the patients. While a physician may not agree to requests for interventions, he or she may acknowledge that the request arises from the deeply held beliefs of the patient and family, which the physician does respect. This expressed respect might mitigate some anger the patient and the family experience if they believe that medicine does not take religious beliefs seriously. Patient or family insistence on therapies because of religious beliefs is not a conversational trump card that shuts down any further discussion. While such insistence may raise the tension between the physician and patient or family, it is reasonable to respectfully respond with further exploration of the meaning of the request [25]. Chaplain attendance at such conversations can be beneficial since the chaplain may be able to provide a more nuanced interpretation [26].

A conversation about the patient's spiritual concerns is not about the meshing of medical interventions with the faith beliefs of the patient although this may become a welcome by-product. The spiritual conversation is about enabling the patient and family to achieve a better understanding and acceptance of the end of life.

The patient may have misunderstandings about what is expected of them as faithful followers of a tradition. Careful discussion about these misunderstandings may be beneficial if the patient expresses some confusion about doctrine and the physician is truly capable of explaining the tradition; it is more appropriate to seek clarification from the patient's personal pastor or the chaplain.

Eck describes three approaches to the issue of religious differences – the exclusivist, inclusivist and pluralistic response [27]. The exclusivists are sure that their tradition of encountering God is the correct approach. The inclusivists believe that there are many paths to encountering God but that their tradition is the apogee of all such paths. The pluralists acknowledge that there are many paths to encountering God and these paths are neither exclusive nor inclusive.

These stances should be reflected upon before embarking on spiritual discussion with patients. If a physician determines himself or herself to be an exclusivist, engaging in spiritual care of the patient at the end of life has to proceed extraordinarily carefully, if at all lest the personal life spills over into the professional life. Chaplains receive significant training in the separation of personal role and professional role. Inclusivists must also guard against smugness when working with the patient and family at the end of life. And of course, pluralists must avoid being so general as to not be particularly helpful to the dying patient. The intent of the interaction is to provide meaningful support for the patient; no other agenda is appropriate. The patient's religious traditions will also influence the roles and responsibilities of the physician in such discussions.

Spiritual Concerns

Proselytizing

Proselytizing is generally understood as attempts to convert a person to a different religion. Proselytizing is unacceptable behavior for any hospital staff member. The hospital is designed to provide healthcare, not religious conversion. Sulmasy explains several of the reasons for the proselytizing prohibition [28]. On occasion, the proselytizing may come from a family member. Although it is difficult, one solution is for ICU staff to monitor and limit the verbal contact between the patient and a proselytizing family member. It is emotionally hard for the medical team to limit visitation when a patient is dying, in rare circumstances it may be necessary. It can be argued that visiting is a privilege, not a right and appropriate behavior is part of the privilege. Proselytizing may also occur if an exclusivist as described by Eck dominates conversation about appropriate spiritual care of the dying patient [27].

What ought a physician do if in his or her opinion the patient is demonstrating significant misunderstandings of the faith tradition? This concern is best resolved by having a chaplain of the patient's faith tradition or better yet have the patient's personal clergy visit with the patient. It is entirely possible that the physician is misinformed about the tradition.

Nuances of traditions can also be of concern. When family members practice in a manner distinct from the patient, and the patient is not able to defend his or her approach, it may be tempting for the family to rearrange the patient's tradition to better align with the family's tradition. Without prior discussion with the patient, it may be difficult for the team to discern the patient's wishes. This speaks to the utility of Advance Directives with information about the patient's spiritual and religious preferences and to the benefit of taking a spiritual history at the time of admission, if possible. When a spiritual history is not possible, talking with the patient's personal pastor will provide the best information about what the patient most values. Families may acknowledge their differences if they are offered a safe, non-judgmental space and place to do so.

Praying with the Patient and Family

The physician may be asked to participate in prayers for the patient by either the patient or family members. Responses to this request may be negative or positive but there should be some consistency to the response. If the physician has previously spent time in self-reflection, then his or her response whatever it is, will be genuine. If the physician has not thought about his or her response to this request, there may be a reflexive refusal based on an assumption that participating in prayer is well beyond the scope of his or her medical practice.

If the physician has determined that participation in prayer is not part of his or her practice, there should be a brief respectful explanation, recognizing that the patient and family members may be hurt by such a refusal. This hurt might be ameliorated by an offer to have the chaplain pray with the family. If the rest of the healthcare team is aware of the physician's stance, they can encourage the use of chaplain services in anticipation of prayer requests so there are fewer hurt feelings.

Patients or families who makes this request are acknowledging the power of the role of physician as healer and are appreciative of their physician's participation. It is of course reasonable for the physician to know what kind of participation is being requested – leading a prayer or being present as prayers are offered. The physician may be comfortable with leading prayer, if asked and if the religious tradition of the patient is the same as or very similar to that of the physician. It is also reasonable to solicit possible prayer content. As the traditions of patient and physician diverge, it may become increasingly difficult to craft a meaningful prayer. The physician might then best serve the patient and family by acknowledging his or her ignorance of appropriate prayers and instead ask either the patient or a family member to lead the prayer or offer to seek assistance from chaplaincy.

When patients or families lead prayers, physicians must be aware that what is prayed for may be in contradistinction from what is either medically possible for the patient or what the physician is willing to do for the patient. On the other hand, if the physician is leading prayer, the patient and or family may not be particularly happy with the content either. If the physician is not leading the prayer, attention to prayer content may provide clues to forging a better patient/family/physician alliance. After a prayer is ended, there may be time for calm exploration of the meaning of the prayer.

If a physician is willing to craft a prayer, time should have been spent learning about the many different kinds of prayers to determine which type would be of most benefit to the patient and family toward the end of life, particularly in the context of the patient's stated concerns. There may be missteps in the prayer but a sincere attempt will likely be appreciated. Praying for guidance through the hard times being experienced by all would be one possible prayer.

The Patient and/or Family Praying for a Miracle

The family may tell the physician that they are praying for a miracle. The physician may find this to be a demonstration of the family's inability to understand or accept the terminal nature of the patient's illness. Several authors have described the meaning of miracles in their faith tradition [29–32]. DeLisser suggests that the miracle expectation may be an expression of hope, a denial of the severity of the patient's illness or an expression of anger at the team [33]. Another possibility is that this expectation indicates that the family really does understand the dire nature of the patient's illness. By making such a statement, the family may be acknowledging the need to seek a cure from some other source – a transcendent source since the therapies provided by the physician have reached their limits without improving the health of the patient. Asking for a miracle may be the recognition that tools outside the domain of scientific medicine are needed to help the patient.

Physician discomfort with this statement may reflect a control issue. Particularly in an ICU, a physician is able to monitor and manipulate many physiologic parameters. This capability may encourage the belief that the physician is in charge of the patient, but of course the physician does not control every aspect of the life of the patient. Prayer is generally not considered to be in the toolbox of medicine but it may be a vital part of the spiritual dimension of the patient and family. Praying can be the most authentically powerful contribution a family can make and it should be appreciated. Prayers for a miracle can be viewed as another dimension of the care of the patient. Prayers do not inherently interfere with the medical care being provided by the healthcare team.

Statements about miracles may require clarification [34]. Attempting such a conversation may be challenging but respectful elucidation of the expectations of the family about the miracle can create an atmosphere of trust [33, 35]. Some questions might include – What is a miracle? Who defines it? Is the only acceptable miracle the recovery of the patient? These questions may be best discussed with the guidance of a chaplain. The physician should attend the meeting with the chaplain in order to hear what the patient and family are anticipating as well as their concerns.

A more difficult problem may arise if the family asks that the patient be kept alive until the miracle occurs. This necessitates a calm and compassionate explanation about what is being done, what can be done and that death may occur in spite of medicine and prayers. If the patient is expected to receive cardiopulmonary resuscitation (CPR), there should be some shared understanding of the guidelines for termination of CPR.

Rituals Near the Time of Death

If a patient has not practiced his religion for many years, it is possible that the leaders of the particular faith no longer consider remembered traditions important. Consultation with a chaplain of the same tradition can provide an update for the patient. On the other hand, unless the requested tradition has been completely removed from the faith, the patient may find significant comfort in following the older tradition. It is common for specific individuals to perform specific rites; this information must be learned as soon as possible so that the correct individual is found in a timely manner. If what the patient requests and what the family requests differ, it is important to remember that the fiduciary relationship is with the patient. Thus, if a patient has made adamant statements about end of life rituals, these statements ought to be respected. The family may have to be reminded that the patient's wishes are of paramount importance. The family may not agree on the appropriate way to mourn the death of their loved one. In this situation, it may be a time for the chaplain or palliative care specialists to help with the sorting out of the emotions surrounding the death as well as the most appropriate traditions to follow.

Rites of Passage at the Time of Death

It is best to have information about expected rites before the actual death. The physician's knowledge does not have to come from the family who might be offended if questions are asked about rites while the patient is still alive. Chaplains, of course, are an excellent resource for the physician as is the patient's own religious leader, if one has been identified. Bedside nurses are also resources for the physician, as well as the family members who have accepted the impending death and who plan on participating in these rites.

If a patient's death becomes a coroner's case, a sensitive explanation to the family expecting to bury the patient within a certain time frame is a necessity. Advocacy on behalf of the family to the coroner to perform the autopsy expeditiously will be appreciated. Foreknowledge of this possibility can help the medical team prepare the family. It is legitimate to inform the family of state laws that may impact time of burial.

Body preparation for burial may also require understanding of the preferences of the patient and family. Sensitive questions can enable the team to observe the traditions. Discerning appropriate preparation is most easily accomplished with discussion with a chaplain or with the patient's personal pastor. Asking family members or the patient is a direct method of obtaining an answer; however, these questions may be interpreted as giving up on the patient with subsequent mistrust.

It may be possible to have a ceremony at the bedside. Sometimes the whole ceremony cannot be accommodated. If there is an understanding of the details of the ceremony, thought can be given to which parts are reasonable in a hospital setting. Symbolic gestures may help the family grieve. There may be space limitations and/or restrictions on the use of fire or alcoholic beverages, but there should be accommodation to the extent possible. Awareness of the appropriate participants in the ceremony is essential.

Theodicy Questions

Patients and families may raise the question, 'why me?' or 'why my loved one?' The patient's personal pastor or a chaplain who has the time for an extended conversation can best answer this very serious and fundamental question.

Conclusion

While more patients are able to achieve the commonly expressed goal of dying at home, there are also many patients who die in an ICU. The impending ICU death is shaped by the spiritual and religious practices of the patient and the family. As there is less that a physician can do medically for the patient, the physician should be willing to focus on the spiritual concerns of the patient. This focus at the end of life is entirely in step with the increasing emphasis on treating the whole patient. Helping a patient and family work through spiritual concerns can be immensely satisfying. This help must start with an educational process about spirituality at the end of life. The physician should become comfortable with his or her own spirituality, develop an understanding of the prevalent religions practiced by the community the hospital serves, recognize his or her personal limitations in such encounters, learn about available resources for difficult questions, and strive to improve communication skills. Enabling a better death for a patient is the ultimate goal of attention to the spiritual concerns of the patient and family.

References

1. Rothman DJ. Where we die. N Engl J Med. 2014;370(26):2457–60.
2. Aslakson RA, Curtis JR, Nelson JE. The changing role of palliative care in the ICU. Crit Care Med. 2014;42(11):2418–28.
3. Cook D, Rocker G. Dying with dignity in the intensive care unit. New Engl J Med. 2014;370(26):2506–14.
4. The Joint Commission. Spiritual assessment. 2008. http://www.jointcommission.org/mobile/standards_information/jcfaqdetails.aspx?StandardsFAQId=290&StandardsFAQChapterId=29. Revised 24 Nov 2008. Accessed 16 May 2015.
5. Davidson JE, Powers K, Hedayat KM, Tieszen M, Kon AA, Shepard E, et al. Clinical practice guidelines for support of the family in the patient-centered intensive care unit: American College of Critical Care Medicine Task Force 2004–2005. Crit Care Med. 2007;35(2):605–22.
6. Jaul E, Zabari Y, Brodsky J. Spiritual background and its association with the medical decision of DNR at terminal life stages. Arch Geron Geriatr. 2014;58(1):25–9.
7. Kinzbrunner BM. Jewish medical ethics and end-of-life. J Palliat Med. 2004;7(4):558–73.
8. United States Conference of Catholic Bishops. Ethical and religious directives for Catholic Health Care services. 5th ed. 2009. http://www.usccb.org/issues-and-action/human-life-and-dignity/health-care/upload/Ethical-Religious-Directives-Catholic-Health-Care-Services-fifth-edition-2009.pdf. Accessed 16 May 2015.
9. Al-Shahri MZ, Al-Khenaizan A. Palliative care for Muslim patients. J Support Oncol. 2005;3(6):432–6.
10. Ankerry RA, Clifford R, Jordens FC, Kerridge IH, Benson R. Religious perspectives on withdrawal of treatment from patients with multiple organ failure. Med J Aust. 2005;183(11/12):616–21.
11. Pew Research Center. "Religious groups" views on end-of-life issues. 2013. http://www.pewforum.org/2013/11/21/religious-groups-views-on-end-of-life-issues/. Accessed 16 May 2015.
12. Bulow HH, Sprung CL, Reinhart K, Prayag S, Du B, Armaganidis A, Abroug F, Levy MM. The world's major religions' points of view on end-of-life decisions in the intensive care unit. Intensive Care Med. 2008;34(3):423–30.
13. Puchalski C, Romer AL. Taking a spiritual history allows clinicians to understand patients more fully. J Palliat Med. 2000;3(1):129–37.
14. Sulmasy DP. Spirituality, religion and clinical care. Chest. 2009;135(6):1634–42.
15. Groopman J. God at the bedside. N Engl J Med. 2004;350(12):1176–8.
16. Richardson P. Spirituality, religion and palliative care. Ann Palliat Med. 2014;3(3):150–9.

17. Pesut B. A conversation on diverse perspectives of spirituality in nursing literature. Nurs Philos. 2008;9(2):98–109.
18. Todres DI, Catlin EA, Thiel MM. The intensivist in a spiritual care training program adapted for clinicians. Crit Care Med. 2005;33(12):2733–6.
19. Saguil A, Phelps K. The spiritual assessment. Am Fam Physician. 2012;86(6):546–50.
20. Sulmasy DP. Spiritual issues in the care of dying patients: "…it's okay between me and God. JAMA. 2006;296(11):1385–92.
21. Fitchett G. Next steps for spiritual assessment in healthcare. In: Cobb M, Pulchalski CM, Rumbold B, editors. Oxford textbook of spirituality in healthcare. New York: Oxford University Press; 2012. p. 299–305.
22. Yardley SJ, Walshe CE, Parr A. Improving training in spiritual care: a qualitative study exploring patient perceptions of professional educational requirements. Palliat Med. 2009;23(7):601–7.
23. Marie Curie Cancer Care. Spiritual and religious care competencies for specialist palliative care. 2003. www.mariecurie.org. Accessed 6 Jan 2015. p. 4–8.
24. Coulehan JL, Platt FW, Egener B, Frankel B, Lin C, Lown B, Salazar WH. "Let me see if I have this right…": words that help build empathy. Ann Intern Med. 2001;135(3):221–7.
25. Quill TE, Arnold R, Back AL. Discussing treatment preferences with patients who want "everything". Ann Intern Med. 2009;151(5):345–9.
26. Brett AS, Jersild P. "Inappropriate" treatment near the end of life: conflict between religious convictions and clinical judgment. Arch Intern Med. 2003;163(14):1645–9.
27. Eck DL. Chapter 7: Is our god listening? In: Encountering god: a spiritual journey from Bozeman to Banaras. Boston: Beacon Press; 1993. p. 166–99.
28. Sulmasy DP. Ethical principles for spiritual care. In: Cobb M, Pulchalski CM, Rumbold B, editors. Oxford textbook of spirituality in healthcare. New York: Oxford University Press; 2012. p. 465–70.
29. Pinches C. Miracles: a Christian theological overview. South Med J. 2007;100(12):1236–42.
30. Yu C. Eye on religion: miracles in the Chinese Buddhist tradition. South Med J. 2007;100(12):1243–5.
31. Khan F. Miraculous medical recoveries and the Islamic tradition. South Med J. 2007;100(12):1246–51.
32. Mackler AL. Eye on religion: a Jewish view on miracles of healing. South Med J. 2007;100(12):1252–4.
33. DeLisser HM. A practical approach to the family that expect a miracle. Chest. 2009;135(6):1643–7.
34. Sulmasy DP. Distinguishing denial from authentic faith in miracles: a clinical-pastoral approach. South Med J. 2007;100(12):1268–72.
35. Orr RD. Responding to patient beliefs in miracles. South Med J. 2007;100(12):1263–7.

Chapter 16
Ethics in Research and Publication

Stephen H. Jackson and Gail A. Van Norman

Abstract Medical research and publication serve to promote the scientific integrity and efficacy of the medical profession. The ethical principles of beneficence and nonmaleficence demand that physicians strive to advance medical knowledge so as to improve patient's lives and avoid harmful or ineffective patient care. The objective of medical research is to seek scientific truths and support these ethical principles. The integrity of clinical investigation involves the just and honest conduct of experimentation, the honest analysis and reporting of data, and then, the fair peer review and publication of these investigations. Research and the publication of research executed dishonestly divert the search for factuality and defile the medical literature. Within the last two decades, several clinical researchers from various specialties whose publications profoundly influenced the practice of anesthesiology were guilty of extensive research fraud and misconduct, and therein, adversely affected the safe practice of anesthesiology.

Keywords Research and Publication Fraud • Research Misconduct • Fabrication and Falsification of Data • Plagiarism • Ghost and Honorary Authorship • Redundant Publication • Ethical Peer Review • Ethical Journal Editorship • Perioperative Beta-Blockade • Quality Performance Measures

---

S.H. Jackson, MD (✉)
Department of Anesthesiology, Good Samaritan Hospital, 2425 Samaritan Drive, San Jose, CA 95124, USA
e-mail: hojacks@gmail.com

G.A. Van Norman, MD
Department of Anesthesiology and Pain Medicine, Department of Biomedical Ethics, University of Washington, 1959 NE Pacific Street, Seattle, WA 98195, USA
e-mail: gvn@uw.edu

B.G. Jericho (ed.), *Ethical Issues in Anesthesiology and Surgery*,
DOI 10.1007/978-3-319-15949-2_16

Case Presentation
Your hospital is vigorous in ascertaining compliance to the Surgical Care Improvement Project (SCIP). In fact, the anesthesia record, newly constructed in 2013, has a specific area for confirming adherence to SCIP measures, including perioperative continuation of beta-adrenergic blocking drugs for patients on chronic therapy. A 78-year-old patient is scheduled for a same-day outpatient bilateral laparoscopic inguinal hernia repair. Other than hypertension treated with a beta-blocker (and one other antihypertensive taken at night) and some mild memory loss, the patient has an otherwise normal history with no cardiac symptoms. The patient was instructed by the pre-anesthesia nurse to take her usual evening dose of antihypertensive medications, including metoprolol. However, on the morning of surgery, she admits to having failed to take her nightly medications, attributing this to her forgetfulness and being distracted by concerns over her surgery. Without any anesthetic premedication, she arrives at the operating room alert and moderately apprehensive, with vital signs unchanged from the admission area – pulse 47 and blood pressure 90/68. Your resident judges that she might be overly beta-blocked and does NOT want to administer any beta blockade drugs in the perioperative period unless indicated. Yet, she knows that she then would not be in compliance with the SCIP beta-blockade measure unless a note documenting the reasons for such were placed in the chart. She suggests that it would be easier and prudent to administer 1 mg of esmolol IV in order to satisfy the SCIP requirement. She and most of her department are unaware of the retirement of this SCIP measure by the Centers for Medicare and Medicaid Services and The Joint Commission as of December 31, 2014. You notify the resident that the establishment of the beta-blocking drug quality measure was largely based on two studies [1, 2] from the 1990s that later were found to be insufficient scientifically, and even of greater concern, in one case, likely fraudulent [2].

Introduction

The "social contract" of physicians obliges them to *demonstrate that they deserve social trust, authority and reward. Societies expect that a physician's primary concern is their patient's well being. Three themes – personal character, interpersonal duty and social responsibility – are recurrent topics of ethical reflection, and constitute the threads that bind medicine and morality. This has come to be known as medical ethics* [3].

The ethics of clinical research may best be understood from three disparate perspectives: (1) the process of obtaining new knowledge; (2) the moral use of that knowledge; and (3) the personal ethics of the scientist pursuing this knowledge [4]. This latter element, that of the personal morality of the clinical investigator, deserves particular attention, as the physician researcher is the ultimate guardian of the design, safety, conduct and analysis of the study, the knowledge gained there from, and its dissemination to the medical profession. The personal ethics of a research scientist is a critical element of the moral quality of human research.

Clinical researchers have potentially conflictive roles as *scientist, physician and private individual*, and each of these roles is commanded by a different ***value*** [4].

For ***science***, the value system is truth – knowledge is good in its own sake – and the discovery of "generalized concepts, theories or laws about human physiognomy or disease" [4]. Scientists must rigorously design studies and examine these experiments for their verifiability and falsifiability. "Observations must be accurate, honestly reported, objectively interpreted, subject to peer review, and shared openly with colleagues and the world at large" [4].

For ***medicine***, the value is *beneficence* toward the patient or patient population – the good of the patient – the helping and healing of human beings. Medicine, therefore, is not purely science, but rather applies science and the truths that science provides for the good of the patient.

For the ***individual***, the primary value likely is self-interest in the form of advancing one's career, economic gain, and the personal satisfactions of patient appreciation/satisfaction, peer approval and societal acknowledgment. Unfettered, this interest can introduce moral obstacles and obfuscate moral sensitivity. The covenants that the physician (clinical investigator) holds with both the patient (experimental subject) and society serve as the foundation for the moral obligation specific to clinical research. These covenants spring from a trust relationship that despite the oversight of governmental regulations and institutional review boards (IRB), ultimately relies on the good character and moral integrity of the physician investigator.

The manner in which physician scientists address these conflicts in value determines the degree to which society will facilitate or restrict the scientific autonomy necessary for fruitful research. Thus the ethical sensitivity and moral integrity of the clinical investigator is paramount in the quest for medical knowledge. A research project, from design to publication, that is void of scientific integrity places knowledge, truth and humans at risk and violates society's expectations of science and scientists.

Institutional hubris is another potentially corrosive element. Competitiveness amongst such institutions can potentially lower an IRB's ethical guardianship, and can, as we shall soon demonstrate, promote overreliance on the supposed moral character of a scientifically prolific or prominent researcher.

Scientific Misconduct [3, 5, 6]

Two prominent ethical principles – beneficence and nonmaleficence – demand that physicians must seek to further medical knowledge with the goal of bettering their patients' lives *while concomitantly* identifying harmful or ineffective treatments.

The integrity of the process of scientific advancement is more than simply the just and honest conduct of scientific investigation. It also includes honest and truthful analysis and synthesis of the experimental results, appropriate attributions for the submitted product, the integrity of the subsequent peer review, and, last but not least, the unbiased and fair publication of the research.

Publication is an important component of academic medicine as it sets scholarly efforts apart from the actual practice of medicine. As an essential factor for achieving a successful academic career, authorship is integral to receiving credit for one's research, creative ideas and other educational forays. Publications influence promotions, enhance job searches, and facilitate future research opportunities, including, importantly, funding for such endeavors.

While investigators and authors of scientific papers have primacy over the ethical conduct, analysis, reporting and submission of their studies, there also are important ethical obligations for those involved with the publication process – that is, the reviewers, editors and publishers.

Medicine and Medical Science as Moral Enterprises

Medicine is a moral enterprise, individually and collectively, and physicians are obligated to exercise moral integrity. This behavior, in turn, builds the public trust and serves as a structurally stabilizing and protective force for the medical profession's interaction with the society it serves. In return, physicians, including researchers, retain considerable authority and privilege to control the critically important aspects of their practice and research. Indeed, medicine's scientific endeavors necessarily are built upon a foundation of trust: "If science is to flourish and attain its appropriate role in aiding human progress, it is incumbent upon … the scientific community to help provide a research environment that, through its adherence to high ethical standards … will attract and retain individuals of outstanding intellect and character" [7].

Researcher-Author Fraudulent Behavior and Misconduct [3, 5, 6]

Fabrication and Falsification

Among the most ethically troublesome categories of research and publication fraud are ***fabrication*** – the invention of false results – and ***falsification*** – the manipulation or omission of key data leading to inaccurate representation of the research.

Research and the publication of research executed dishonestly divert the search for factuality and defile the medical literature, ultimately diminishing the quality of care delivered to patients, or potentially even leading to the endorsement of actually harmful treatments. Research fraud also *prevents beneficence* by dissuading physicians from utilizing beneficial therapies. Moreover, corrupted information can divert other investigators from pursuing a truthful path of scientific research. Fabrication and falsification, when exposed, damage the image of scientific investigation as a noble undertaking. The social contract that physician investigators hold with the society they serve demands a bedrock of honesty and a spirit of selfless service to the public.

How frequent is such misbehavior? Although likely underreported, evidence points to a significant frequency. One study found about one in 50 researchers admitted to at least one episode of fabrication during their career, but of interest, about 14% claimed to know of colleagues who did such [8]. Another survey reported almost 5% of authors admitted to having been participant to research that involved fabrication or misrepresentation, and, again not surprisingly, a larger number (more than one-sixth) claimed to be aware of such behavior in colleagues [9].

Misbehavior in research has been exposed in all specialties. Historically, perhaps the most potentially harmful to society may be the now discredited false claim published in 1998 linking regressive autism and measles-mumps-rubella (MMR) vaccinations [10]. The subsequent MMR vaccine scare later was determined to be based on a deliberate fraud. Appallingly, the researcher's claims followed his retention by a law firm to assist with lawsuits against manufacturers of the vaccine [11]! The worldwide consequences of this moral and ethical transgression in terms of morbidity and mortality due to arousing scientifically unfounded parental fears of vaccinating their children with MMR vaccine is huge and ongoing 17 years later. Regrettably, the process of reversing such egregious dishonesty, which involves retraction and expunging from the literature, inevitably will be incomplete.

But, we need not wander from anesthesiology to find examples of some of the largest individual research and publication fraud [3, 5, 6]. American anesthesiologist Scott Reuben was found by the medical center in which he conducted his research to have published a number of fraudulent research articles [12]. These studies promoted the routine worldwide clinical administration of "replacement" drugs for postoperative narcotic therapy with theoretically detrimental effects on bone healing in orthopedic patients. The editor-in-chief of the journal *Anesthesia and Analgesia* (A&A) listed 21 journal articles (ten from *A&A* and three from *Anesthesiology*) that had been based on the fraudulent data, and then correctly predicted their retraction [13]. Moreover, research findings from numerous studies that had relied upon Reuben's articles for their design and comparisons were called into question. The culprit was fined and imprisoned.

Not confined to the United States, extensive cases of scientific fraud in anesthesia and surgery research have been identified in Germany and Japan. German anesthesiologist Joachim Boldt misrepresented major aspects of a published study, involving fabricated data on the deployment of hydroxyethyl starch as a priming agent for cardiopulmonary bypass [14]. Moreover, the researcher failed to seek institutional review board (IRB) approval for his investigations as well as to obtain informed consent from the patients. Unprecedented widespread publication of his ubiquitously published work necessitated an international collaboration of the editors of 16 medical journals to publish a collective letter acknowledging that 88 of his 102 studies had failed to adhere to basic ethical standards for human experimentation [15]. Many of the study files were missing or incomplete, and false data were published in at least 10 of the 91 studies examined, thus further setting the stage for retractions. The researcher had his academic position removed and was subject to both monetary fines as well as imprisonment. In stark contradistinction to the United States, in Germany the state medical association holds jurisdiction over physician misbehavior and misconduct [16].

A Japanese anesthesiologist, Yoshitake Fujii, likely holds a "Guinness-type" world record for the number of fraudulent publications thus far [17]. A retraction of virtually all of his extensive research papers has ensued. Interestingly, an initial question regarding the integrity of his investigations arose a decade earlier [18], but was not pursued in depth [19]. It now has been determined that there was consistent violation of obtaining IRB approval, adhering to ethical standards for human investigation, and veracity of data. Furthermore, for some articles he named co-authors who were unaware of such and whose signatures on submission letters had been forged! Again, there was an international collaboration of editors from prominent anesthesiology journals to prompt investigation of these misdeeds and deception at the host institutions as well as to correct and retract, as much as feasible, the falsified literature. The editors were "*completely engaged with the process of coordinating our efforts to identify and reduce research fraud. … It is a team effort. … Everyone is on board*" [20–22]. The researcher was fired by his university.

Interestingly, to identify falsified data, statistical techniques to identify unusual patterns of categorical and continual variables have been developed. As a result, in addition to earlier methodology to detect plagiarism [23], editors now have substantial technology to detect research and publication dishonesty [24, 25].

Plagiarism

Plagiarism is the "appropriation of someone else's words and/or ideas as one's own" [5]. Because science and scholarship involve new knowledge and creative ideas, the wording utilized might be less important than the ideas that the words convey for the determination of whether a scientific thesis has been plagiarized. Plagiarism is an ethical violation because it harms the true authors by not giving them credit and not recognizing their work. But, plagiarism also damages the reader by deception and obfuscation of the pathway taken in the development of an idea. Furthermore, trust of the body of work of the plagiarist inevitably surfaces. In 1998, it was determined that complaints (likely underreported) involving medical authorship such as the plundering of non-credited work of junior faculty had risen precipitously, and moreover, appeared to disproportionately involve females and non-United States citizens as victims [26]. Perhaps the most infamous example of scientific plagiarism involved the unauthorized acquisition of Rosalind Franklin's unpublished research on DNA – as well as her confidential research progress report – by Watson and Crick. The latter of these famed biologists later acknowledged that the double helix model was based on her data, by which time Franklin, tragically, was deceased [27, 28].

Plagiarism is antithetical to the principles of nonmaleficence and justice. Nonetheless, identifying plagiarism is difficult. Editors now have within their armamentarium reliable methodology to detect plagiarism. This notwithstanding, words, when compared with ideas, do not in every circumstance hold equal weight in determining originality [29].

"Ghost" Authorship and "Honorary" Authorship

The International Committee on Medical Journal Editors defines an author as someone who has made a substantial contribution to a scientific publication. This would include participating in all of the following arenas of the scientific project: concept, design and acquisition of data, drafting or critical revision of the publication, and final approval of the version that is published.

"Ghost" authorship involves the acceptance of credit for a publication written by another ("ghost") individual. Industry, for example, often provides a professional writer (the "ghost" who is not identified or acknowledged) to compose a substantial portion of a publication to which is attached the name of an "author" who did not actually write the piece. "Honorary" authorship constitutes the assignment of credit to an individual (usually a senior academic or industry leader, or even government regulator or administrator) who did not participate to a meaningful degree in the research, analysis, review and/or synthesis of ideas upon which the publication is based. Both of these behaviors are commonplace, particularly in industry-financed publications [30, 31].

Such dishonest attribution of authorship is deleterious to the publication process in several ways. The attachment of the name of a well-respected researcher or prominent policy-maker to a paper might falsely give more significance and credibility of an investigation. Ghostwriters can conceal conflicts of interest that could influence the credibility of a publication as, for example one extolling the value of a new drug or medical device. Identification of the true author(s)/researcher(s) is key with respect to accountability and the ability to retrospectively investigate data of past publications that may have come into question. Pure and simply: authors who knowingly permit their name to be attributed to a publication in which they did not participate are engaging in fraud.

Redundant Publication

Redundant or duplicative publication is publication of the same results of one research project in more than one journal, or publishing a review of such results nearly at the same time in another journal, or the deliberate division of results from one study into several publications. This practice spuriously inflates academic "achievements," but unfortunately, is commonplace [32]. Inflating an already oversized medical literature and publication process is disingenuous and misleading. Self-plagiarism is a form of duplicative publication.

Ethical Duties of Peer Reviewers [5, 6]

As a fundamental segment of the process of medical publications, appropriately conducted peer review is, in the end, a major determinant for safe, quality patient care. Peer review determines whether research has been properly and ethically designed and conducted, and also accurate in its analysis, discussion and conclusions. It therefore affirms and confirms research as being a credible origin of new scientific information. Review articles as well as research also fall under the protective canopy of peer review.

Peer review serves to maintain professional autonomy for evaluating professional performance, impacts career development, and determines directions for the generation of new knowledge. Given the aforementioned examples, it becomes evident that there are numerous opportunities for unethical behavior. As such, peer review assuredly is a challenging task and invaluable filtering service to scientific advancement. Indeed, we believe it to be overlooked and not fully valued and appreciated by the medical profession.

Peer reviewers assuredly must have the expertise to serve in such a role. Far too often, incompetent review hampers the process, but this situation is not restricted to the scientific realm as it also occurs in the humanities and social sciences. In fact, over half of polled researchers complained that they had experienced what they believed to be incompetent reviews, which included inadequate familiarity of the subject matter, failure to diligently read the article, or making mistakes of fact and/or reasoning [33].

Peer reviewers are trusted to be fair and balanced in their application of their knowledge and expertise, free of bias and conflicts of interest, guardians of the confidentiality of submitted data, and shields against fraud and misconduct. Breaches of confidentiality, plagiarism and even theft, while infrequent, do occur and abuse the ethical duty of protecting the work and attribution of the author(s). The peer review process also serves to guard against inordinate delays of dissemination of scientific knowledge [33]. Although difficult to believe, there even have been instances of abusive reviews in the form of personal and retributive attacks on authors!

Ethical Duties of Journal Editors [5, 6]

Last, but certainly not least, we visit the gatekeepers of the publication process, journal editors. These powerful and influential individuals carry a huge responsibility, once again underappreciated and overlooked by the scientific community. Their value and obligation is to ensure, as much as is feasible, that the process of scientific publication is transparent and that the manuscripts published are original, truthful, accurate and ethically achieved. When one considers all the potential for misconduct as described heretofore, we should appreciate that editors carry the herculean burden of a determinedly diligent and courageous stewardship of the advancement of medical science.

External Safeguards [5]

As we have seen, scientific misconduct is a serious international problem – and recognized as such. However, only a dearth of countries have regulatory mechanisms in place to mitigate against such fraud. Even prior to the aforementioned examples, the United States Congress did respond to a then mounting amount of investigative misbehavior with potential for far-reaching adverse consequences to human health by establishing the Office of Scientific Integrity (now the Office of Research Integrity) in 1989. In the United Kingdom, all medically related fraud is referred to the General Medical Council. In the early 1990s Norway, Sweden, Denmark and Finland instituted formal review councils for examining scientific fraud. Encouragingly, there does exist a voluntary "international" agency to review instances of misconduct, the Committee on Publication Ethics (COPE), which has a membership of the editors and publishers of over 300 journals in Europe and Asia. The less enthralling aspect of COPE is that it serves only as an advisory board and has no authority to sanction or punish the detected miscreants. It would seem that federal regulatory agencies are needed to deal with this class of violations of medical ethics. Absent this vehicle, the reporting, investigation, and, when indicated, sanctioning of research and publication miscreants will continue to remain in the perhaps overwhelmed laps of fellow professionals, research institutions, peer reviewers, and journal editors.

Henry K. Beecher and Unethical Human Experimentation

Over a half a century ago, Harvard Professor of Anesthesia, Henry K. Beecher published a landmark paper that forever altered the conduct of human scientific exploration and publication [34]. In that article he described 22 examples of research abuse in human experimentation. With this and other publications, Beecher largely single-handedly initiated a transition from an insulated research community without any meaningful internal or external oversight to a medical community mandating informed consent and public oversight (such as institutional review boards) of both standard and research medical procedures. He was a staunch supporter of researchers having an understanding and adherence to the rules governing morality. Interestingly, in none of the cases he reported did he believe there was fabrication or falsification of data, but rather that of ethical transgressions in "thoughtlessness and carelessness" (not "willful" acts) in experimental conduct that showed no regard or respect for patient autonomy and rights. Beecher staunchly believed, however, that the integrity of medical knowledge and advances in clinical medicine rely on the truthful pursuit of ethically designed and conducted research, on "the presence of an intelligent, informed, conscientious, compassionate investigator," that is, *on the integrity of individual researchers* [34, 35].

Returning to the Case Presentation

Establishing quality performance measures in anesthesia and surgery has become a high priority item for institutional and system-wide quality improvement programs, regulators and payors (both private and government). We now shall focus on our case involving perioperative beta-blocking drugs.

Largely based on the results of two 1990s investigations (that later would be called in question) [1, 2], in 2001, the US Agency for Healthcare Research and Quality labeled preoperative beta-blockade as a "major advance in perioperative medicine" for which "wider use … should be promoted" [36]. This soon was followed by an enthusiastic recommendation by the American College of Cardiology/American Heart Association (ACC/AHA) that beta-blockers should be used for high-risk patients similar to those of the 1999 Poldermans study [2], and a somewhat lesser level of endorsement for use in moderate to high-risk patients like those in the 1996 Mangano [1] study [37]. The Leapfrog Group, a juggernaut of public and private healthcare purchasers, soon adopted beta-blockade use for high-risk surgical patients.

The ensuing two decades witnessed the waxing prominence of employing beta-blocking drugs for prevention of adverse post-surgical cardiac events *despite* the fact that *from its inception* the evidence supporting such practice had been highly debatable and controversial. Several credible randomized studies in the ensuing decade failed to support the beta-blockade quality measure [38–41]. Indeed, there now is widespread agreement that there is *no* valid scientific evidence-base for the beta-blocker measure as a "best practice."

In retrospect, within only a couple of years of publication of the Mangano study there appeared the first of numerous criticisms for its being poorly designed for demonstrating benefit in the *immediate and/or early* perioperative period. Immediate deaths were excluded from the statistical analysis, and the major benefit was detected only *months* following surgery [42, 43].

More importantly and pertinent to this chapter, the 1999 Poldermans study [2] and a multitude of his other articles contained what still remains as an unquantified but significant amount of fraudulent research and publication (including failure to obtain informed consent, fabricating data and dishonestly manipulating analyses). Poldermans, a highly regarded, prolific Dutch researcher (over 500 papers in respected peer-reviewed journals) ultimately was dismissed from his academic position at Erasmus University [44]. His "research" had been the basis for worldwide evidence-based guidelines, medical policies, and, ultimately, the care of millions of patients. His data, like that of Fujii mentioned earlier, were considered "too good to be true" [45]. His reputation and belief in his publications were so widespread and ingrained that even when his misconduct was exposed, extensive research efforts by others continued to try to validate his discredited work [41].

While we now know that beta-blockade can diminish the incidence of non-fatal myocardial ischemia and/or infarction, it also *increased* the incidence of clinical stroke and 30-day mortality [46, 47].

Looking back, it now is frightening that the beta-blockade guidelines of both the European Society of Cardiology (ESC) (Poldermans chaired its committee) and the ACC/AHA relied heavily on information dominated by Poldermans' now known to be "non-secure" work [46, 47]. For well over a decade, beta-blockade has been harming an untold (but assuredly huge) number of patients undergoing *noncardiac* surgery.

The ESC guidelines, constructed in 2009, advocated initiation of a course of perioperative beta-blockade in three classes of patients: (1) with known ischemic heart disease or myocardial ischemia according to preoperative stress testing; (2) scheduled for high-risk surgery; and (3) scheduled for intermediate risk surgery. All of these groups' recommendations were classified as Class I. Poldermans' studies dominated the meta-analysis "conclusion that beta-blockers had a neutral effect on mortality and allowed them [cardiologists] to focus on the reduction of non-fatal myocardial infarctions as a surrogate endpoint" [46, 47]. Appallingly, all of these recommendations are taking a long time to modify [48, 49].

The ACC/AHA guidelines, initially written in 2007, endorsed perioperative beta blockade in patients: (1) undergoing vascular surgery and coronary ischemia demonstrated on preoperative testing – Class I evidence base; (2) having vascular surgery and with already documented coronary artery disease – class IIa; (3) scheduled for vascular surgery with more than one risk factor for coronary arterial disease – Class IIa; (4) to undergo intermediate risk surgery with established coronary artery disease and/or more than one risk factor [50].

A 2013 meta-analysis of the secure trials (eliminating those of Poldemans' unsecure data) detailed that initiation of beta-blockers prior to surgery caused a 27% risk *increase* in 30-day all cause mortality [46, 47]. The Poldermans family of studies had heavily out-weighted and mal-influenced the meta-analysis of the *secure* trials with respect to mortality. While the secure trials showed that beta-blockade reduced *nonfatal* myocardial infarction, these drugs concomitantly increased stroke and hypotension – likely contributing to the cause of the high mortality.

Quality Performance Measures: From There to Here and Back to There

The National Quality Forum (NQF) is a nonprofit, nonpartisan, public service organization committed to transforming the US healthcare system to be "safe, equitable, and of the highest value" [51]. The NQF "reviews, endorses, and recommends" use of quality performance measures that are "tools used to evaluate how well healthcare services are being delivered." They supposedly "have undergone a rigorous review by a panel of *providers*, *measurement experts*, and *consumer representatives*." The Centers for Medicare and Medicaid Services (CMS) has chosen to be a "steward" of some of these NQF quality measures, one of them being "surgery patients on beta-blocker therapy prior to arrival who received a beta-blocker during the perioperative period" (NQF, #0284).

Another entity, the Surgical Care Improvement Project (SCIP), is a national quality partnership of organizations whose collective goal is to enhance surgical care by reducing surgical complications. SCIP is an element in the US government-sponsored effort to introduce evidence-based strategies into the clinical care of patients undergoing anesthesia and surgery [52]. The Joint Commission has aligned with the CMS with respect to the so-called core measures for surgical patients. It defines quality measures, adopting some created by the NQF, that then are tracked by institutions where surgery is performed. For over a decade the SCIP quality measure for beta-blocking drug use in noncardiac surgical patients tracked those patients who had, previous to their surgery, been on beta-blocking therapy, and the percentage of "surgery patients on beta-blockade therapy prior to arrival who receive a beta-blocker during the perioperative period." The perioperative period was defined as either the day before or the day of surgery, and also either the first or second postoperative day. Exclusion populations were defined, necessitating documentation of a reason for *not* administering the beta-blocker.

Compliance with SCIP is supported by the American Society of Anesthesiologists (ASA): "*The ASA is firmly committed to high-quality patient care and supports SCIP's goal to reduce the incidence of postoperative complications. Anesthesiologists play a key role in providing the clinical services that are embodied in the SCIP evidence-based recommendations for improving perioperative care.* Furthermore, *The ASA encourages anesthesiologists to consider the SCIP recommendations for all patients and to implement them when appropriate for patients under their care*" [53].

As clinical guidelines are offered as vehicles to improve quality of care and enhance cost effectiveness, the durability of these recommendations over time is critical for informing clinical practice and healthcare policy. Recommendations arrived at prematurely can lead not only to ineffective care, but even to morbidity and/or mortality, a violation of the ethical obligation of physician beneficence and nonmaleficence [54-56]. The ACC/AHA have been held as the gold standard for construction of credible guidelines, yet even the durability of Class 1 ("procedure/treatment should be performed/administered") "varied significantly across individual guidelines and levels of evidence, with recommendations that were based on multiple clinical trials being the most likely to endure over time" [56]. Of interest, although only 1% of recommendations were reversed, 9% were downgraded and 11% omitted at the time the guidelines were next revised. Performance measures based on single trial observational studies, consensus opinions or a standard of care were threefold less durable than those based on multiple randomized trials.

Another report reviewed the guidelines of "interventional medicine subspecialties" (*non* anesthesia-related or those of the ASA), which tend to have much less rigorous review and oversight by the Federal Drug Administration than do pharmaceuticals. Startling as is may seem, only 11% of these invasive specialties' guidelines deployed evidence that included randomized controlled trials and meta-analysis, and perhaps worse, almost half were based solely on case studies or expert opinion [57]! Possible conflicts of interest were not mentioned in the majority of these guidelines.

An eye-opening, informative and thoughtful analysis of the mistakes that can be made with clinical practice guidelines recants the beta-blockade saga [58]. In fact, the beat-blocker fiasco is only one of several recent examples in which expert, well-intentioned endorsements changed dramatically when newer evidence alerted clinicians of the potential harms that had been overlooked. This "story shows how the prestige that medical researchers and clinicians afford to randomized controlled trials can obscure important uncertainties surrounding new treatments, particularly when placed in political contexts that prioritize the rapid translation of research into practice. … [These] guidelines went wrong not because they overlooked the need for randomized trials but because of experts' very faith in such trials" [58].

In the dust storm of the final days of the beta-blockade quality performance measurements, the Joint Commission has quietly "retired" this SCIP requirement as of the last day of 2014. No fanfare, no acknowledgements, no clinical alerts by any of the involved specialties. At the time of writing this chapter, many if not most anesthesiologists and surgeons are unaware of this retraction and continue to practice according to guidelines that now no longer are supported by any base of scientific evidence, and antithetically, now are considered potentially unsafe and even harmful.

And, finally, with respect to the case, even if beta-blockade were a best practice (which it is not), it is *un*ethical to play the 'guideline adherence and compliance' game by administering small (homeopathic) doses of a short acting beta-blocking drug (esmolol). Even when clinical guidelines are "proven" to be "secure" and "valid" according to *existing* evidence, physicians always should employ their clinical judgment so as to care and treat each patient as a unique individual with a unique physiognomy and needs.

References

1. Mangano DT, Layug EL, Wallace A, Tateo I. Effect of atenolol on mortality and cardiovascular morbidity after noncardiac surgery. Multicenter Study of Perioperative Ischemia Research Group. NEJM. 1996;335:1713–20.
2. Poldermans D, Boersma E, Bax JJ, Thomson IR, van de Ven LL, Blankensteijn JD, et al. The effect of bisoprolol on perioperative mortality and myocardial infarction in high-risk patients undergoing vascular surgery. Dutch Echocardiograph Cardiac Risk Evaluation Applying Stress Echocardiography Study Group. NEJM. 1999;341:1789–94.

3. Jackson S, Van Norman G. Anesthesia, anesthesiologists and modern medical ethics. In: Eger II E, Saidman L, Westhorpe R, editors. The wondrous story of anesthesia. New York: Springer; 2014. p. 205–18.
4. Pelligrino E. Beneficence, scientific autonomy, and self-interest. Camb Q Healthc Ethics. 1992;4:361–9.
5. Van Norman G, Jackson S. Publication ethics: obligations of authors, peer reviewers, and editors. In: Van Norman G, Jackson S, Rosenbaum S, Palmer S, editors. Clinical ethics in anesthesiology. Cambridge: Cambridge University Press; 2011. p. 209–25.
6. Jackson S, Van Norman G. Ethical issues in the publication of medical research. ASA Newsl. 2011;75:14–6.
7. Alberts B. Promoting scientific standards. (Editorial). Science. 2010;327:12–3.
8. Fanelli D. How many scientists fabricate and falsify research? A systematic review and meta-analysis of survey data. PLoS One. 2009;4:e5748.
9. Gardner W, Lidz C, Hartwig K. Authors' reports about research integrity problems in clinical trials. Contemp Clin Trials. 2005;26:244–51.
10. Wakefield AJ, Murch SH, Anthony A, Linnell J, Casson DM, Malik M, et al. Ileal lymphoid nodular hyperplasia, non-specific colitis, and pervasive developmental disorder in children [RETRACTED]. Lancet. 1998;351:637–41.
11. Godlee F, Smith J, Marcovitch H. Wakefield's article linking MMR vaccine and autism was fraudulent. BMJ. 2011;342:c7452.
12. Borell B. A medical Madoff: anesthesiologist faked data in 21 studies. Scientific American. 2009. http://www.scientificamerican.com/article.cfm?id=a-medical-madoff-anesthesiologist-faked-data. Accessed 5 July 2015.
13. White P, Carl R, Shafer S. The Scott Reuben saga: one last retraction. Anesth Analg. 2011;112:512–5.
14. Retractions Watch. http://retractionwatch.wordpress.com/2011/02/28/22-papers-by-joachim-boldt-retracted-and-67-likely-on-the-way/. Accessed 10 Aug 2012.
15. Yentis S. Lies, damn lies, and statistics. Anaesthesia. 2012;67:455–6.
16. Wagner E. Who is responsible for investigating suspected research misconduct? Anaesthesia. 2012;67:462–6.
17. Normile D. A new record for retractions? Science Insider (American Association for the Advancement of Science). 2 July 2012.
18. Kranke P, Apfel C, Roewer N. Reported data on granisetron and postoperative nausea and vomiting by Fujii et al. are incredibly nice! Anesth Analg. 2000;90:1004–7.
19. Moore R, Derry S, McQuay H. Fraud or flawed: adverse impact of fabricated or poor quality research. Anesthesia. 2010;65:327–30.
20. Shafer S. Anesthesia and Analgesia policy on institutional review board approval and informed consent for research. Anesth Analg. 2011;112:494–5.
21. Yentis S. Research, audit, and journal policies. Anes Analg. 2011;112:496–7.
22. Shafer S. Personal communication to Stephen Jackson. 1 Nov 2012.
23. Shafer S. You will be caught. Anesth Analg. 2011;112:491–3.
24. Carlisle J. The analysis of randomised controlled trials to test data integrity. Anaesthesia. 2012;67:521–37.
25. Pandit J. On statistical methods to test if sampling in trials is genuinely random. Anaesthesia. 2012;67:456–62.
26. Wilcox L. Authorship. The coin of the realm, the source of complaints. JAMA. 1998;280:216–7.
27. Fuller W. Who said 'helix'? Nature. 2003;424:876–8.
28. Zallen D. Despite Franklin's work. Wilkins earned his Nobel. Nature. 2003;425:15.
29. Bouville M. Plagiarism: words and ideas. Sci Eng Ethics. 2008;14:311–33.
30. Flanagin A, Carey LA, Fontanarosa PB, Phillips SG, Pace BP, Lundberg GD, et al. Prevalence of articles with honorary authors and ghost authors in peer-reviewed medical journals. JAMA. 1998;280:222–4.
31. Gotzsche PC, Hrobjartsson A, Johansen HK, Haahr MT, Altman DG, Chan A-W. Ghost authorship in industry-initiated randomized trials. PLoS Med. 2007;4:e19.

32. Khanyile TD, Duma S, Fakude LP, Mbombo N, Daniels F, Sabone MS. Research integrity and misconduct: a clarification of the concepts. Curationis. 2006;29:40–5.
33. Resnick D, Gutierrez-Ford C, Peddada S. Perceptions of ethical problems with scientific journal peer review: an exploratory study. Sci Eng Ethics. 2008;14:305–10.
34. Beecher H. Ethics and clinical research. NEJM. 1966;274:1354–60.
35. Freidenfelds L. Recruiting allies for reform: Henry Knowles Beecher's "Ethics and Clinical Research". Int Anes Clinic. 2007;45:79–103.
36. Shojania KG, Duncan BW, McDonald KM, Wachter RM. Making health care safer: a critical analysis of patient safety practices (Evidence Report/Technology Assessment, No. 43). Rockville: U.S. Agency for Healthcare Quality and Research; 2001. p. 1–8.
37. Eagle KA, Berger PB, Calkins H, Chaitman BR, Ewy GA, Fleischmann KE, et al. ACC/AHA guideline update for perioperative cardiovascular evaluation for noncardiac surgery – executive summary: a report of the American College of Cardiology/American Heart Association Task Force on Practice Guidelines (Committee to Update the 1996 Guidelines on Perioperative Cardiovascular Evaluation for Noncardiac Surgery). J Am Coll Cardiol. 2002;39:542–53.
38. Brady AR, Gibbs JS, Greenhalgh RM, Powell JT, Sydes MR. Preioperative beta-blockade (POBBLE) for patients undergoing infrarenal vascular surgery: results of a randomized double-blind controlled trial. J Vasc Surg. 2005;41:602–9.
39. Yang H, Raymer K, Butler R, Parlow J, Roberts R. The effects of perioperative beta-blockade: results of the Metoprolol after Vascular Surgery (MaVS) study, a randomized controlled trial. Am Heart J. 2006;152(5):983–90.
40. Juul AB, Wetterslev J, Gluud C, Kofoed-Enevoldsen A, Jensen G, Callesen T, et al. Effect of perioperative β blockade in patients with diabetes undergoing major non-cardiac surgery: randomised placebo controlled, blinded multicentre trial. BMJ. 2006;332:1482.
41. Devereaux PJ, Yang H, Yusuf S, Guyatt G, Leslie K, Villar JC, et al. Effects of extended-release metoprolol succinate in patients undergoing non-cardiac surgery (POISE trial): a randomised controlled trial. Lancet. 2008;371:1839–47.
42. Leung J. Diabetes and not lack of treatment with atenolol predicts decreased survival after noncardiac surgery. Anesthesiology. 1999;90:1226–7.
43. Chopra V, Plaisance B, Cavusoglu E, Flanders SA, Eagle KA. Perioperative beta-blockers for major noncardiac surgery: Primum Non Nocere. Am J Med. 2009;122:222–9.
44. Erasmus Medical Center fires Dr. Don Plodermans. www.medscape.com/viewarticle/753941. Accessed 17 Apr 2015.
45. Montori VM, Devereaux PJ, Adhikari NK, Burns KE, Eggert CH, Briel M, et al. Randomized trials stopped early for benefit: a systematic review. JAMA. 2005;294:2203–9.
46. Bouri S, Shun-shin MJ, Cole GD, Mayet J, Francis DP. Meta-analysis of secure randomised controlled trials of β-blockade to prevent perioperative death in non-cardiac surgery. Heart. 2014;100:456–64.
47. Chopra V, Eagle K. Perioperative mischief: the price of academic misconduct. Am J Med. 2102;125:953–5.
48. Fleisher LA, Beckman JA, Brown KA, Calkins H, Chaikof EL, Fleischmann KE, et al. 2009 ACCF/AHA focused update on perioperative beta blockade incorporated into the ACC/AHA 2007 guidelines on perioperative cardiovascular evaluation and care for non-cardiac surgery. J Am Coll Cardiol. 2009;54:e13–118.
49. Shekelle PG, Wachter RM, Pronovost PJ, et al. Making health care safer II: an updated critical analysis of the evidence for patient safety practices. (Evidence report/technology assessment No. 211). Rockville: U.S. Agency for Healthcare Research and Quality; 2013. p. 169–71.
50. Fleisher LA, Fleischmann KE, Auerbach AD, Barnason SA, Beckman JA, Bozkurt B, Davila-Roman VG, et al. 2014 ACC/AHA guideline on perioperative cardiovascular evaluation and management of patients undergoing noncardiac surgery: executive summary. Journal of Nuclear Cardiology. 2015;22(1):162–215.
51. National Quality Forum. http://qualityforum.org.
52. Joint Commission/SCIP – Specification Manual for National Hospital Inpatient Quality Measures. http://jointcommission.org/specifications*manual*for_national_inpatient_quality_measures.aspx. Accessed 17 Apr 2015.

53. American Society of Anesthesiologists. Statement on the surgical care improvement project (SCIP). 2010. http://www.asahq.org/Search.aspx?q=care+improvement+project+scip. Accessed 17 Apr 2015.
54. Prasad V, Cifu A, Ioannidis JPA. Reversals of established medical practices: evidence to abandon ship. JAMA. 2012;307:37–8.
55. Prasad V, Vandross A, Toomey C, Cheung M, Rho J, Quinn S, et al. A decade of reversal: an analysis of 146 contraindicated medical practices. Mayo Clin Proc. 2013;88:790–8.
56. Neuman MD, Goldstein JN, Cirullo MA, Schwartz JS. Durability of Class I American College of Cardiology/American Heart Association clinical practice guideline recommendations. JAMA. 2014;311:2092–100.
57. Feuerstein JD, Akbari M, Gifford AE, Hurley CM, Leffler DA, Sheth SG, et al. Systematic analysis underlying the quality of the scientific evidence and conflicts of interest in interventional medicine subspecialty guidelines. Mayo Clin Proc. 2014;89:16–24.
58. Neuman MD, Bosk CL, Fleisher LA. Learning from mistakes in clinical practice guidelines: the case of perioperative β-blockade. BMJ Qual Saf. 2014;23:957–64.

Chapter 17
Ethics and Evidence Regarding Animal Subjects Research: Splitting Hares–or Swallowing Camels?

Gail A. Van Norman

Abstract Nonhuman animals are the subject of medical research, industrial testing and educational projects in human efforts. Modern biological research has produced information that challenges assumptions that animals lack characteristics that make them deserving of moral standing, and the success of modern animal subjects research in medicine is commonly overstated. Public opinion in favor of animal research is conditional and waning. This chapter will discuss the ethical principles surrounding use of nonhuman animal subjects, research that challenges basic assumptions about the utility of nonhuman animal subjects research, and ethical obligations of researchers, editors and reviewers with regard to nonhuman animal subjects research.

Keywords Animal Research • Ethics

Case Presentation

Thalidomide became an over-the-counter drug in 1957 after extensive testing in rodents, dogs and primates. Marketed as a sedative and anxiolytic, the drug quickly became a treatment for morning sickness in pregnant women. Shortly after the drug was released in Germany, 5000–7000 infants were born with amelia (absence of arms) or phocomelia (rudimentary or short arm or leg bones). About 40% of infants survived. When suspicions arose that the fetal malformations and deaths were due to thalidomide, doctors were reluctant to embrace the association, and the drug stayed on the market for another 4 years. During that time an estimated 10,000–20,000 cases of severe birth

G.A. Van Norman, MD
Department of Anesthesiology and Pain Medicine, Department of Biomedical Ethics, University of Washington, 1959 NE Pacific Street, Seattle, WA 98195, USA
e-mail: gvn@uw.edu

B.G. Jericho (ed.), *Ethical Issues in Anesthesiology and Surgery*,
DOI 10.1007/978-3-319-15949-2_17

deformities associated with thalidomide use were reported worldwide, and fewer than half of the affected infants survived. Other birth defects also associated with maternal use of thalidomide included deformities of the eyes, heart, gastrointestinal and genitourinary tracts and deafness.

Introduction

Experiments conducted in nonhuman animals have been a foundation of biomedical inquiry for hundreds of years. Protection of human research subjects has been reliant on animal testing. The Nuremberg Code, for example, stated explicitly that all medical experimentation should be based on prior animal studies [1]. There is no doubt that some animal experiments have proven beneficial to human health. Because of a border collie named Marjorie and ten other dogs, we have insulin therapy for diabetes, for example [2]. How do we measure the lives of a handful of animals against potentially millions of human lives saved?

Despite a long history of acceptance, growing numbers of scientists and an increasing proportion of the public question the utility and morality of using animals in industrial testing and medical experimentation. Many decry animal experimentation as an unacceptable practice that retains a false credibility based on repeated citations of a few notable successes, rather than objective examination of its efficacy–and perpetuated in ignorance of the suffering that it causes and its frequent and often shocking failures to predict human responses.

Researchers themselves have increasingly joined the chorus of skeptics, pointing out that *past* practices do not necessarily justify *continuing* practices, and suggesting that the morality of research, like the knowledge it has brought, must evolve. In the words of Dr. Neal Barnard:

> Let's say that it's true, that animals were indispensable to the discovery of insulin. That was a long time ago. I think [that] to say, 'It was done this way and there's no other way it could have been done' is a bit of a leap of faith, but let's say that at the time there was no other way. You could also say that you couldn't have settled the South without slavery. Would you still do it that way today? Just because something seemed necessary or acceptable at the time is not to say that we should do it in our time [2].

Animal experimentation takes place in a complex moral landscape, and researchers must not ignore the problems it poses, whether or not they agree with its critics. It is imperative that all investigators, editors, reviewers, and publishers of animal research have a thorough understanding of the ethical questions involving animal research, and of the directions that our changing knowledge and understanding of nonhuman animals and their interests are likely to take biomedical research in the future.

At its core, the conflict over the use of animals in research asks but a single moral question: Are humans *morally justified* in using animals in this way? Arguments favoring animal experimentation are that humans have a higher moral standing than animals and a right to further their own interests at the cost of animal lives and suffering, and that benefits of animal experimentation outweigh the moral harms we incur.

In this chapter, we will explore evolving moral concepts regarding animals, discuss widely held assumptions about the efficacy of animal experimentation, and review basic ethical principles of animal research.

Moral Standing of Nonhuman Animals

The philosophical relationship between man and nonhuman animals has been predominantly shaped by religious philosophy and not scientific principles. Most if not all religions express not only principles of how humans should treat each other, but also how humans should treat animals. Western culture is steeped in Judeo-Christian principles that present animals as being bequeathed to Adam, to do with as he wished. Early principles of scientific inquiry were heavily influenced by the philosophy of Descartes in the 1500s, who argued that animals are automata that might *look* as though they are conscious, reasoning and reacting, but are not so. All animal behavior could be explained in mechanistic terms [3]. In the famous words of philosopher Nicholas Malebranche, "They eat without pleasure, cry without pain, grow without knowing it; they desire nothing, fear nothing, know nothing" [4]. Without consciousness, animals could have no interests, no experiences, and no moral standing.

Twentieth century religious scholars, however, were sorely challenged with regard to scientific theories and man's relationship to the world and its other inhabitants. New scientific disciplines such as paleontology and the theory of evolution gained ground, suggesting that man not only was *not* truly different from the animals, but may have actually arisen from them. Such developments test the very structure of scientific inquiry, which relies heavily on the concept that man is separate from, and greater than his experimental subjects. In the words of primatologist Fran De Waal, "Our culture and dominant religion have tied human dignity and self-worth to our separation from nature and distinctness from other animals" [5]. He goes on to point out that scientists are biased against acknowledging uncomfortable similarities between human and nonhuman animals, because such acknowledgement weakens arguments for the moral superiority of man.

The scientific study of animals no longer supports the Cartesian paradigm, and few biologists seriously argue that animals can be clearly distinguished from humans on the basis of many traditionally held concepts. Rigorous research demonstrates that animal consciousness and abilities show startling parallels to those previously thought to be uniquely human. Tool manufacture and use is now well described in primate, nonprimate and even nonmammalian animals [6]. Great apes appear to be capable of using symbolic language [7], and nonhuman animals have been shown to work with numbers–both strong markers of abstract thinking [8]. Animals demonstrate "culture," in which uniquely individual and adaptive behaviors are passed within social groups by observation rather than instinct or genetic programming [9]. "Episodic recall," believed to be an important marker of sentience, is seen in meadow voles [10]. Cetaceans have knowledge of symbolic representations and exhibit an awareness of self [11], which has also been demonstrated in primates, elephants [12], and magpies [13]. Recent studies in dogs indicate an extensive abstract vocabulary, and the ability to extrapolate names [14].

Nevertheless, many scientists are still reluctant to relinquish Cartesian ideals. Bioethicist Bernard Rollin poses that scientists have evolved an "ideology" of their own–one that asserts, "science might provide society with the facts relevant to making moral decisions, but it steers clear of any ethical debate" [15]. This belief is self-evidently false: if there is no moral component to scientific efforts, then there would be no need to report the breach of moral principles with the cruel experimentation on research subjects. In fact, such an "ideology" asserts that scientific studies can be performed without the consideration for the treatment of its research subjects-be it human or animal. Thankfully, the idea that medical research does not answer to moral considerations has thoroughly been disparaged, as the Doctor's Trial at Nuremberg after World War II clearly demonstrated.

Most bioethicists now agree that animals do have moral standing, but *which* animals and how much moral standing are subjects of debate. There is agreement that deliberately causing animal suffering is a moral harm to be prevented or mitigated and must be weighed heavily against any perceived benefits it might provide. Furthermore, Kantian philosophy holds that cruelty toward an animal is contrary to man's duty to himself, because he who is cruel to animals will likely be cruel to humans as well [16].

There are many moral "theories" by which animal rights and moral standing are discussed, but it is useful to consider three basic types of arguments. The first two are based on the idea that "rights" belong to "persons" and "persons" are defined as any being that has sentience or consciousness.

The first theory is a simplified view of a "conservative"[1] moral philosophy that humans and only humans have sentience or consciousness and that therefore only humans have "rights." Philosopher Christina Korsgaard suggests that humans not only have perceptions and desires (which she concedes animals do too) but also are uniquely able to reflect on those perceptions and desires, and that it is this reflection that sets us apart from other nonhuman animals [17]. Thus nonhuman animals do not necessarily have "rights." However, even if they do not have "rights" per se, she points out that this does not imply that humans do not have explicit moral duties towards them. A second more "expansive" moral view is that morally important qualities such as rationality exist in some, if not most animals, and that therefore animals have moral standing in their own right. This point of view argues that some animals (e.g., great apes) have sentience and rationality, while some humans (e.g., infants and those with dementia) have only partial or potential rationality, and still other humans (e.g., permanently comatose individuals) lack rationality altogether. If

[1] The term "conservative" in this context is meant merely to convey a theory that is more restrictive and is not related to any political ideology or framework.

rationality and sentience are the necessary and sufficient conditions for "personhood" and "rights," then actually some animals do have "personhood" and "rights", and some humans clearly do not. Finally, a third, "moderate" approach to moral obligations in our treatment of animals does not address the question of "personhood" and "rights" at all, but asks simply if it is ever morally acceptable to cause nonhuman animals to suffer. Peter Singer argues that animals have "interests" whether or not they have rights, and that all animals have an interest in avoiding suffering. Therefore, it is almost always morally wrong to willfully cause animals to suffer. He does *not* argue, for example, that using animals for food is wrong, so long as they are humanely treated and killed. However, using animals in ways that cause suffering must be seriously weighed against any human need it answers. He further argues that a great deal of animal research causes suffering without satisfying any direct or urgent purpose and answers only minor human interests when weighed against the animal's more serious interest in avoiding suffering. In many (but not necessarily all) cases, Singer argues, we should end animal research [18].

Obviously, to weigh the morality of animal research, we need to attempt to quantify the role of animal research in the safety and efficacy of medical treatments and whether animal research is beneficial.

The story of thalidomide is an important one in the annals of animal research. Although it is often cited as a reason supporting animals studies, it actually illustrates a spectacular *failure* in basic assumptions about animal studies: that the mechanisms of action of a drug will be similar in animal models to that of humans, and that use in animal subjects will disclose dangers of a drug prior to its use in humans.

When human birth defects first began to appear in the offspring of women who had ingested thalidomide during pregnancy, researchers pointed out that animal studies had failed to demonstrate any teratogenic potential of thalidomide in rats and that therefore thalidomide could not be the culprit. In fact, as J.L Schardien has observed, "in approximately 10 strains of rats, 15 strains of mice, 11 breeds of rabbit, 2 breeds of dogs, 3 strains of hamsters, 8 species of primates, and other such varied species as cats, armadillos, guinea pigs, swine and ferrets in which thalidomide has been tested, teratogenic effects have been induced only occasionally" [19]. Ultimately, similar birth defects to those seen in humans were found when high doses of thalidomide were administered to the New Zealand White rabbit after the fact, but only to a lesser extent than in other strains of rabbits. Schardein goes on to say, "Trying to justify the performing of animals studies, however, is a somewhat frustrating exercise in futility. Despite the extensive testing in animals prior to human use, the labeling of marketed drugs does not fully reflect the results of such studies, nor does it indicate the clinical experience with a drug that may have had many years of apparent safe use…" [19].

The United States largely escaped the tragedy of thalidomide compared to other Western countries. Only 17 cases were ever reported [19]. Why? Because Frances Oldham Kelsey–a reviewer for the Food and Drug Administration (FDA)–on her very first assignment in her first month with the agency, had grave doubts about thalidomide that were based ironically on neuropathic side effects shown in *human* studies, but had been largely ignored. She halted the approval of the drug in the

United States (U.S.) only one day before approval was to automatically go into effect [20].

Is the thalidomide story a unique example of how animal studies fail? Unfortunately, the answer is no.

The Quality and Predictive Value of Animal Studies in Human Therapies

How much do animal experiments contribute to medical advancements? Do animal experiments accurately predict human responses?

In many cases, medical treatments commonly cited as depending for their success on animal studies were in fact actually *impeded or contradicted* by animal research. Even the Center for Disease Control (CDC), on its "Overview of Animals in Scientific Research Fact Sheet" lists smallpox vaccine (cow), and penicillin (mouse), as among the "tangible benefits" of animal research to medicine [21], yet Jetsy and Jenner actually each tested their smallpox vaccines in *human* subjects and not cows, and Fleming decided based on rabbit experiments that penicillin *wouldn't work*. He shelved the drug and only found it to be effective years later when he used it to treat a human infection because he had run out of all other options. Only *after* the human success did he test the drug in mice. We are all fortunate that Fleming did not choose to test it in guinea pigs–in which it is toxic [22].

Possibly two of the most spectacular recent failures of animal studies were the infamous trials of TGN1412, a monoclonal antibody developed to treat leukemia and autoimmune disorders, and Fialuridine, an antiviral drug with activity against Hepatitis B.

Animal studies in mice, rabbits and monkeys supported TGN1412's safety. But when the drug was administered to six human volunteer subjects during 1 day in March of 2006 in a dose 1/500th of that used in animals, all volunteers suffered catastrophic reactions within minutes [23]. All volunteers survived the initial experience after receiving intensive medical support, but one required the amputation of all fingers and toes and a second volunteer was diagnosed within several months with a rare hematologic cancer believed to be secondary to receiving TGN1412 [24].

In the case of Fialuridine, preclinical testing in mice, rats, dogs, monkeys and woodchucks indicated that the drug was safe in doses that were hundreds of times higher than those to be used in humans. However, the administration of the drug during human Phase II clinical trials lead to the deaths of 5 healthy volunteers due to liver failure. Two other volunteers survived, but only after undergoing liver transplantation [23].

Many other well-known examples of research in which animal studies may have mislead researchers or impeded scientific advances include studies of the role of asbestos exposure in lung disease, AIDs research, and cancer treatments [25].

Systematic Reviews of Animal Studies

Simply stating "research involving animals has played a vital role in virtually every major medical advance of the last century" does not make it so. Nor is the report of a few admittedly spectacular failures sufficient to discount the value of animal research. Just as other elements of medical practice must be based on real evidence, so too must our understanding of the role that animal research plays now and that it should play in the future be based on sound evidence and not conjecture. Disciplined analysis of the translatability of published animal subjects research is a relatively new, but growing field of inquiry in the medical literature, and these reviews pose unsettling, but important questions about the true utility of animal research.

In a recent analysis of systematic reviews of animal studies to determine if they had informed clinical research in humans, Pound and colleagues [26] found the following problems:

- Several systematic reviews found that animal studies were frequently conducted *concurrently* with the human studies, and thus the animal study was irrelevant with regard to the conduct of the human trial or human outcomes.
- Human clinical trials proceeded even when the animal studies indicated no benefit to the therapy being studied–i.e., results in animal subjects were not used to inform the human trial.
- The quality of animal subject trials was generally poor, with common problems being lack of randomization of animals, lack of blinded assessments, and failure to measure outcomes beyond the acute phase.
- Numbers of animal studies were often too small to draw stable conclusions, and pooled data analysis was not used to amplify the results prior to human studies.
- Statistical analysis of animal studies was often simplistic and did not account for confounding variables, nor did it follow intention-to-treat principles.
- Researchers were biased in citing animal studies, often only citing supportive studies rather than presenting a balanced view that included negative studies.

Roberts et al. systematically reviewed 44 randomized controlled trials of fluid resuscitation experiments in traumatized animals [27]. Three large trials could not be included in the analysis because they had no control group, multiple studies compared different blood pressure targets, mortality was not reported in 2 of the 44 trials, and reanalysis of trial data using appropriately sophisticated statistical techniques to account for confounding variables demonstrated statistical heterogeneity [27]. The authors suggest that continuing systematic reviews of animal studies are needed to ensure that animal experiments do not set out to answer questions that have already been answered, and that they will actually provide generalizable results.

In a review of 76 animal studies that was reported in the Journal of the American Medical Association in 2006, the authors reached a number of troubling conclusions [28]. Almost half of the experiments were never confirmed in human studies, dead-ending their usefulness. In 18%, human results contradicted animal studies.

In 221 studies reviewed by Perel, et al., agreement between animal and human studies occurred only about 50% of the time–essentially randomly [29].

A number of scientists have analyzed the probability that animal testing will predict human adverse effects in drugs and the results are eye-opening. As early as 1962, Litchfield compared testing results in rats, dogs and humans for 6 drugs [30]. He found that the predictive value of a positive test (PPV) in the animal models (for similar reactions in humans) was 0.49 and 0.55, respectively–roughly random chance (PPV 0.5) [30]. Heywood found a 20% correlation between toxicity tests results in rodents and non-rodents [31]. He concluded that interspecies extrapolation of toxicology tests was unrealistic [31]. Salsburg also reported low correlations between animal models and human responses in carcinogen testing [32]. He commented that "a lifetime feeding study in rodents has less probability of finding known human carcinogens than tossing a coin" [32]. In 1990, Heywood reported on drugs that had been withdrawn from clinical trials or the general market due to severe human toxicity, and found that the animal data correlated with human data less than 14% of the time [33].

Another important failure of animal experimentation has been that animal studies have at times prevented drugs from coming to market that may be beneficial to human beings even though the probability that adverse effects seen in the animal model would predict human outcomes is so poor [34]. The National Cancer Institute concludes that effective cancer-fighting drugs have been lost because of animal studies [35].

An interesting question to ask based on what are now numerous analyses of the translational value of animal studies is whether performing animal studies is unethical because of the *danger* they actually present to humans. As Greek and colleagues point out: (1) Due to the low PPV of animal toxicity studies, telling human volunteers that the drug has tested safe in animals is falsely reassuring, since such tests do not correlate well for reactions in humans, and therefore citing animal studies in the informed consent process is misleading and unethical, and (2) drugs that could be helpful in human disease are being denied development because of animal toxicity testing that is simply not correlated with human response in any meaningful way [36]. As academic physician Robert Burns comments, "As physicians, researchers, and educators, we must take a long-overdue objective look at how and why we use animals in research and education. A great deal of animal-based research adds very little to our understanding of the diagnosis and treatment of our patients" [37].

Venerable scientific institutions have begun to critically evaluate the use of animals in medical research and are slowly beginning to conclude that skepticism is warranted: in a landmark report in 2011, the Institute of Medicine declared that most current use of chimpanzees in biomedical research is unnecessary. Furthermore, they enjoined that, any animals that might be retained for essential research should be maintained in appropriate physical and social environments–as would happen in natural habitats [38]. As a result of the report, the National Institutes of Health (NIH) Director Dr. Francis Collins announced that the NIH would reduce the number of chimpanzees held for research in the U.S. to 50, retiring all remaining animals [39]. This decision brought the U.S. in alignment with steps already taken by many Westernized countries to ban or strictly limit medical research involving great apes [40].

Laws and Animal Research

Most Western nations now have explicit laws governing the use and treatment of animals in research and industrial testing. In the US, the Animal Welfare Act (AWA) was passed in 1966. The Health Research Extension Act in 1985 and amendments to the AWA required the establishment of Institutional Animal Care and Use Committees (IACUCs), to inspect the animal facilities of institutions; review and approve, modify, or disapprove the proposed use and care of laboratory animals; investigate concerns and review research facilities' use of animals and the care of animals; ensure that veterinary medical care is provided; and educate and train laboratory personnel in the ethical care and use of animals including the appropriate use of anesthetic and analgesic agents as well as methods of euthanasia [41]. Parallel action in Great Britain included the passing of the Animals (Scientific Procedures) Act of 1986 (ASPA) that regulates animal research that might cause "pain, distress, suffering or lasting harm" [42]. Furthermore, at a local level, the United Kingdom (UK) in 1999 subsequently required local ethical review committees to review research involving animals. These precedents lead to the member states of the European Union (EU), including the UK, adopting the 1986 European Convention for the Protection of Animals used for Experimental and Other Scientific Purposes [43].

The Magnitude of Animal Research

How many animals are used in laboratories in the United States annually? The United States Department of Agriculture (USDA) reveals that the number of "reportable" animals in research has trended downward, from over 2 million animals in 1992, to just over 1 million in 2013 [44]. Yet, a 2002 amendment to the Animal Welfare Act (AWA) did not require laboratories to report research on birds, rats and mice, and USDA statistics therefore do not include research on these animals. Thus, the actual number of animals utilized in research is unknown, yet it is estimated that over 30 million animals every year are utilized in research across the world [45]. In 2013, the Home Office of Great Britain reported approximately 4 million procedures were done on animals in research in 2013 with over 70% of the *reported* experiments not providing anesthesia and causing "pain, suffering, distress, or lasting harm to the animal" [46]. An accurate number regarding how many animals that are exempted from USDA reporting are subjected to untreated pain during research protocols is unavailable, but presumed to be in the millions.

The 3 Rs

It has now been 56 years since the publication of the seminal work *The Principles of Humane Experimental Technique* [47] by William Russell and Rex Burch. They concluded that the most humane possible treatment of animals in research was not merely a moral requirement, but a requisite for good science [47]. This sentiment was echoed by J. Edward Gates from the University of Maryland: "*Pain and stress can add an uncontrollable variable into an experiment and so it is in the interest of good science to control pain and distress whenever possible*" [48]. Russell and Burch put forth the 3 Rs of animal experimentation:

- ***R****eplace* animals in experiments whenever possible.
- ***R****educe* the number of animals to the minimum needed.
- ***R****efine* scientific procedures and husbandry to improve the welfare of animals used in research and attenuate existing or potential pain, stress, or lasting injury.

While the 3Rs are alluded to in most professional organizations and scientific bodies dealing with animal research, evidence that scientific journals hold researchers accountable to these standards is lacking. Furthermore, in a 2009 review of 271 published animal research studies, even basic scientific rigor was missing from many [49]. Less than 60% of these studies stated all of the following: the hypothesis they were testing; the number of animals utilized in the study; and the sex, strain, and weight or age of the animals in the experiment [49]. Only 12% used randomization and only 14% used blinding to reduce bias [49]. Furthermore, 30% did not identify the statistical methods they used in analysis with a variation or error measure [49].

In another review of 236 randomly selected English language journals that contained animal research studies, over half had no editorial policy regarding publication of animal research [50]. Only 1 out of 111 journals that did have such policies mentioned the 3Rs, and only 1 journal stated that adherence to their policies was required for publication–a finding that may help explain the dismal results of the systematic reviews of animal studies previously cited [50].

Laws and regulations in the European Union, US, UK, and other nations have recognized the importance of enforcing the 3Rs, and animal welfare committees and/or IACUCs have been established to help oversee animal research, much as Institutional Review Boards oversee human subjects research proposals. These committees potentially could enforce standards of animal research and not give approval to studies that do not meet the ethical standards of animal research. Yet, many IACUCs members prefer not to review potential animal research studies to assess if they meet scientific standards and, furthermore, many members do not have a thorough knowledge of the ethics of animal research to serve in this capacity [51, 52]. Some have proposed that the composition of IACUCs is often highly skewed towards animal researchers themselves and institutional veterinarians, both of whom have vested interests in continuing animal research [53].

Public Opinion Regarding Animal Research

Gates asserts that, "A research institution that receives money and support from the public is responsible for conducting research according to the limits set by society…the use of animals in research is a <u>privilege</u>, and not a <u>right</u>. The consensus at this time in the United States is that animals should be treated humanely and that pain and distress should be minimized when animals are used for research or teaching purposes" [48].

Medical research, like clinical care, falls under a "social contract" extended to physicians and researchers; in return for acting in the public interest, society extends them both special privileges and prestige. This is a contract that society can withdraw when it is no longer perceived to be in the public interest. The researcher is not permitted to pursue research that does not meet the standards and the needs that society sets forth. It is this "social contract" that prevents researchers from being able to pursue unregulated research for personal ends without moral oversight. And the interest of society in animal research is slowly, but steadily waning.

An international comparison in 1994 of the public's opinion of animal research in 15 nations indicated that most of the European countries studied, particularly France (almost 70%), disagreed or strongly disagreed with the following statement: "Scientists should be allowed to do research that causes pain and injury to animals like dogs and chimpanzees if it produces new information about human health problems" [54]. In a 2008 US survey, public concern about treatment of animals was high; 97% believed that animals require protection, and 25% believed that "animals deserve the exact same rights as people to be free from harm and exploitation" [55]. Thirty-five percent of respondents indicated that they would ban all medical research on animals and 39% would ban all testing of products on research animals [55]. According to the Gallup organization's annual Survey of Values and Beliefs, the number of people opposing animal research has been climbing. The rise in opposition is largest in the younger age groups, suggesting that as the baby boomer generation exits, opposition to animal subjects research is likely to continue to grow [56].

Public pressure to restrict animal research has had concrete results: in response to public pressure US commercial airlines have ceased all shipments of research primates within the US [57]. Laws limiting the use of primates in research have been discussed or passed in a number of European countries. In fact, in the year 2000 in Switzerland, the constitution was amended to protect the dignity of animals–with Swiss courts subsequently ruling to limit the use of primates in medical investigation to translational research. Unfortunately, such restrictions in Europe motivated by the public's desire to improve animal welfare may have had the paradoxical effect of pushing primate research outside of Europe to countries that have lower levels of concern for animal welfare [57].

Summary

Medical therapies headed for use in humans have been tested in nonhuman animals for hundreds of years. The legitimacy of this practice is based in Western theological origins that give humans moral supremacy over nonhuman animals. This belief was further advanced by Cartesian philosophies among scientists, who assumed that animals did not have sentience or other characteristics that make them deserving of moral consideration. Modern biological studies have proven earlier assumptions about the intellectual and emotional lives of animals to be mistaken and rooted in cultural and theological bias. Modern ethicists generally agree that animals have moral standing and cannot be treated as mere objects in the pursuit of human health.

Many researchers firmly believe that modern medicine would not have had the same potential to advance without animal research. Whether or not that is true, it does not necessarily follow that future medical advances must or even should be based on prior animal research. Analyses of animal experimentation show that scientists have not always followed the "animals first, then humans" rule of testing–often running simultaneous human and animal studies concurrently. Animal studies have frequent basic procedural flaws, and have not been subject to the same rigorous review as human studies.

For the last several decades, well-respected researchers have been increasingly skeptical about the translational value of animal studies, which have poor positive predictive value of revealing problems in human use. Many believe that animal studies have actually prevented progress on important treatments that would have been valuable in humans. Other authors have raised the question of whether animals studies increase the risk to humans by falsely reassuring researchers in a significant number of cases that treatments will be safe when they are not. Furthermore, citation of animal studies in recruiting human volunteers for safety and efficacy studies may be unethical, because the literature has been shown to be biased towards positive results in animals studies, and because human volunteers may not be fully informed of the poor predictive value of preceding animal experiments.

Public opinion, scientific communities and biomedical ethicists agree that researchers have moral obligations to reduce or eliminate animal suffering in research, and to strive to eliminate animal experimentation altogether. Scientific publications have been slow to enforce widely recognized ethical rules for animal testing, such as the 3 Rs, and IACUCs have largely failed to provide ethical guidance on research design. Both problems need to be addressed if the quality and relevance of animal studies is to improve.

In the meantime the public is slowly withdrawing support for animal experimentation, and many Western nations have restricted animal research, particularly in great apes. This public trend can be expected to continue as the current generation and its views become predominant in society.

References

1. National Institute of Health. Regulations and ethical guidelines. Reprinted from Trials of War Criminals before the Nuremberg Military Tribunals under Control Council Law No. 10, vol. 2. Washington, DC: U.S. Government Printing Office; 1949. p. 181–2.
2. Lauerman JF. Animal research. Harvard Magazine, Jan–Feb 1999;48. http://harvardmagazine.com/1999/01/mice.html. Accessed 26 Apr 2015.
3. Harrison P. Descartes on animals. Philos Quart. 1992;42:219–27.

4. Nicholas Malebranche. In: Rodis-Lewis G, editor. Oeuvres completes, vol. II. Paris: J. Vrin; 1958–1970. p. 394.
5. De Waal F. The ape and the sushi master; reflections of a primatologist. New York: Basic Books; 2001.
6. Taylor AH, Hunt GR, Holtzhalder C, Gray RD. Spontaneous metatool use by new Caledonian crows. Curr Biol. 2007;17:1504–7.
7. Tanner JE, Patterson FG, Byrne RW. The development of spontaneous gestures in zoo-living gorillas and sign-taught gorillas: from action and location to object representation. J Devel Process. 2006;1:69–122.
8. Pepperberg IM, Carey S. Gray parrot number acquisition: the inference of cardinal value from ordinal position on the numeral list. Cognition. 2012;125:219–32.
9. Byrne RW, Barnard PJ, Davidson I, Janik VM, McGrew WC, Miklosi A, et al. Understanding culture across species. Trends Cogn Sci. 2004;8:341–6.
10. Ferkin MH, Combs A, delBarco-Trillo J, Pierce AA, Franklin S. Meadow vòles, Microtus pennsylvanicus, have the capacity to recall the "what", "where", and "when" of a single past event. Anim Cogn. 2008;11:147–59.
11. Marino L, Connor RC, Fordyce RE, Herman LM, Hof PR, Lefebvre L, et al. Cetaceans have complex brains for complex cognition. PLoS Biol. 2007;5:e139.
12. Plotnik JM, de Waal FB, Reiss D. Self-recognition in an Asian elephant. Proc Natl Acad Sci U S A. 2006;103(45):17053–7.
13. Prior H, Schwarz A, Gunturkun O. Mirror-induced behavior in the magpie (Pica pica): evidence of self-recognition. PLoS Biol. 2008;6:e202.
14. Pilley JW, Reid AK. Border collie comprehends object names as verbal referents. Behav Processes. 2010;86:184–95.
15. Rollin BE. Animal research: a moral science. Talking point on the use of animals in scientific research. EMBO Rep. 2007;8:521–5.
16. Kant I. The groundwork for the metaphysics of morals (trans: Gregor MJ). Cambridge: Cambridge University Press; 1998. p. 428.
17. Korsgaard C. Fellow creatures: kantian ethics and our duties to animals. Tanner Lectures Human Values. 2005;25:77–110.
18. Jecker NS. Animal subjects research part I. Do animals have rights? In: Van Norman G, Jackson S, Rosenbaum S, Palmer S, editors. Ethics in anesthesiology: a case-based textbook. Cambridge: Cambridge University Press; 2011. p. 168–73.
19. Schardein JL. Drugs as teratogens. Cleveland: CRC Press; 1976. p. 5, 49.
20. Changing the face of medicine: Dr. Frances Kathleen Oldham Kelsey. U.S. National Library of Medicine, Bethesda. Last reviewed 5 Dec 2013. http://www.nlm.nih.gov/changingthefaceofmedicine/physicians/biography_182.html. Accessed 27 Apr 2015.
21. Overview of animals in scientific research fact sheet. Nov 16, 2006. Department of Health and Human Services Center for Disease Control and prevention: CDC in the News. http://www.cdc.gov/news/2006_11/animal_care/factsheet_ar_general.htm. Accessed 16 May 2015.
22. Steffee CH. Alexander Fleming and penicillin. The chance of a lifetime? NC Med J. 1992; 53:308–10.
23. Attarwala H. TGN1412: from discovery to disaster. J Young Pharm. 2010;2:332–6.
24. NatureNews. TGN1412 drug trial leaves patient with terminal cancer. 2006. http://www.naturalnews.com/019928_drug_trials_TGM1412.html. Accessed 21 Apr 2015.
25. Dennis C. Cancer: off by a whisker. Nature. 2006;442:739–41.
26. Pound P, Ebrahim S, Sandercock P, Bracken MB, Roberts I, et al. Where is the evidence that animal research benefits humans? Observations from a systematic review of international animal experiments on fluid resuscitation. BMJ. 2004;328:514–7.
27. Roberts I, Kwan I, Evans P, Haig S. Does animal experimentation inform human healthcare? BMJ. 2002;324:474.
28. Hackam DG, Redelmeier DA. Translation of research evidence from animals to humans. JAMA. 2006;296:1731–2.

29. Perel P, Roberts I, Sena E, Wheble P, Briscoe C, Sandercock P, et al. Comparison of treatment effects between animal experiments and clinical trials: systematic review. BMJ. 2007;334:197–203.
30. Litchfield Jr JT. Symposium on clinical drug evaluation and human pharmacology. XVI. Evaluation of the safety of new drugs by means of tests in animals. Clin Pharmacol Ther. 1962;3:665–72.
31. Heywood R. Target organ toxicity II. Toxicol Lett. 1983;18:83–8.
32. Salsburg D. The lifetime feeding study in mice and rats–an examination of its validity as a bioassay for human carcinogens. Fundam Appl Toxicol. 1983;3:63–7.
33. Heywood R. Clinical toxicity–could it have been predicted? Post-marketing experience. In: Lumley CE, Walker S, editors. Animal toxicity studies: their relevance for man. Lancaster: Quay; 1990. p. 57–67.
34. Sankar U. The delicate toxicity balance in drug discovery. Scientist. 2005;19:32.
35. Gura T. Cancer models: systems for identifying new drugs are often faulty. Science. 1997;278:1041–2.
36. Greek R, Pippus A, Hansen LA. The Nuremberg Code subverts human health and safety by requiring animal modeling. BMC Med Ethics. 2012;13:16.
37. Burns R. Animals in research. Acad Med. 1989;62:780.
38. Institute of Medicine and National Research Council committee on the use of chimpanzees in biomedical and behavioral research. Principles guiding the use of chimpanzees in research. In: Altevogt BM, Pankevich DE, Shelton-Davenport MK, et al., editors. Chimpanzees in biomedical and behavioral research: assessing the necessity. Washington, DC: National Academic Press; 2011. p. 27.
39. National Institutes of Health news and events. Statement by NIH director Dr. Francis Collins on the Institute of Medicine report addressing the scientific need for the use of chimpanzees in research. 2011. http://www.nih.gov/news/health/dec2011/od-15.htm. Accessed 16 May 2015.
40. Institute of Medicine (US) and National Research Council (US) committee on the use of chimpanzees in biomedical and behavioral research. International policies guiding chimpanzee use. In: Altevogt BM, Pankevich DE, Shelton-Davenport MK, Kahn JP, editors. Chimpanzees in biomedical and behavioral research: assessing the necessity. Washington, DC: National Academy of Sciences Press (US); 2011. Table 3. p. 18–9.
41. Anderson LC, Ballinger MB, Bayne K, Bennett BT, Bernhardt DB, Brown MJ, et al. In: Pitts M, Bayne K, Anderson LC, et al., editors. Institutional animal care and use committee guide book. Applied research ethics national association/office of laboratory animal welfare; 2002. p. 17–8, 27–30, 43–51, 53–7, 65–70, 87–90. http://grants.nih.gov/grants/olaw/guidebook.pdf. Accessed 30 May 2015.
42. Animal (Scientific Procedures) Act 1986. Great Britain. http://www.archive.official-documents.co.uk/document/hoc/321/321.htm. Accessed 27 Apr 2015.
43. European convention for the protection of vertebrate animals used for experimental and other scientific purposes. Strasbourg, 18.III.1986 (amended Dec 2, 2005 to reflect formation of the European Union). http://www.conventions.coe.int/Treaty/en/Treaties/Html/123.htm. Accessed 27 Apr 2015.
44. United States department of agriculture animal and plant health inspection service. Research Facility Annual Reports. Last modified 11 Dec 2014. http://www.aphis.usda.gov/wps/portal/banner/help/!ut/p/a1/04_Sj9CPykssy0xPLMnMz0vMAfGjzOK9_D2MDJ0MjDwtzD0MDDzd_L28nVyCjQ1cDIEKIpEVuAdbuhp4-oW5-Vr4mBt7e5kTp98AB3A0IKQ_XD8KVQkWF4AV4LGiIDc0wiDTUREAfqAG8w!!/?1dmy&urile=wcm%3apath%3a%2FAPHIS_Content_Library%2FSA_Our_Focus%2FSA_Animal_Welfare%2FSA_Obtain_Research_Facility_Annual_Report%2F. Accessed 27 Apr 2015.
45. Bishop LJ, Nolen AL. Animals in research and education: ethical issues. Kennedy Inst Ethics J. 2001;11(1):91–112.
46. Statistics of scientific procedures on living animals: Great Britain 2013. Home Office. Ordered by the House of Commons to be printed. London. 2014. https://www.gov.uk/government/uploads/system/uploads/attachment_data/file/327854/spanimals13.pdf. Accessed 30 May 2015.

47. Russell W, Burch R. The principles of humane experimental technique. London: Methuen & Co. Ltd; 1959.
48. Gates JE. Committee Chair, Appalachian Laboratory, University of Maryland Center for Environmental Science. Lecture: Institutional animal care and use committee, general information. 2013. http://slideplayer.com/slide/3729983/. Accessed 16 May 2015.
49. Kilkenny C, Parsons N, Kadyszewski E, Festing MF, Cuthill IC, Fry D, et al. Survey of the quality of experimental design, statistical analysis and reporting of research using animals. PLoS One. 2009;4:e7824.
50. Osborne NJ, Payne D, Newman ML. Journal editorial policies, animal welfare, and the 3Rs. Am J Bioeth. 2009;9:55–9.
51. Rowan AN. Animals, science, and ethics—section IV. Ethical review and the animal care and use committee. Hastings Cent Rep. 1990;20:s19–24.
52. Houde L, Dumas C, Leroux T. Ethics: views from IACUC members. Altern Lab Anim. 2009;37:291–6.
53. Hansen LA. Institutional animal care and use committees need greater ethical diversity. J Med Ethics. 2013;39:188–90.
54. Pifer L, Shimizu K, Pifer R. Public attitudes toward animal research: some international comparisons. Soc Animals. 1994;2:95–113.
55. Post derby tragedy, 38 % support banning animal racing. The Gallup Organization. 2008. http://www.gallup.com/poll/107293/PostDerby-Tragedy-38-Support-Banning-Animal-Racing.aspx. Accessed 30 May 2015.
56. Wilke J, Saad L. Older Americans' moral attitudes changing. The Gallup Organization. 2013. http://www.gallup.com/poll/162881/older-americans-moral-attitudes-changing.aspx. Accessed 30 May 2015.
57. Abbot A. Biomedicine: the changing face of primate research. Nature. 2014;506:24–6.

Index

B.G. Jericho (ed.), *Ethical Issues in Anesthesiology and Surgery*,
DOI 10.1007/978-3-319-15949-2

MIX
Papier aus verantwortungsvollen Quellen
Paper from responsible sources
FSC® C105338

If you have any concerns about our products,
you can contact us on
ProductSafety@springernature.com

In case Publisher is established outside the EU,
the EU authorized representative is:
Springer Nature Customer Service Center GmbH
Europaplatz 3, 69115 Heidelberg, Germany

Printed by Libri Plureos GmbH
in Hamburg, Germany